The Greenberg Rapid Review

Thieme

The Greenberg Rapid Review

A Companion to the 7th Edition

Leonard I. Kranzler, MD, JD, LLM, FACS
Chief of Neurosurgery
Advocate Illinois Masonic Hospital
Clinical Professor of Surgery (Neurosurgery)
University of Chicago
Chicago, Illinois

Justin M. Kranzler, BA
Contributing Editor

Thieme
New York • Stuttgart

Thieme Medical Publishers, Inc.
333 Seventh Ave.
New York, NY 10001

Executive Editor: Kay Conerly
Editorial Assistant: Lauren Henry
Editorial Director, Clinical Reference: Michael Wachinger
International Production Director: Andreas Schabert
Vice President, International Sales and Marketing: Cornelia Schulze
Chief Financial Officer: James W. Mitos
President: Brian D. Scanlan

Compositor: Friedhelm Hübner Electronic Publishing GmbH
Printer: Transcontinental Printing

Cover image adapted from *Handbook of Neurosurgery*, 7th Edition, with permission from Mark S. Greenberg, MD

Library of Congress Cataloging-in-Publication Data is available from the publisher.

Printed in Canada

5 4 3 2 1

ISBN 978-1-60406-366-0

Contents

Contents vii
Preface ix
Acknowledgments. xi
  1 Neuroanesthesia 1
  2 Neurocritical Care 3
  3 General Care. 14
  4 Neurology. 29
  5 Neuroanatomy and Physiology. 44
  6 Neuroradiology. 70
  7 Operations and Procedures 83
  8 Developmental Anomalies. 106
  9 Neuroendovascular Intervention 129
10 Electrodiagnostics 130
11 Neurotoxicology. 134
12 Coma 138
13 Brain Death 145
14 Cerebrospinal Fluid 146
15 Hydrocephalus 152
16 Infections. 165
17 Seizures 179
18 Spine and Spinal Cord. 195
19 Functional Neurosurgery 230
20 Pain. 239
21 Tumor. 248
22 Radiation Therapy 325
23 Stereotactic Surgery 328
24 Peripheral Nerves. 330
25 Neuro-ophthalmology 366
26 Neurotology. 379
27 Head Trauma 385
28 Spine Injuries 426
29 Stroke. 463
30 SAH and Aneurysms 476
31 Vascular Malformations. 508
32 Intracerebral Hemorrhage 519
33 Occlusive Cerebrovascular Disease 529
34 Outcome Assessment 547
35 Differential Diagnosis (DDx) by Location 548

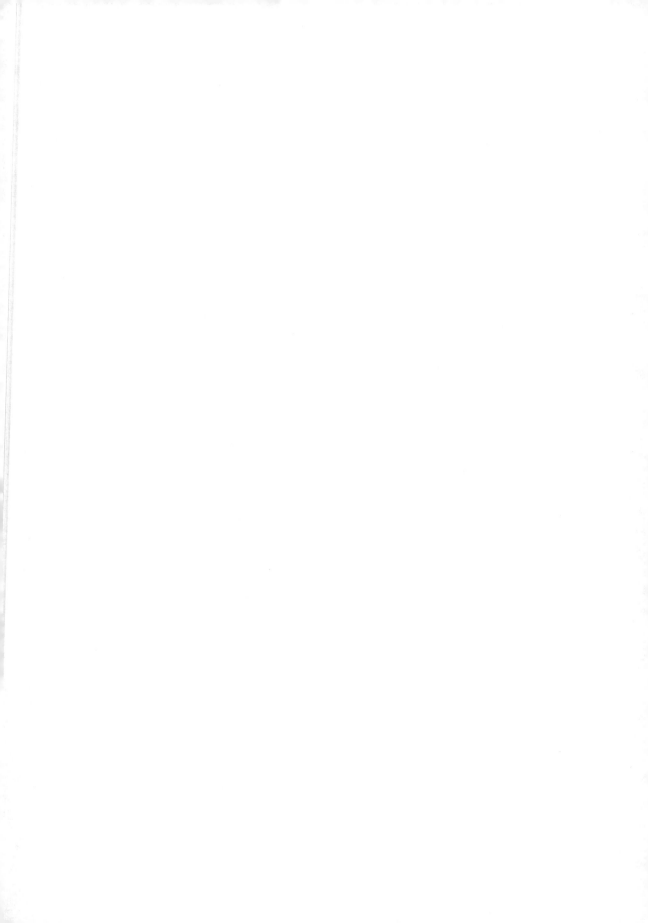

Preface

This offering is a study and review aid. It is to be used in conjunction with *Handbook of Neurosurgery*, 7th Edition, by Mark S. Greenberg. It permits the user, after reading a page, section, or chapter in Greenberg, to test retention of the details of that portion. Every question is directly referenced to Greenberg's text where background information and context is readily available. An effort has been made to highlight the important facts in neurosurgical practice by posing questions to the reader that forces active involvement in the learning and review process.

The purpose is to pinpoint for clinicians what they should expect to know using a rapid review format. It will help identify what the student already knows, what is not known, and provide a method by which an individual can verify that fact has been learned. The reader can also have confidence that what has been highlighted as valuable has been identified by peers and by an editor who has been involved in neurosurgical education as coordinator of the Chicago Review Course in Neurological Surgery since 1974. Many questions were contributed by enrollees in the Chicago Review Course in Neurological Surgery over a three-year period and therefore represent questions from individuals at all levels of neurosurgical sophistication similar to those who might use this book.

It is expected that the reader will review the material multiple times until success in responding to the questions has been achieved. The question formats take advantage of the established ideas in learning theory:

- complex subjects broken into small bits
- fill-in-the-gap exercises in sentences and words
- progressive withdrawal of cues forcing the user to recall more and more of the details
- mnemonics or hints (some material has been arranged in "study charts" to aid mnemonic teaching techniques)
- humor
- alternate arrangements of the material (the same facts presented in different formats)
- repetition

Each question and answer is referenced to the millimeter from the top of the page in Handbook of Neurosurgery, 7th Edition by Greenberg where confirmation and further information can be found. For example, the reference "G7 p.2:145mm" means that the answer can be found 145 mm down on page 2 of Greenberg, 7th edition. Please note that some references to the 6th edition of Greenberg have been made in order to include additional valuable factual material. Moreover, this study guide is designed with answers appearing directly after the questions (we recommend that users cover the answers in the outer page margin with a piece of paper) so that additional time is not wasted searching for correct answers in the back of the book. This format should further facilitate rapid review.

Please note that literature references and the index are present in the parent volume *Handbook of Neurosurgery*, 7th Edition. Knowledge of this material demonstrated by correct responses to the questions can give confidence to the reader that much of the current scientific foundation of the specialty of neurosurgery has been mastered. This reassurance of a strong, up-to-date knowledge base should be helpful to the resident, the instructor, the neurosurgeon in practice, and those who are planning to take written, oral, or recertification examinations.

Note to the Reader

Please call to my attention any mistakes that you identify. Please suggest any additional mnemonic devices that might help others in the field of neurosurgery. Be aware that medical knowledge is ever changing and that some items and opinions conveyed in these pages are controversial.

Contact the author at likranzlermd@hotmail.com.

Acknowledgments

I would like to acknowledge with appreciation the cooperation and encouragement of Dr. Mark S. Greenberg. Our generation of neurosurgeons is fortunate that Dr. Greenberg has collated the literature of our field and presented it to us in such a concise, authoritative, well-balanced, and wise manner.

This project could not have been done without the pleasant and efficient efforts of Maria Peña who typed many iterations of this manuscript. I also appreciate the support for this project by my nurse of 33 years, Judith Borchers, and our chief secretary Lucy Salgado.

The team at Thieme Publishers has been wonderful to work with. Their efforts improved this offering greatly. My young students and colleagues, Dr. Mahua Dey and Javid Khader Eliyas, proofread and greatly added to the manuscript's accuracy. Thank you all.

1

Neuroanesthesia

■ General Information

1. **Provide general information on neuroanesthesia.**
   a. Name the most potent cerebral vaso dilator. — CO_2 — G7 p.1: 85mm
   b. Effect of hyperventilation on — G7 p.1: 85mm
      i. $PaCO_2$ — reduces
      ii. CBV — decreases
      iii. CBF — decreases
      iv. Goal is end tidal CO_2 of ($ETCO_2$) _____ — 25 to 30 mm Hg
      v. Correlates with a PCO_2 of _____ — 30 to 35 mm Hg
   c. For every _____ degree change in temperature — 1 — G7 p.1: 110mm
   d. there is a change in cerebral metabolic rate of oxygen by _____%. — 7%
   e. The effect that hyperglycemia has on ischemic deficits is to make them _____. — worse — G7 p.1: 115mm
   f. Elevating the patient's head will have the following effect on: — G7 p.1: 127mm
      i. arterial blood flow — decreases
      ii. ICP — reduces
      iii. venous blood outflow — improves

■ Drugs Used in Neuroanesthesia

2. **Inhalation anesthesia agents have the following effects:** — G7 p.1: 177mm
   a. cerebral vessels _____ — dilate
   b. auto-regulation is _____ — disturbed
   c. cerebral blood volume is _____ — increased
   d. CSF volume is _____ — increased
   e. Reactivity of vessels to CO_2 is _____ — increased

3. **What anesthetic drug may come out of solution and aggravate pneumocephalus?** — nitrous oxide — G7 p. 2:45mm

4. To reduce the risk of tension pneumocephalus you would   G7 p. 2:52mm
a. fill any space with _____   fluid
b. and turn off _____   agent
c. _____ minutes before closing the dura.   10

5. Complete the following regarding barbiturates: G7 p.2:147mm
a. Most are anticonvulsants but there is an exception that actually lowers the seizure threshold called B_____.   Brevital
b. They cause peripheral vaso _____   dilatation
c. which may cause _____   hypotension
d. and _____ the CPP.   reduce

6. True or False. Morphine and Demoral   G7 p.3:42mm
a. release histamine   true
b. produce hypotension   true
c. cause vasodilation   true
d. increase ICP   true
e. compromise CPP   true
f. Demoral can cause seizures.   true

7. Characterize synthetic narcotics.   G7 p.3:72mm
a. Have the advantage that they don't cause h_____ r_____.   histamine release
b. An example is f_____.   fentanyl   G7 p.3: 85mm

8. Benzodiazepines are _____ agonists.   GABA   G7 p.3:115mm

9. Characterize pancuronium (Pavulon).   G7 p.4:40mm
a. Potentially, _____ minutes are necessary for full reversal of pancuronium (Pavulon).   20
b. True or false. Due to its long action it is indicated for intubation.   false

10. Answer the following questions concerning anesthesia requirements for evoked potential monitoring: G7 p. 4:177mm
a. What technique is preferred?   total IV anesthesia
b. Second best is _____.   nitrous/narcotic
c. Are muscle relaxants permitted?   yes
d. How should fentanyl be infused?   continuously as opposed to intermittent injections

11. The antiepileptic drugs that do not effect SSEP are   G7 p.5:25mm
a. c_____   carbamazepine
b. p_____   phenytoin
c. p_____   phenobarbital

2

Neurocritical Care

■ Fluids and Electrolytes

1. **The diagnosis is hyponatremia if the serum sodium is less than _____ mEq/l.**

   135

   G7 p.7:107mm

2. **The syndrome is SIADH**

   G7 p.7:107mm

   a. if the serum osmolality is less than _____ mOsm/l

   275

   b. and the urine osmolality is more than _____ mOsm/l.

   100

3. **The syndrome is CSW if the urinary sodium is greater than _____ mEq/l.**

   20

   G7 p.7:123mm

4. **Severe hyponatremia is considered a sodium lower than _____ mEq/l.**

   125

   G7 p.7:142mm

5. **Hyponatremia is considered**

   G7 p.7:145mm

   a. mild if sodium is_____ mEq/l

   135

   b. moderate if sodium is_____ mEq/l

   130

   c. severe if sodium is_____ mEq/l

   125

6. **Matching. For Na metabolism, match the conditions with their characteristics and treatment.**
   Characteristics and treatment:
   ① hyponatremia; ② increased intravascular volume; ③ treat with volume restriction; ④ volume depletion; ⑤ treat with Na + volume replacement; ⑥ symptoms made worse by fluid restriction
   Conditions:

   G7 p.7:145mm

   a. inappropriate antidiuretic hormone (ADH)

   ①, ②, ③

   b. cerebral salt wasting

   ①, ④, ⑤, ⑥

7. **Complete the equation to calculate serum osmolality.**

   G7 p.8:175mm

   a. Effective serum osmolality = measured osmolality − [ ]mg/dl

   BUN

   2.8

2

8. **Matching. Match symptoms with severity of hyponatremia.**   G7 p.9:150mm
   Hyponatremia:
   ① mild hyponatremia is less than 130 mEq/l, ② severe hyponatremia is less than 125 mEq/l
   Symptoms:
   a. headache   ①
   b. cerebral edema   ②
   c. anorexia   ①
   d. nausea vomiting   ②
   e. muscle weakness   ①
   f. muscle twitching   ②
   g. seizures   ②
   h. respiratory arrest ②
   i. difficulty concentrating ①

9. **List the symptoms of hyponatremia.**   G7 p.9:158mm
   Hint: c^6natremia
   a. cep_____   cephalgia
   b. cer_____ e_____   cerebral edema
   c. com_____   coma
   d. con_____   confusion
   e. conv_____   convulsions
   f. c_____   cramps
   g. n_____   nausea
   h. a_____   anorexia
   i. t_____   twitching
   j. r_____ a_____   respiratory arrest
   k. e_____   excitability
   l. m_____ w_____   muscle weakness
   m. i_____   irritability
       a

10. **SIADH criteria are**   G7 p.10:115mm
    a. NA is _____   low
    b. Urine osmolality is_____ high
    c. Volemia is_____   high
    d. Due to release of _____   ADH
        i.   without _____ stimuli   osmotic
        ii. creates _____hyponatremia dilutional
    e. The release of ADH without a stimulus is   inappropriate
        what makes the release_____

11. **One of the major effects of antidiuretic hormone is to**   G7 p.11:155mm
    a. _____ the permeability of the   increase
    b. _____ renal tubule. This results in   distal
    c. _____ _____ of water.   increased reabsorption
    d. Its effects on the circulating blood?   dilutes it
    e. Its effect on urine volume?   reduces urine volume
    f. Its effect on urine concentration?   increases urine concentration

2

12. **True or False. SIADH stands for syndrome of inappropriate antidiuretic hormone.**

true

G7 p.10:115mm

13. **SIADH can also stand for s_____ i_____ a_____ d_____ h_____.**

sodium is abnormal dilutionally hyponatremic

G7 p.10:115mm

14. **Complete the following regarding the treatment of hyponatremia:**

G7 p.10:140mm

a. Avoid _____ correction.

rapid

b. Avoid _____ correction.

over

c. Do not exceed _____ mEq/l per hour.

1

d. Do not exceed _____ mEq/l per 24 hours.

8

e. Do not exceed _____ mEq/l per 48 hours.

18

15. **Matching. Diagnosis of SIADH depends on three diagnostic criteria. Match the laboratory value with the appropriate test.**

G7 p. 11:28mm

Test:
① serum Na; ② serum K; ③ serum osmolality; ④ urinary osmolality; ⑤ urinary Na; ⑥ urinary K; ⑦ blood urea nitrogen (BUN) creatinine
Laboratory value:

a. low

①

b. high

④

c. normal

⑦

16. **Give the expected result for each test in the diagnosis of SIADH.**

G7 p.11:35mm

a. serum Na _____ _____ _____

low—below 134 mEq/l

b. serum osmol _____ _____ _____

low—below 280 mOsm/L

c. urinary Na _____ _____ _____

high—above 18 mEq/l

d. urinary Na may be as high as _____

50 to 150 mEq/l

e. serum BUN below _____

10

f. serum creatinine _____

normal

17. **Na at what level is always symptomatic?**

120 to 125 mEq/l

G7 p.11:95mm

18. **Characterize the symptoms of SIADH.**

G7 p11:95mm

a. Symptoms are almost always present at a Na of _____ to _____

120 to 125mEq/l

b. May treat if asymptomatic with _____ restriction

fluid

c. Avoid too rapid _____

correction

2

19. Central pontine myelinolysis (CPM) is   G7 p.11:150mm
   a. aka o_____ d_____ syndrome   osmotic demyelination
   b. due to r_____ c_____ of   rapid correction
      hyponatremia
   c. a disorder of p_____ w_____   pontine white matter
      m_____
   d. Its symptoms are
      i.   f_____ q_____   flaccid quadriplegia
      ii. m_____ s_____ changes   mental status
      iii. c_____ n_____ abnormalities   cranial nerve
      iv. p_____ p_____ appearance   pseudobulbar palsy

20. Features common to patients who   G7 p.11:178mm
   develop CPM are
   Hint: rodi
   a. r_____ c_____   rapid correction
   b. o_____ c_____   over correction
   c. d_____ in d_____ for more than   delay in diagnosis, 48
      _____ hours
   d. increase in NA by more than   25; 48
      _____ mEq/l within _____ hours

21. To treat mild SIADH you could modify   G7 p.13:100mm
   the following by:
   a. H$_2$O _____ _____   restrict fluid
   b. Salt _____ _____   use 3% NaCl (to increase Na)

22. To treat cerebral salt wasting (CSW)   G7 p.14:65mm
   you could modify the following by:
   a. H$_2$O _____ _____   give fluid
   b. Salt _____ _____   give salt (Hint: CSW—cure
      with salt and water.)

23. What is the treatment of severe   G7 p.12:140mm
   hyponatremia?
   a. Correct hyponatremia that is below   125
      _____ mEq/l.
   b. Start with a _____% correction.   10%

24. Do not exceed a correction of   G7 p.13:15mm
   a. more than _____ mEq/l/hr   1.3
   b. more than _____ mEq/l/24/hrs   10
   c. use _____% NaCl   3%
   d. this has _____ Eq/NaCl   513
   e. start with _____ cc/hr   25
   f. simultaneously administer _____   furosemide

25. List the expected patient laboratory   G7 p.14:20mm
   result when comparing SIADH with
   CSW.
   a. water: in SIADH _____, in   SIADH: hypervolemic, CSW:
      CSW_____   hypovolemic
   b. Na (serum): in SIADH _____, in   SIADH: low, CSW: low
      CSW_____
   c. osmol (serum): in SIADH _____, in   SIADH: low, CSW: high
      CSW_____

   d. osmol (urine): in SIADH _____, in   SIADH: high, CSW: high
      CSW _____

   e. Na (urine): in SIADH _____, in   SIADH: high, CSW: high
      CSW _____

   f. Hct: in SIADH _____, in   SIADH: low, CSW: high
      CSW _____

26. What is the treatment of CSW?   G7 p.14:70mm
   a. Hydrate
      i. with _____% _____ saline   0.9%, normal
      ii. at _____ cc/hr   100 to 125
   b. Use furosemide (yes or no?)   no
   c. Avoid _____ correction   rapid

27. In neurosurgical patients   G7 p.14:140mm
hyponatremia is seen in
   a. c_____ s_____ w_____   cerebral salt wasting
   b. and S_____.   SIADH

28. In neurological patients   G7 p.14:144mm
hypernatremia is seen in
   a. d_____ i_____.   diabetes insipidus
   b. Define hypernatremia.   Na above 150 mEq/l

29. Characterize diabetes insipidus.   G7 p.15:40mm
   a. Due to low level of _____.   ADH
   b. Urine output is > _____ cc/hr.   200
   c. Specific gravity of urine is < _____.   1.003
   d. Serum osmolarity is normal or _____.   high
   e. Serum sodium is _____.   high

30. In diabetes insipidus is the following   G7 p.15:40mm
low or high?
   a. ADH is _____.   low
   b. Urine specific gravity is _____.   low
   c. Urine output is _____.   high
   d. Serum osmolality is _____.   high
   e. Serum sodium is _____.   high

31. Diabetes insipidus features: G7 p.15:40mm
   a. Urine output is _____.   high
   b. Urine mOsm/l is below _____.   200
   c. Specific gravity is below _____.   1.003
   d. Serum osmol is _____.   high or normal
   e. Normal serum osmol is between   282 and 295 mOsm/l
      _____ and _____ mOsm/l.

32. Diabetes insipidus etiology: G7 p.15:80mm
   a. neu_____   neurogenic
   b. nep_____   nephrogenic

33. Diagnosis of diabetes insipidus occurs   G7 p.16:110mm
when
   a. urine output is above _____.   250 cc/hr
   b. urine osmol is below _____.   200 mOsm/l
   c. specific gravity is below _____.   1.003

34. Characterize serum osmolality.   G7 p.19:30mm
  a. Normal range is between _____ to   282 to 295
      _____ mOsm/l
  b. Dangerous if below _____ mOsm/l   240
  c. Dangerous if above _____ mOsm/l   320
  d. Risk of renal failure if above _____   320
      mOsm/l
  e. Seizures can occur if above _____   400
      mOsm/l

■ Blood Pressure Management

35. List the effects of labetalol on the   G7 p.20:50mm
following:
  a. ICP   no change
  b. pulse   no change
  c. cardiac output   no change
  d. coronary ischemia   no change
  e. renal failure   no change

36. List the plasma expanders that are   G7 p.22:50mm
useful cardiovascular agents for
treating shock.
  a. cr_____   crystalloids
  b. co_____   colloids
  c. bl_____ p_____   blood products

37. Describe the method of dosage for an   G7 p.20:70mm
intravenous (IV) drip of labetalol.
  a. add _____ ml (200 mg)   40
  b. to _____ ml volume to create a   160
      volume
  c. of _____ ml and infuse   200
  d. at _____ ml/min until   2
  e. _____ mg is given or the desired   300
      blood pressure (BP) is achieved.

38. For the listed pressors complete the
following statements to describe the
cautions required.
  a. Neo-Synephrine: avoid in s_____   spinal cord injuries   G7 p.22:170mm
      c_____ i_____
  b. Dopamine: may cause h_____   hyperglycemia   G7 p.22:100mm
  c. Dobutamine: may cause dysfunction of   platelets   G7 p.22:127mm
      p_____

■ Sedatives and Paralytics

39. The Richmond Scale: Rass quantitates   agitation and sedation   G7 p.23:90mm
_____ and _____ levels.

40. **True or False. Indicate whether the following statements are true or false:**

G7 p.24:25mm

a. Methohexital (Brevital) is more potent and shorter acting than thiopental.

true

b. Fentanyl causes dose-dependent respiratory depression.

true (also causes chest wall rigidity if given rapidly)

c. Propofol has better neuroprotection than barbiturates (during aneurysm surgery).

false (barbiturates are better)

d. Haldol can cause neuroleptic malignant syndrome.

true

41. **True or False. The following sedatives may induce seizures:**

G7 p.24:30mm

a. thiopental

false

b. methohexital

true

c. fentanyl

false

d. propofol

false

e. haloperidol

false

42. **True or False. The drug that can produce a neuroleptic malignant syndrome as a secondary effect is**

G7 p.24:47mm

a. propofol

false

b. benzodiazepines

false

c. fentanyl

false

d. haloperidol

true

e. thiopental

false

43. **Complete the following statements about the neuroleptic malignant syndrome:**

G7 p.24:47mm

a. Characterized by
   Hint: neuroleptic

   i. n_____ — motor, mutism

   ii. e_____ — elevation of temperature

   iii. u_____ — unconsciousness

   iv. r_____ — rigid muscles, rapid heart rate, respiratory failure

   v. o_____ — opisthotonus

   vi. l_____ — lethargy, leucocytosis

   vii. e_____ — elevated CPK

   viii. p_____ — potentially lethal

   ix. t_____ — trembling

   x. i_____ — imbalance of autonomic system

   xi. c_____ — coma

2

44.   True or False. Regarding thiopental: G7 p.24:86mm
a.   It's a long-acting barbiturate.   false (Thiopental is a short-acting barbiturate with consciousness returning after 20 to 30 minutes.)
b.   It causes dose-related respiratory depression.   true
c.   It causes myocardial depression.   true
d.   It is an antianalgesic.   true
e.   It causes hypotension in hypovolemic patients.   true

45.   True or False. The following sedative causes necrosis when injected intraarterially: G7 p.24:94mm
a.   thiopental   true
b.   fentanyl   false
c.   propofol   false

46.   True or False. Choose the correct order from long-acting to short-acting for the following neuromuscular blocking agents: G7 p.24:120mm
a.   succinylcholine, vecuronium, pancuronium, nocuronium   false
b.   vecuronium, pancuronium, succinylcholine, rocuronium   false
c.   pancuronium, vecuronium, rocuronium, succinylcholine   true—pancuronium (Pavulon)—60 to 180 minutes vecuronium (Norcuron)—40 to 60 minutes rocuronium (Zemuron)—40 to 60 minutes (but shorter onset) succinylcholine (Anectine)—20 minutes
d.   rocuronium, succinylcholine, pancuronium, vecuronium   false
e.   vecuronium, pancuronium, rocuronium, succinylcholine   false

47.   True or False. The following is always required in a conscious patient simultaneously with a paralytic agent and as ventilation is being established: G7 p.25:100mm
a.   arterial line   false
b.   Swan-Ganz catheter   false
c.   sedation   true
d.   intracranial pressure (ICP) monitor   false
e.   all of the above   false

48. True or False.   G7 p.25:165mm
  a. Pancuronium is a long-acting agent.   true
  b. Rocuronium is a short-acting agent.   true
  c. Succinylcholine is a competitive blocker   false (Succinylcholine is a
     and is short acting.   noncompetitive blocker and
                                              is considered the only
                                              depolarizing ganglionic
                                              blocker. It has been linked to
                                              malignant hyperthermia.)
  d. Sedation is required for conscious   true
     patients.

49. True or False. The only depolarizing   G7 p.26:25mm
ganglionic blocker among the
following paralytics is
  a. succinylcholine   true
  b. rapacuronium   false
  c. mivacurium   false
  d. rocuronium   false

50. True or False. Possible side effects of   G7 p.26:53mm
succinylcholine include
  a. elevated serum K+   true (Succinylcholine can
                                              cause elevated K+, especially
                                              in patients with neuronal
                                              [spinal cord injury,
                                              hemiparesis] or muscular
                                              pathology, causing
                                              hyperkalemia.)
  b. cardiac arrest in adolescents and children   true (Adolescents and
                                              children with undiagnosed
                                              cardiac myopathies may
                                              arrest.)
  c. sinus bradycardia   true (It causes dysrhythmia,
                                              mainly sinus bradycardia.)
  d. malignant hyperthermia   true (It has been linked to
                                              malignant hyperthermia.)

51. True or False. The following paralytic   G7 p.26:60mm
is contraindicated in the acute phase
of injury because of the risk of
hyperkalemia:
  a. succinylcholine   true
  b. metocurine   false
  c. doxacurium   false
  d. pancuronium   false
  e. vecuronium   false

52. True or False. The shortest-acting   G7 p.26:162mm
nondepolarizing neuromuscular
blocking agent (NMBA) is
  a. mivacurium   false
  b. rocuronium   false
  c. vecuronium   true
  d. metocurine   false
  e. doxacurium   false

53. **True or False. The nondepolarizing paralytic that does not affect ICP or CPP is**   G7 p.26:168mm
    a. vecuronium   true
    b. pancuronium   false
    c. succinylcholine   false
    d. rapacuronium   false
    e. rocuronium   false

54. **True or False. The main difference between cisatracrium and its isomer atracurium is**   G7 p.27:40mm
    a. cost   false
    b. onset of action   false
    c. duration   false
    d. cisatracrium does not release histamine   true
    e. none of the above   false

55. **The complete reversal of Pavulon's effect takes _____ minutes.**   G7 p.27:55mm
    20

56. **True or False. It is true about pancuronium that**   G7 p.27:55mm
    a. it is not reversible   false (It is reversible with anticholinesterases.)
    b. it is not a competitive paralytic   false (It is a competitive paralytic.)
    c. it increases cardiac output, pulse rate, and ICP   true
    d. it is eliminated through the liver   false (It is eliminated through the kidneys.)

57. **True or False. Regarding atracurium:**   G7 p.27:60mm
    a. It is a nondepolarizing (competitive) blocker.   true
    b. It can produce hypotension.   true
    c. It is reversible with neostigmine.   true
    d. It is metabolized in the kidneys and liver.   false

■ Neurogenic Pulmonary Edema

58. **True or False. Which of the following statements about neurogenic pulmonary edema are true and which are false?**

   a. relatively common condition in the neurosurgical patient — false

   b. caused by intracranial pathologies such as subarachnoid hemorrhage (SAH), seizure (Sz), head injury — true

   c. mechanism caused in part by slow increase in intracranial pressure (ICP) — false

   d. surge of catecholamine disrupts capillary endothelium with increase in alveolar permeability — true

G7 p.28:30mm

59. **True or False. For treatment of neurogenic pulmonary edema, you should use high levels of positive end expiratory pressure (PEEP) to keep alveoli distended.**

false—low levels of PEEP

G7 p.28:55mm

60. **True or False. For neurogenic pulmonary edema, dobutamine does *not* reduce cerebral perfusion.**

true—and therefore is better than á or â blockers to treat neurogenic pulmonary edema

G7 p.28:67mm

3

General Care

■ Endocrinology

1. **True or False. The following has to be replaced in adrenal failure:**
   a. mineralocorticoids   true
   b. glucocorticoids   true

   G7 p.31:100mm

2. **True or False. The following has to be replaced in pituitary failure:**
   a. mineralocorticoids   false
   b. glucocorticoids   true

   G7 p.31:100mm

3. **Matching.**
   ① glucocorticoids;
   ② mineralocorticoids; ③ none
   a. In primary adrenocortical insufficiency   ①
   you must replace _____ and
   b. _____.   ②
   c. In secondary adrenocortical insufficiency   ①
   you must replace _____ and
   d. _____.   ③

   G7 p.31:100mm

4. **True or False. The following meds should be used for primary adrenocortical insufficiency:**
   a. cortisone   true
   b. cortisol   true
   c. Solu-Cortef   true
   d. prednisone   true
   e. methylprednisolone   false
   f. dexamethasone   false

   G7 p.31:165mm

5. **True or False. The following meds should be used for secondary adrenocortical insufficiency:**
   a. cortisone   false
   b. cortisol   false
   c. Solu-Cortef   false
   d. prednisone   false
   e. methylprednisolone   true
   f. dexamethasone   true

   G7 p.31:165mm

6. **If you use mineralocorticoids when they are not needed, you risk developing the following:**
   Hint: pawnb

   a. p_____ a_____

   potassium—hypokalemia altered

   b. w_____

   water retained—fluid retention

   c. N_____

   Na retained—salt retention

   d. b_____ p_____

   blood pressure (BP) elevated—hypertension

G7 p.31:165mm

7. **Hypothalamic—pituitary—adrenal suppression can occur if a dose of**

   a. 40 mg of prednisone is given for _____ days.

   7

   b. 10 mg of Decadron is given for _____ days.

   7

   c. If steroids are given for less than 7 days taper _____.

   not needed

   d. If given for 7 to 14 days taper over _____.

   1 to 2 weeks

   e. You should taper prednisone by reducing 5 mg every _____ days.

   5 (3 to 7)

   f. You should taper Decadron by reducing 0.75 mg every _____ days.

   5 (3 to 7)

   g. After a month on steroids HPA axis may be depressed for as long as _____.

   1 year

   h. HPA = _____ _____ _____ axis

   hypothalamic pituitary adrenal

G7 p.32:30mm
G7 p.32:85mm
G7 p.32:52mm

8. **Stress (supplemental) doses of steroids may be needed**

   a. if patient is on steroids

      i. c_____ or was on them during the

   chronically

      ii. past _____ years

   1 to 2

G7 p.32:165mm

9. **Study Chart. List the possible deleterious effects of steroids.**

   a. A

   alkalosis, amenorrhea, avascular necrosis (hip)

   b. B

   bone loss

   c. C

   cushingoid features, cataracts, compression fractures, reactivation of chickenpox

   d. D

   diverticular perforation, diabetes

   e. E

   epidural lipomatosis

   f. F

   fungal infections, fetal adrenal hypoplasia

   g. G

   growth suppression in children, gastrointestinal bleed, gastritis, glaucoma

G7 p.33:45mm

3

h. H   hypertension: hypokalemia,
                            hirsutism, hyperlipidemia,
                            hypercoagulopathy, hiccups
i. I   impaired wound healing,
                            immunosuppression

j. J
k. K
l. L   lipomatosis, spinal epidural
m. M   mental agitation, muscle
                            weakness, steroid myopathy
n. N   nonketotic coma, nitrogen
                            metabolism is disturbed
o. O   obesity, osteoporosis
p. P   progressive multifocal
                            leukoencephalopathy (PML),
                            pseudotumor cerebri,
                            pancreatitis
q. Q   Q.
r. R   reactivation of tuberculosis
                            (TB)
s. S   sodium retention, steroid
                            psychosis
t. T   tissue plasminogen activator
                            inhibition
u. U   U.
v. V   V.
w. W   water retention

10. What are the symptoms of addisonian   G7 p.34:75mm
     crisis?
     Hint: claw
a. c_____   confusion
b. l_____   *l*ethargy
c. a_____   *a*gitation
d. w_____   *w*eakness

11. What are the signs of Addisonian   G7 p.34:75 mm
     crisis? Choose hypo- or hyper-.
a. BP   hypotension (shock)
b. Na   hyponatremia
c. K   hyperkalemia
d. glucose   hypoglycemia
e. temperature   hyperthermia

■ Hematology

12. Complete the following concerning platelets: G7 p.34:165mm

a. Normal platelet count is _____ to _____. 150 k to 400 k/mm³

b. Delay surgery if platelets are below _____. 50,000/mm³

c. Transfuse if:
   i. surgery is _____ urgent
   ii. patient is on _____ or _____ and can't wait _____ days. Plavix or ASA / 5 to 7

d. Usual transfusion is _____ of platelets. an eight-pack (= 6 to 10 U)

e. One U raises platelets by _____. 10 k

13. Complete the following regarding platelet therapy: G7 p.35:20mm

a. 1 unit of platelets has a volume of approximately _____ cc. 50

b. Platelet count can be checked in _____ hours. 2

c. Re-transfusion will be needed in _____ days. 3 to 5   G7 p.35:120mm

14. Complete the following concerning fresh frozen plasma: G7 p.35:130mm

a. One bag equals _____ cc. 250

b. Risk of acquired immunodeficiency syndrome (AIDS) or hepatitis is the same as _____. a unit of blood

c. Use to reverse Coumadin:
   i. prothrombin time (PT) greater than _____ 18 seconds
   ii. international normalized ratio (INR) greater than _____ 1.6
   iii. von Willebrand disease unresponsive to _____ DDAVP
   iv. multiple coagulation dysfunction such as in
       h_____ _____ hepatic dysfunction
       v_____ _____ _____ vitamin K deficiency
       D_____ DIC

15. In regard to the use of anticoagulation in a patient who has: G7 p.37:60mm

a. An incidental aneurysm < 4mm, anticoagulation is _____ ok

b. A drug eluting cardiac stent—continue _____ Plavix

c. At onset of SAH we should _____ anticoagulation reverse

d. Postoperative craniotomy may start on day _____ to _____ weeks after surgery 3 to 5

16. **In regard to anticoagulation in preparation for surgery, if a patient has:**

G7 p.37:145mm

a. a mechanical heart valve
  i. stop warfarin _____ days before surgery   3
  ii. and use _____   Lovenox
b. chronic A-fib
  i. stop warfarin _____ days before surgery   4 to 5

17. **Complete the following concerning anticoagulation:**

G7 p.37:167mm

a. May resume anticoagulation _____ days after craniotomy   3 to 5
b. Annual risk of nonanticoagulation for a patient with
  i. mechanical heart valve is _____% per year   6%
  ii. chronic atrial fibrillation is _____% per year   4 to 6%
c. If patient is on Plavix or acetylsalicylic acid (ASA) delay surgery for _____.   5 to 7 days

18. **Provide coagulation factors for neurosurgery.**

G7 p.38:20mm

a. PT should be below _____ seconds.   13.5
b. INR should not be above _____.   1.4
c. For emergencies give _____ _____ units   FFP 2
d. and _____ _____.   vitamin K

19. **Both Plavix and ASA inhibit platelet function for how long?**   permanently

G7 p.38:90mm

20. **Plavix is a more dangerous drug than ASA because it remains**

G7 p.38:130mm

a. _____ for up to   active
b. _____ after the last dose and   several days
c. can inhibit even those _____ _____ given as treatment.   transfused platelets

21. **Complete the following concerning warfarin (Coumadin):**

G7 p.39:42mm

a. Don't start Coumadin until a _____ _____ _____ _____ has been achieved on heparin   therapeutic partial thromboplastin time (PTT)
b. to reduce the risk of _____ _____.   Coumadin necrosis
c. For the first 3 days of Coumadin therapy patients are actually _____;   hypercoagulable
d. therefore continue _____ for a few _____.   heparin days

3

22. **Possible heparin side effects include**   G7 p.39:95mm
    a. t_____   thrombosis
    b. t_____   thrombocytopenia
    c. These are due to:
       i.   _____ in heparin-induced   consumption
            thrombosis
       ii. _____ formed against a heparin– antibodies
            platelet protein complex
    d. In such cases of heparin-induced   lepirudin (Refludan)
       thrombocytopenia, treat with _____.

23. **Low molecular weight heparin should**   G7 p.39:135mm
    have
    a. fewer _____ complications   hemorrhagic
    b. more predictable _____ levels   plasma
    c. less need to _____ biologic activity monitor
    d. a longer _____ life   half
    e. need for _____ doses per day   fewer
    f. a lower incidence of _____   thrombocytopenia
    g. more effective in _____ prophylaxis DVT
       than warfarin

24. **A serious side effect could be spinal**   G7 p.39:170mm
    _____ _____.   epidural hematoma

25. **Complete the following concerning**   G7 p.40:170mm
    coagulopathy:
    a. To reverse Coumadin anticoagulation in 2 to 3 units fresh frozen
       a patient who is at the usual therapeutic plasma
       levels use _____.
    b. For severely prolonged coagulation use 6 units fresh frozen plasma
       _____.
    c. To reverse PT from Coumadin use
       i.   _____   vitamin K aqua mephyton
       ii. administered by what route?   IM
       iii. Administration may be fatal if given intravenously
            _____.
       iv. Why?
            h_____   hypotension
            a_____   anaphylaxis

26. **Matching. Use the numbers of the**   G7 p.41:20mm
    listed terms to complete the following
    statements.
       ① prothrombin complex concentrate;
       ② protamine sulfate; ③ vitamin K;
       ④ AquaMEPHYTON
    a. Coumadin is reversed by:
       i.   p_____ c_____ c_____   ①
       ii. v_____ k_____   ③
       iii. A_____   ④
    b. Heparin is reversed by p_____   ②
       s_____

3

27. **Complete the following concerning thromboembolism:**   G7 p.42:35mm
a. Risk of embolism from calf deep-vein thrombosis (DVT) is _____%.   1%
b. Extends to proximal deep veins in _____%.   30 to 50%
c. Embolism from thigh veins is _____.   40 to 50%
d. Mortality of DVT of legs is _____.   9 to 50%
e. DVTs in NS (neurosurgical) patients occur in _____.   19 to 50%

28. **Conditions that make NS patients prone to DVTs are**   G7 p.42:50mm
Hint: clot
a. c_____ _____   concomitant sludging
b. l_____-_____ _____   long-time immobility (i.e., bed rest, paralysis)
c. o_____ _____/d_____   operating room/dehydration
d. t_____ _____   thromboplastin release

29. **The best prophylaxis against DVTs is**   G7 p.42:110mm
a. PCBs is the abbreviation for _____ _____ _____   pneumatic compression boots
b. low _____ _____   dose heparin (5000 IU subcutaneous every 8 to 12 hours start first postop day)

30. **Matching. One can diagnose DVT with the following tests. Match the finding with its appropriate diagnostic value.**   G7 p.43:80mm
Diagnostic value:
① gold standard; ② associated with PE and DVT; ③ only 50% accurate; ④ 99% specific
Clinical finding or procedure:
a. hot swollen tender calf with positive Homan sign   ③
b. contrast venography   ①
c. Doppler ultrasonography   ④
d. D-dimer   ②

31. **What is the treatment of DVT?**   G7 p.43:135mm
a. b_____ _____   bed rest
b. e_____ i_____ leg   elevate involved leg
c. h_____, L_____ or   heparin, Legoparin
d. L_____ plus   Lovenox
e. C_____   Coumadin
f. Consider G_____ f_____   Greenfield filter
g. a_____   ambulate
h. after _____ to _____ days   7 to 10
i. wear _____-_____ _____   anti-embolic stockings
j. For how long ? _____   indefinitely

32. **Extramedullary hematopoiesis can result in**   G7 p.43:170mm
   a. abnormal skull x-ray called _____   hair on end
      _____ _____
   b. spinal cord compression due to   vertebral body thickening
      _____ _____ _____

33. **Extramedullary hematopoiesis can be treated with**   G7 p.43:170mm
   a. r_____ and/or   radiotherapy
   b. s_____   surgery

■ Pharmacology

34. **True or False. Prostaglandins sensitize A-delta and C fibers.** true   G7 p. 44:140mm

35. **True or False. Metastatic cancer pain can be desensitized by**   G7 p.44:140mm
   a. steroids   true
   b. aspirin   true
   c. nonsteroidal anti-inflammatory drugs (NSAIDs) true
   d. acetaminophen (Tylenol)   false

36. **How do NSAIDs work?**   G7 p.44:170mm
   a. They inhibit _____   cyclooxygenase
   b. which thereby interferes with the synthesis of p_____   prostaglandins
   c. and t_____.   thromboxanes
   d. This inhibits the function of _____   platelets
   e. and prolongs _____ _____.   bleeding time
   f. They may also injure _____ (_____). kidneys (nephrotoxicity)

37. **Complete the following concerning NSAIDs and platelet function:**   G7 p.45:50mm
   a. The NSAID that results in irreversible binding is _____.   aspirin
   b. Which NSAID results in reversible inhibition of platelet function?   most NSAIDS
   c. The NSAID that does not interfere with platelet function is _____.   Relafen (nabumetone)

3

38. **List the dosages for the following substances:**   G7 p.45:148mm
   a. NSAIDs to use
      i. Naprosyn loading: _____ then   500 mg, then 250 mg every
         _____ every _____ to   6 to 8 hours
         _____ hours.
      ii. Motrin no loading: Start dose   Start dose 400 to 800 mg,
         _____ to _____mg then   then 4 times a day
         _____ times a day.
   b. opioids to use (moderate to severe pain)
      i. Percodan no loading: Start dose   1 to 2 pills every 3 to 4 hours
         _____ to _____ pill(s) every
         _____ to _____ hours.
      ii. Vicodin no loading: Start dose   1 pill every 6 hours
         _____ pill(s) every _____   8 pills every 24 hours
         hours. Limit _____to _____
         every _____ hours per day.
   c. opioids to use (mild to moderate pain)
      i. codeine loading? Start dose   no loading 30 to 60 mg at
         _____ to _____ mg at   3 hours
         _____ hours, to _____ mg at   60 mg at 3 to 5 hours
         _____ to _____ hours.

39. **How much Tylenol is safe?**   G7 p.46:145mm
   a. comes in dosages of _____ or   650 or 1000 mg
      _____
   b. safe up to _____ mg per day   4000
   c. has a ceiling effect at _____ mg/day   1300
   d. has hepatic toxicity above _____   10,000
      mg/day

40. **A serious side effect of Tylenol is**   hepatic toxicity   G7 p.46:160mm
   _____ _____.

41. **True or False. Regarding opioid analgesics:**   G7 p.46:180mm
   a. They are only indicated for the treatment   false
      of acute pain.
   b. Tolerance develops with chronic use.   true
   c. Potential for respiratory depression is   false
      limited.
   d. Seizures are not a known adverse effect.   false

42. **True or False. Regarding opioid analgesics:**   G7 p.47:18mm
   a. They have no ceiling effect.   true
   b. With chronic use, tolerance develops.   true
   c. Overdose is possible with severe   true
      respiratory depression.
   d. Treatment of overdose includes   true
      administration of naloxone.
   e. Flumazenil helps in treatment of   false (Flumazenil is useful in
      overdose.   treatment of overdose from
                   benzodiazepines not from
                   opioids.)

43.	**True or False. Regarding narcotics:**	G7 p.47:18mm
a.	Some opioids may cause seizures.	true
b.	Physical and psychological tolerance develops with chronic use.	true
c.	There is a ceiling effect with increasing dosage.	false (There is *no* ceiling effect with opioids. Increasing dosage *does* increase effectiveness, but side effects may limit higher doses.)
d.	Overdose can cause respiratory depression.	true

44. Complete the following mnemonic about opioids: G7 p.47:28mm

a. o_____ — *o*verdose is possible
b. p_____ — *p*otential for respiratory depression
c. i_____ — *i*ncrease dosage = increase effect—no ceiling effect
d. o_____ — small pupils—miosis—*o*
e. i_____ — *i*ntoxication: treat with Narcan
f. d_____ — *d*evelops tolerance with chronic use

45. To what type of opioid receptor subtype does tramadol (Ultram) bind? μ (MU) opioid receptor   G7 p.47:103mm

46. Ultram acts centrally to inhibit re-uptake of   G7 p.47:105mm
a. n_____ and — norepinephrine
b. s_____. — serotonin

47. True or False. OxyContin tablets should never be taken crushed, divided, or chewed. true   G7 p.48:40mm

48. What is the intramuscular:per os (IM:PO) potency for morphine?   G7 p.49:20mm
a. single dose — 1:6
b. chronic dosing — 1:2 to 3

49. What metabolite of meperidine might cause delirium and seizures? normeperidine   G7 p.49:22mm

50. True or False. When taken with monoamine oxidase inhibitors (MAOIs), meperidine may cause   G7 p.49:30mm
a. severe encephalopathy — true
b. death — true

51. Tricyclic antidepressants elevate levels of what endogenous analgesic? endorphin   G7 p.548:150mm

3

52. **Indicate the following adjuvant medications' characteristic actions:**

   a. tricyclic   blocks serotonin uptake   G7 p.48:150mm
   b. tryptophan   precursor of serotonin   G7 p.50:40mm
   c. antihistamines   anxiolytic   G7 p.50:50mm
   d. phenothiazine   tranquilizing   G7 p.50:75mm

53. **What craniofacial pain syndromes are responsive to carbamazepine (Tegretol)?**   G7 p.50:62 mm

   a. t_____ n_____   trigeminal neuralgia
   b. g_____ n_____   glossopharyngeal neuralgia
   c. p_____-h_____ n_____   post-herpetic neuralgia

54. **Matching. Match each adjuvant pain medication with each description.**   G7 p.50:80mm
   Description:
   ① increases serotonin by blocking reuptake; ② increases serotonin by being a substrate for its production; ③ anxiolytic and hypnotic, helps with nociceptive pain; ④ tranquilizing, helpful with other adjuvants in neuropathic pain
   Pain medication:

   a. tryptophan   ② Amino acid precursor for serotonin, a potentiator for analgesic effects of endorphin. Warning: Daily use depletes vitamin B_6—use multivitamins. Give 1.5 to 2.0 mg h.s.

   b. phenothiazines   ④ Example is fluphenazine (Prolixin). Give with tricyclic for neuropathic (diabetic) pain. May reduce seizure threshold.

   c. tricyclic antidepressant ① Elavil (75 mg q.d.), desipramine (10 to 25 mg q.d.), or doxepin (75 to 150 mg q.d.), more effective than norepinephrine reuptake blockers.

   d. antihistamine   ③ Histamine plays a role in nociception. Hydroxyzine 50 mg every a.m. and 100 mg every h.s.

55. True or False. Regarding antispasmodics/muscle relaxants: G7 p.50:110mm

a. Robaxin (methocarbamol) is contraindicated in patients with peptic ulcer disease because of its aspirin content.   true

b. Parafon Forte (chlorzoxazone) should not be used because of its risk of fatal hepatotoxicity.   true

c. All of these act as central nervous system sedatives and have proven efficacious with acute low back problems.   false (Although they act centrally, their efficacy for acute low back problems is dubious.)

d. Soma (carisoprodol) may produce euphoria and has abuse potential.   true

e. Taken for "night cramps," quinine sulfate is an abortifacient, can cause thrombotic thrombocytopenic purpura (TTP), and can also result in cinchonism.   true

◼ Benzodiazepines

56. True or False. Regarding benzodiazepines: G7 p.51:92mm

a. Effective for treatment of anxiety and insomnia   true

b. Safe in the first trimester of pregnancy   false (Not safe in the first trimester of pregnancy; BZDs are contraindicated during first trimester—teratogenic.)

c. Shorter-acting agents are more likely to cause rebound depression or withdrawal symptoms.   true

d. Longer-acting agents result in cumulative sedation and impairment of psychomotor function.   true

57. True or False. The following group of benzodiazepines is more prone to cause rebound depression or withdrawal syndrome: G7 p.51:100mm

a. long duration   false
b. intermediate duration   false
c. short duration   true
d. all of the above   false
e. none of the above   false

58. True or False. A contraindication to the use of benzodiazepines is   G7 p.51:115mm

a. second trimester of pregnancy   false
b. first trimester of pregnancy   true
c. third trimester of pregnancy   false
d. alcohol use   false (but adds no sedation)
e. hypoglycemia   false

3

59. True or False. Regarding midazolam (Versed): G7 p.51:140mm
a. more potent than diazepam (Valium)   true
b. crosses blood–brain barrier   true
c. has good amnestic effect   true
d. has good anticonvulsant effect   true
e. is associated with respiratory arrest true

60. You have been called in consultation to see a head-injured patient who is intubated, sedated, and paralyzed. How long must you wait to do your examination? G7 p.51:150mm
a. if Pavulon has been used _____   about 60 minutes
b. if Norcuron has been used _____   about 60 minutes
c. if Versed has been used _____   about 2 hours

61. True or False. The following benzodiazepine has a greater amnestic effect: G7 p.51:150mm
a. oxazepam   false
b. alprazolam   false
c. midazolam   true
d. temazepam   false
e. diazepam   false

62. True or False. The mechanism of action of flumazenil is to G7 p.52:80mm
a. stimulate adenosine monophosphate (AMP)   false
b. inhibit AMP   false
c. hyperpolarize postganglionic neurons   false
d. competitively inhibit benzodiazepines at receptor sites   true

63. The correct order for the following oral benzodiazepines from long-acting to short-acting duration of action is: G7 p.52:40mm
a. diazepam, flumazenil, alprazolam   false
b. flumazenil, alprazolam, diazepam   false
c. alprazolam, flumazenil, diazepam   false
d. alprazolam, diazepam, flumazenil   false
e. diazepam, alprazolam, flumazenil   true (Diazepam [Valium] is long acting. Alprazolam [Xanax] is intermediate acting. Flumazenil [Romazicon] is intermediate to short acting.) G7 p.52:80mm

64. Complete the following statement about the previous answer. Therefore it is used for _____.   reversing benzodiazepine (BDZ) that had been used for conscious sedation or general anesthesia   G7 p.52:80mm

65. **Unusual concerns with flumazenil are**   G7 p.52:80mm
  a. c_____ in p_____   contraindicated in pregnancy
  b. works for only 10 to 60 minutes;   resedation may occur
     therefore, r_____ may o_____

66. **True or False. Regarding flumazenil**   G7 p.52:80mm
     (Romazicon):
  a. resedation may occur if large amounts of   true
     benzodiazepines (BZDs) have been given
  b. reversal of BZD-induced respiratory   true
     depression is partial or nil
  c. duration of action is shorter than most   true
     BZDs
  d. binds BZDs to stop/inhibit their action   false (Flumazenil
                                                 competitively inhibits BZDs at
                                                 receptor sites.)
  e. may provoke panic attack   true

67. **True or False. The recommended**   G7 p.52:100mm
     initial dose of flumazenil to reverse
     benzodiazepines used for conscious
     sedation or general anesthesia is
  a. 5 mg IV over 15 seconds   false
  b. 0.5 mg IV over 1 minute   false
  c. 2 mg IV over 1 minute   false
  d. 0.1 mg IV over 5 minutes   false
  e. 0.2 mg IV over 15 seconds   true

68. **True or False. How long before brain**   G6 p.37:140mm
     magnetic resonance imaging (MRI) is
     scheduled do you give chloral hydrate
     to a child?
  a. 5 minutes   false
  b. 12 hours   false
  c. 30 to 60 minutes   true
  d. it is not relevant   false
  e. 3 hours   false

69. **True or False. The following drugs are**   G6 p.37:160mm
     used in the "DPT" lytic cocktail:
  a. meperidine, promethazine,   true
     chlorpromazine   meperidine (Demerol)
                                                  promethazine (Phenergan)
                                                  chlorpromazine (Thorazine)
  b. meperidine, atenolol, flumazenil   false
  c. propofol, promethazine, thiopental   false
  d. haloperidol, propofol, methohexital   false
  e. midazolam, atracurium, chlorpromazine   false

70. **True or False. Examples of central**   false (Spinal cord injury is a   G7 p.52:137mm
     nervous system (CNS) factors that   CNS risk factor for stress ulcer
     increase the risk of stress ulcers are   also.)
     brain tumors and intracerebral
     hemorrhage (ICH) but not spinal cord
     injury.

3

71. **True or False. Extra CNS factors that increase the odds of stress ulcer are the following:**

G7 p.52:143mm

a. burns covering > 25% of body surface area   true

b. hypotension   true

c. renal failure   true

d. coagulopathies   true

72. **When is the peak time for acid and pepsin production after head injury?**   3 to 5 days after injury

G7 p.52:155mm

73. **There is a medication better than H2 antagonists to reduce incidence of stress ulcer.**

G7 p.52:171mm

a. It is called _____.   sucralfate

b. The brand name is _____.   Carafate

74. **Name the histamine (H2) antagonists you can prescribe.**
Hint: TAPPZ

G6 p.41:20mm

a. T_____   Tagamet

b. A_____   Axid

c. P_____   Pepcid

d. Z_____   Zantac

75. **Should prophylactic use of H2 blockers be used if steroids are given?**   no—usually not warranted

G7 p.52:175mm

4

Neurology

■ **Dementia**

1. What is the definition of dementia? — G7 p.56:50mm
a. Loss of i_____ abilities — intellectual
b. Severe enough to interfere with _____ — social
c. or o_____ functioning — occupational
d. Cardinal feature is m_____ d_____ — memory deficit
e. plus at least one additional i_____ — impairment
f. Affects _____% of persons over 65 — 3 to 11%

2. Risk factors for dementia include — G7 p.56:70mm
Hint: afA
a. a_____ a_____ — advanced age
b. f_____ h_____ — family history
c. A_____ _____ _____ a_____ — Apoli protein E4 allele

3. True or False. Because delirium is distinct from dementia, patients with dementia are not at increased risk of developing delirium. — false (Patients with dementia are at increased risk of developing delirium.) — G7 p.56:75mm

4. True or False. Fifty percent of patients with delirium die within 2 years. — true — G7 p.56:85mm

■ **Headache**

5. In regard to a unilateral headache, if it persists — G7 p.57:90mm
a. for > a year an _____ _____ is recommended — MRI scan
b. because this is _____ for migraine — atypical
c. and may be a hint of an underlying _____ — AVM

4

6. **Matching. Match symptoms with category of migraine.** G7 p.57:135mm
   Symptoms:
   ① Episodic H/A; ② N/V; ③ Photophobia;
   ④ Aura; ⑤ Focal neurological deficit
   (a) that resolves within 24 hrs; (b) slow
   march—like progression of deficit; (c)
   that resolves within 30 days; ⑥ No
   headache; ⑦ Mostly seen in children;
   ⑧ Hemiplegia; ⑨ Mostly seen in
   adolescents; ⑩ Vertigo, ataxia,
   dysarthria, severe HA
   Category of migraine:

   a. Common migraine   ①-②-③
   b. Classic migraine   ①-②-③-④-⑤-⑤a-⑤b
   c. Complicated migraine   ⑤-⑤c-⑥
   d. Migraine equivalent   ②-⑥-⑦
   e. Hemiplegic migraine   ①-⑧
   f. Basilar artery migraine   ⑨-⑩

7. **True or False. Neurological deficits seen in classic migraine typically resolve within** G7 p.57:145mm

   a. 1 hour   false
   b. 1 day   true
   c. 1 week   false
   d. 1 month   false
   e. They are permanent.   false

8. **True or False. Regarding cluster headaches:** G7 p.58:45mm

   a. may include partial Horner and autonomic symptoms — true (ptosis, miosis, tearing, nasal stuffiness)
   b. are more common in women — false (5 men to 1 woman)
   c. occur almost daily — true
   d. last 30 to 90 minutes — true
   e. continue for a 6- to 9-month period — false (1 to 3 months)
   f. may have a period of remission for ~1 year — true

9. **List the drugs for treatment of migraine headaches.** G5 p.61:30mm

   a. M_____ — Midrin (isometheptane mucate, methysergide)
   b. I_____ — Inderal
   c. F_____ — Fiorinal Fioricet
   d. r_____ — rizatriptan (Maxalt)
   e. a_____ — aspirin, amitriptyline (Elavil)
   f. I_____ — (Imitrex) sumatripan (Inderal) propranolol

g. n_____   nonsteroidal antiinflammatory drugs, naproxen (Anaprox)

h. e_____   ergotamine tartrate (Cafergot)

i. S_____   (Sansert) methysergide, serotonin antagonists, steroids

10. True or False. Basilar artery migraines are essentially restricted to   G7 p.58:95mm

a. geriatric patients   false
b. postmenopausal women   false
c. adolescents   true
d. men   false

11. True or False. Patients suffering basilar artery migraine attacks usually have a family history of migraine.   true (86%)   G7 p.58:95mm

12. Most postlumbar puncture headaches occur within _____ after the lumbar puncture.   3 days   G7 p.58:145mm

13. The incidence of postpuncture headaches is _____%.   2 to 40%, typically 20%   G7 p.58:145mm

14. A treatment for post puncture headache that is effective in 90% of cases is _____ _____ _____.   epidural blood patch   G7 p.59:55mm

■ Parkinsonism

15. Matching. Match the symptoms with type of parkinsonism.   G7 p.59:150 mm

Symptoms:
① Gradual onset of bradykinesia;
② Asymmetric tremor; ③ Responds well to levodopa;④ Rapid progression of symptoms; ⑤ Equivocal response to levodopa; ⑥ Early midline symptoms (i.e., ataxia, gait , balance); ⑦ Early dementia; ⑧Orthostatic hypotension; ⑨ Extraocular movement abnormalities
Types of parkinsonism:

a. Primary idiopathic paralysis agitans (IPA)   ①-②-③
b. Secondary parkinsonism   ④-⑤-⑥-⑦-⑧-⑨

16. In parkinsonism, degeneration of substantia nigra cells (pars compacta) results in   G7 p.59:177mm

a. _____ D2 dopamine receptors projecting to the globus pallidus interna (GPi)   ↓

b. _____ D1 receptors projecting to globus pallidus externa (GPe) and subthalamic nucleus (STN)   ↑

17. This results in increased activity by   G7 p.60:15mm

a. _____, causing   GPi

b. _____ of the thalamus, which then suppresses activity in the   inhibition

c. _____ _____ _____.   supplemental motor cortex

18. Provide parkinsonism pathophysiology.   G7 p.59:170mm

a. Degeneration of pigmented _____ neurons   dopaminergic

b. Of the pars compacta of the _____ _____   substantia nigra

c. This reduces the levels of _____ in the   dopamine

d. neostriatum; that is, the:

   i. c_____   caudate

   ii. p_____   putamen

   iii. g_____ p_____   globus pallidum

e. This reduces inhibitory D2 receptors to _____   GPi

f. and causes the loss of inhibitory D1 receptors to _____   GPe

g. and the s_____ n_____.   subthalamic nucleus

h. The net result is an _____ in activity   increase

i. of _____.   GPi

j. GPi has inhibitory projections to the t_____.   thalamus

k. Inhibiting the thalamus also suppresses the s_____ m_____ c_____.   supplemental motor cortex

19. A hallmark of Parkinson disease   G7 p.60:25mm

a. is _____ _____,   Lewy bodies

b. which are

   i. e_____ i_____   eosinophilic intraneuronal

   ii. h_____ i_____   hyaline inclusions

20. **List secondary parkinsonism examples.**
    Hint: P4 secondary

G7 p.60:35mm

a.	P	phenothiazine antiemetics, Compazine
b.	P	progressive supra nuclear palsy
c.	P	poisoning CO_2, manganese
d.	P	Parkinson dementia complex of Guam
e.	S	strial nigral degeneration, Shy-Drager
f.	E	(post)-encephaletic parkinsonism
g.	C	Compazine (phenothiazine antiemetics) carbon monoxide
h.	O	olivo-ponto-cerebellar degeneration
i.	N	neoplasms near substantia nigra
j.	D	dementia pugilistica (boxing—post traumatic parkinsonism)
k.	A	anti psychotic drugs
l.	R	Reglan reserpine, Riley Day (familial dysautonomia)
m.	Y	

21. **Multisystem atrophy (MSA) (i.e., Shy-Drager syndrome) is parkinsonism plus**

G7 p.60:180mm

a. _____ _____ _____ dysfunction — autonomic nervous system (ANS)
b. plus _____ hypotension. — orthostatic
c. Most don't respond to _____ _____. — drug therapy

22. **List the distinguishing features of the progressive supranuclear palsy (PSP) triad.**

G7 p.61:40mm

a. _____ (vertical gaze) — ophthalmoplegia
b. _____ dystonia — axial
c. _____ palsy — pseudobulbar

23. **Characteristics of the early stage of progressive supranuclear palsy (PSP) (i.e., Steele-Richardson-Olszewski) include**

a. falling due to _____ _____ palsy (can't see floor) — downward gaze   G7 p.61:87mm
b. difficulty eating due to _____ _____ palsy (can't see plate) — downward gaze (supranuclear ophthalmoplegia), vertical gaze   G7 p.61:103mm

24. **Fill in the blank to summarize surgical treatment for Parkinson disease.** G7 p.61:122mm

a. The target site was _____ _____.   ventrolateral nucleus

b. True or False. The surgery worked best for which of the following symptoms:
   i.   bradykinesia   false
   ii. tremor   true

c. Which is the more disabling symptom?
   i.   bradykinesia   true
   ii. tremor   false

d. The operation cannot be done bilaterally because of risk to _____ _____.   speech function

e. Current treatment site is the p_____ p_____.   posteroventral pallidum   G7 p.533:168mm

4

■ Multiple Sclerosis

25. **Study Chart.** G7 p.61:150mm

a.	M	(de) myelinating
b.	U	urinary symptoms
c.	L	latitudes (northern latitudes affected)
d.	T	time and space dissemination
e.	I	inter-nuclear ophthalmoplegia (INO)
f.	P	paresthesias, peri-ventricular plaques
g.	L	lymphocytes
h.	E	enhancing lesions on MRI
i.	S	scars of the glia
j.	C	cortico spinal tracts involved
k.	L	la belle indifference (euphoria)
l.	E	equator spared
m.	R	remissions
n.	O	optic atrophy
o.	S	sensory loss
p.	I	inflammatory response, IgG elevated
q.	S	shower test (hot causes exacerbation)

26. **Prevalence of multiple sclerosis (MS) per 100,000 is variable.** G7 p.62:45mm

a. Near the equator it is _____ per 100,000.   1

b. In Canada and the northern United States it is _____ per 100,000.   30 to 80

27. **The most common category is r_____-r_____.**   relapsing-remitting (Acute course with recovery, but 50% become secondarily progressive.) G7 p.62:80mm

28. Name the clinical categories of MS corresponding to their definition.
G7 p.62:60mm

a. r _____-r_____ (acute episodes with recovery)   relapsing-remitting recovery

b. s_____-p_____ (gradual deterioration)   secondary-progressive

c. p_____-p_____ (continuous deterioration)   primary-progressive

d. p _____-r_____ (gradual deterioration with superimposed relapses)   progressive-relapsing

e. Deficits persist if they remain > _____ _____   6 months
G7 p.62:100mm

29. Conditions found in the differential diagnosis for multiple sclerosis include
G7 p.62:115mm

a. _____, generally monophasic   ADEM (acute disseminated encephalomyelitis)

b. CNS _____   lymphoma

30. Matching. Match multiple sclerosis signs and symptoms with anatomic location.
G7 p.62:135mm

Symptoms:
① visual acuity; ② diplopia; ③ extremity weakness; ④ quadriplegia; ⑤ spasticity; ⑥ scanning speech; ⑦ loss of proprioception
Anatomic location:

a. optic nerve   ①
b. retro-bulbar region   ①
c. MLF   ②
d. pyramidal tract   ③-④-⑤
e. cerebellum   ⑥
f. posterior columns   ⑦

31. Matching. Match anatomic location with multiple sclerosis signs and symptoms.
G7 p.62:137mm

Anatomic location:
① optic nerve; ② retro bulbar region; ③ MLF; ④ pyramidal tract; ⑤ cerebellum; ⑥ posterior columns
Symptom:

a. visual acuity   ①-②
b. diplopia   ③
c. extremity weakness   ④
d. quadriplegia   ④
e. spasticity   ④
f. scanning speech   ⑤
g. loss of proprioception   ⑥

4

4

32. Provide the frequency of multiple sclerosis signs and symptoms.
G7 p.62:140mm

a. Visual symptoms are among the presenting symptoms of multiple sclerosis in _____%   15%

b. and occur in multiple sclerosis patients during their course of illness in approximately _____%.   50%

c. In addition, abdominal cutaneous reflexes are lost in _____%.   70 to 80%

33. A multiple sclerosis plaque in the medial longitudinal fasciculus (MLF) will cause
G7 p.62:155mm

a. _____ _____, which will result in   internuclear ophthalmoplegia

b. _____.   diplopia

c. This is important because _____ rarely occurs in other diseases.   INO

34. Indicate the presence or absence of the following reflexes in MS:
G7 p.63:27mm

a. hyperactive muscle stretch reflexes   present

b. Babinski   present

c. abdominal cutaneous reflexes   absent

35. True or False. In multiple sclerosis the more MRI lesions, the higher the likelihood of the diagnosis of MS.   true (MRI is very specific for MS plaques; specificity is 94%.)
G7 p.64:60mm

36. Provide MRI criteria for MS.
G7 p.64:100mm

a. gadolinium: acute lesions _____   enhance

b. size: at least _____ in diameter   3 mm

c. white matter abnormalities: _____%   80%

d. T2-weighted image _____ _____ _____ _____   lesions are high signal

e. periventricular lesions best seen on _____ _____ images   proton density

f. criterion for dissemination is a _____ _____ _____   new enhancing lesion

g. or a _____ _____ _____   new T2WI lesion

37. True or False. Focal tumefactive demyelinating lesions (TDL) can be mistaken for neoplasms because they
G7 p.64:135mm

a. Enhance   true

b. Show perilesional edema   true

c. Can be solitary   true

d. Can be in patients known to have MS   true

e. Can be distinguished from MS   false

f. Biopsy may be necessary   true

g. Biopsy results may be confusing   true

38. **What is CNS analysis for MS?**   G7 p.65:20mm
  a. It should include q_____ _____   qualitative IgG
     testing.
  b. In 90% of MS patients the CSF _____   IgG
     is high.

■ Amyotrophic Lateral Sclerosis

39. **Complete the following regarding**   G7 p.65:145mm
     amyotrophic lateral sclerosis:
  a. aka m_____ n_____ disease   motor neuron
  b. aka L_____ G_____ disease   Lou Gehrig
  c. A mixed _____ and _____   upper and lower
  d. m_____ n_____ disease   motor neuron
  e. Degeneration of alpha motor neurons in
     brain stem
     i.   Therefore _____ m_____   upper motor
          neuron disease
     ii. and in spinal cord, therefore   lower motor
          _____ m_____ neuron
          disease

40. **True or False. In ALS, there is no**   true   G7 p.65:140mm
     cognitive, sensory, or autonomic
     dysfunction.

41. **True or False. ALS spares voluntary eye** true   G7 p.66:22mm
     muscles and urinary sphincter.

42. **The common condition that must be**   cervical myelopathy   G7 p.66:55mm
     distinguished from ALS is _____
     _____.

43. **In ALS, two causes of major disability**   G7 p.65:105mm
     include
  a. a_____   aspiration
  b. s_____   spasticity

■ Guillain-Barré Syndrome

44. **True or False. Guillain-Barré involves**   G7 p.66:158mm
     areflexia and progressive muscle
     weakness
  a. proximally   true (more severely)
  b. distally   false

45. **True or False. Guillain-Barré shows**   G7 p.66:177mm
  a. albuminocytologic dissociation   true (↑ prot > 55 mg/dL, < 10
                                              cells)
  b. little or no sensory involvement   true (but paresthesias are not G7 p.66:167mm
                                              uncommon)

46. **In Guillain-Barré, what infectious**   *Campylobacter jejuni* G7 p.67:40mm
     organism is involved?

47. True or False. In Guillain-Barré, there is   true   G7 p.67:83mm
     progressive motor weakness that is
     relatively symmetric.

48. Features casting doubt on the   G7 p.67:160mm
     diagnosis
  a. asymmetry of _____   weakness
  b. dysfunction of _____   bladder
  c. more than 50 _____ in CSF   monocytes
  d. any _____ in CSF   PMNs
  e. sharp _____ level   sensory

49. Complete the following about CIDP: G7 p.68:95mm
  a. True or False. CIDP is also known as   true
     chronic relapsing Guillain-Barré
     syndrome.
  b. CIDP stands for c_____ i_____   chronic immune
     d_____ p_____.   demyelinating
                                                      polyradituloneropathy
  c. For CIDP, symptoms must be present for   2 months
     more than _____.
  d. CSF findings are similar to _____-   Guillain-Barré
     _____.

50. The Miller-Fisher variant of Guillain-   G7 p.68:15mm
     Barré syndrome includes
  a. a _____   ataxia
  b. a _____   areflexia
  c. o _____   ophthalmoplegia

51. True or False. In Guillain-Barré,   true   G7 p.68:165mm
     plasmapheresis hastens recovery and
     reduces residual deficit.

■ Myelitis

52. True or False. In acute transverse   true   G7 p.69:62mm
     myelitis (ATM), the animal model is
     EAE.

53. Complete the following: G7 p.69:62mm
  a. EAE stands for _____ _____   experimental allergic
     _____.   encephalomyelitis
  b. It requires central or peripheral MBP?   central NS MBP (myelin basic
                                                     protein, not peripheral MBP)

54. True or False. The most common   true (68% thoracic sensory   G7 p.70:53mm
     sensory level in acute transverse   level in ATM)
     myelitis is thoracic.

55. True or False. Acute transverse   true (66% reach maximal   G7 p.70:70mm
     myelitis progresses rapidly.   deficit by 24 hours)

56. **True or False. In acute transverse myelitis, MRI/CT/myelography is often performed to rule out compressive lesions.**

true (no characteristic imaging findings in ATM)

G7 p.70:86mm

57. **True or False. In acute transverse myelitis, symptoms include**

G7 p.70:95mm

   a. paresthesia — true (paresthesia 100%)
   b. weakness — true (weakness 97%)
   c. sphincter disturbance — true (sphincter disturbance 94%—hesitancy, retention, overflow)

58. **Characterize myelitis.**

G7 p.70:120mm

   a. Diagnose with _____. — MRI
   b. If not available use _____. — myelogram
   c. And treat with _____. — steroids

G7 p.70:140mm

59. **True or False. Regarding acute transverse myelitis:**

G7 p.70:160mm

   a. There is 15% mortality. — true (15% mortality by 4 months)
   b. 62% of survivors are ambulatory. — true (62% ambulatory by 3 to 6 months)
   c. Recovery occurs between 1 month to 2 years. — false (1 to 3 months)
   d. No improvement occurs after 3 months. — true

■ Neurosarcoidosis

60. **The most common neurologic**

G7 p.71:38mm

   a. manifestation is _____ _____. — diabetes insipidus
   b. Treat with _____. — corticosteroids

61. **Complete the following statements about neurosarcoidosis:**

G7 p.71:76mm

   a. Pathology characteristic: m_____-e_____ of the s_____ a_____ of the t_____ v_____ and hy_____. May produce d_____ i_____. — meningo-encephalitis of the subependymal area of the third ventricle and hypothalamus / diabetes insipidus
   b. Serum test that is positive in 83% of cases is _____. — ACE

G7 p.71:152mm

   c. Cerebrospinal fluid (CSF) test that is helpful is _____. — ACE
   d. How frequently positive? — 55%
   e. CSF analysis suggests _____. — meningitis
   f. ACE stands for _____ _____ _____. — angiotensin converting enzyme

4

62. Complete the following regarding neurosarcoidosis: G7 p.71:87mm

a. Microscopically we see features of   non-caseating granulomas
    n_____ g_____
b. Clinical findings include:
    i.   c_____ n_____ palsies   cranial nerve
    ii. p_____ n_____   peripheral neuropathy
    iii. m_____   myopathy
    iv. h_____   hydrocephalus
c. Diabetes insipidus from involvement of   hypothalamus
    the _____

63. List the test performed with the results in sarcoidosis.   G7 p.72:15mm

a. Chest x-ray
    i.   h_____ a_____   hilar adenopathy
    ii. m_____ l_____ n_____   mediastinal lymph nodes
b. MRI
    i.   enhancement of l_____   leptomeninges
    ii. enhancement of o_____   optic nerve
         n_____
    iii. best seen on _____ sequence   flair
c. Gallium scan (nuclear medicine). Useful
    in neurosurgery for:
    i.   s_____   sarcoidosis
    ii. c_____ v_____ o_____   chronic vertebral
                                               osteomyelitis

■ Vascular and Dysautoregulatory Encephalopathy

64. You have been called in consultation to see a 6 days post-partum woman complaining of headaches, seizures, and blindness. CT shows occipital intracerebral hemorrhage and bilateral vasogenic edema.   G7 p.73:35mm

a. Diagnosis: _____ stands for   PRES, posterior reversible
    p_____ r_____ e_____   encephalopathy syndrome
    s_____
b. Blood pressure will show _____   hypertension
c. True or False. Other causes beside
    pregnancy could be
    i.   malignant hypertension   true
    ii. eclampsia   true
    iii. infection   true
    iv. auto-immune disease   true
    v.   chemotherapy   true
    vi. transplantation   true

65. **A patient develops blindness. Imaging studies reveal infarctions of both occipital lobes. You should consider**

G7 p.73:107mm

a. the diagnosis of v_____ d_____ r_____ e_____.   vascular dysauto regulatory encephalopathy
b. The blindness may be _____.   temporary
c. Treat with _____ _____ pressure control.   tight blood
d. Without control of BP _____-_____ _____ could occur.   intra-cerebral hemorrhage (ICH)
e. In a non-pregnant patient this syndrome could occur due to a drug toxicity with _____.   cyclosporine

66. **The treatment of vascular dysautoregulatory encephalopathy is to**

G7 p.73:650mm

a. treat b_____ p_____,   blood pressure
b. hold _____ _____, and   immune suppressives
c. remove the p_____.   placenta

67. **Uremic encephalopathy**

G7 p.73:180mm

a. has a site of characteristic edema in the b_____ g_____.   basal ganglia
b. In severe cases, it can develop f_____ i_____.   focal infarcts

68. **Crossed cerebellar diaschisis**

G7 p.74:38mm

a. is h_____ of the cerebellum   hypometabolism
b. due to a
     i.   c_____   contralateral
     ii. c_____ h_____ lesion   cerebral hemisphere
c. Theory is that this occurs because the
     i.   c_____-p_____-c_____ pathway   cerebro-ponto-cerebellar
     ii. becomes _____   disconnected
     iii. resulting in reduced: o_____ and g_____ consumption.   oxygen and glucose
     iv. Decreased _____ production causes CO_2
     v.   local arterial _____   constriction
     vi. and reduced _____ blood flow.   cerebellar

4

■ Vasculitis and Vasculopathy

69. Giant cell arteritis (formerly called temporal arteritis)   G7 p.74:182mm

a. involves branches of the _____ _____ _____.   external carotid artery

b. Most helpful laboratory study is _____.   ESR

c. Most serious consequence is _____.   blindness

d. How frequently?   7%   G7 p.75:133mm

e. Once it occurs is it reversible?   no

f. Which vessels are involved?

    i.   o_____ a_____   ophthalmic artery

    ii.   p_____ c_____ b_____   posterior ciliary branches

g. The warning symptom that precedes permanent visual loss   G7 p.75:125mm

    i.   is _____ _____.   amaurosis fugax

    ii.   How frequently? _____% of the time   44%

h. GCA is associated with another   G7 p.75:160mm

    i.   serious condition: t_____ a_____ a_____.   thoracic aortic aneurysms

    ii.   This condition is _____ times as likely in GCA.   17

i. Sed rate above _____ is suspicious.   40 mm/hr   G7 p.76:40mm

j. Sed rate above _____ is highly suggestive.   80 mm/hr

k. ESR is normal in up to _____% of patients with GCA.   22.5%

l. Temporal artery palpation is normal in _____%.   33%

70. True of False. Proper technique for biopsy of the superficial temporal artery (STA) includes: G7 p.76:105mm

a. Plan to remove the parietal branch of the STA   false

b. Spare the main trunk of the STA   true

c. Make the incision perpendicular to the STA   false

d. Optimal length of STA biopsy is 4 to 6 cm   true

71. Treatment that might prevent blindness

a. is the use of _____.   steroids   G7 p.76:148mm

b. Follow patterns closely for _____.   2 years   G7 p.77:26mm

72. **Behçet syndrome consists of the following:**

G7 p.78:130mm

Hint: Behcets

a. B — Behçet
b. e — eye lesions
c. h — headache
d. c — cerebellar signs, CSF pleocytosis
e. e — erosions of mouth and genitalia
f. t — thrombophlebitis, thrombosis of dural sinuses
g. s — skin lesions, seizures, use steroids

73. **Complete the following statements about fibromuscular dysplasia:**

G7 p.79:114 mm

a. Most common vessels involved are
   i. r_____ a_____ — renal artery
   ii. c_____ a_____ — carotid artery
b. What other abnormality of vessels occurs with FMD? — aneurysms
c. How frequently? — 20 to 50%
d. The gold standard of diagnosis is _____. — angiography
e. The recommended treatment is _____. — aspirin

74. **Complete the following regarding presentation of fibromuscular dysplasia:**

G7 p.80:32mm

a.
   i. h_____ in _____% — headache, 78%
   ii. u_____ — unilaterally
   iii. can be mistaken for t_____ m_____ — typical migraine
b.
   i. s_____ in _____% — syncope, 31%
   ii. due to involvement of the c_____ s_____ — carotid sinus
c.
   i. T_____ changes in _____% — T wave, 33%
   ii. Due to involvement of c_____ a_____ — coronary arteries
d. H_____ syndrome in _____% — Horner, 8%

5

Neuroanatomy and Physiology

■ Surface Anatomy

G7 p.84:65mm

1. **Characterize the lateral cortical surface.**
   a. The pre-central sulcus is not _____. — complete
   b. The middle frontal gyrus connects with the _____ gyrus through this _____. — precentral, isthmus
   c. The central sulcus is separated from the sylvian fissure _____% of the time. — 98%
   d. The tissue separating them is called the _____ _____. — sub-central gyrus
   e. The inferior and superior parietal lobules are separated by the _____ sulcus. — intra-parietal
   f. The inferior parietal lobule is composed of
      i. the s_____ m_____ g_____ — supra marginal gyrus (SMG)
      ii. and the a_____ g_____. — angular gyrus
   g. The sylvian fissure
      i. terminates in the _____, — SMG
      ii. which is the Brodmann area #_____. — 40
   h. The superior temporal gyrus
      i. terminates in the _____, — AG
      ii. which is the Brodmann area #_____. — 39

2. **Complete the following regarding surface anatomy:**
   G7 p.84:80mm
   a. The middle frontal gyrus often connects with the _____ _____. — pre-central gyrus
   b. The central sulcus joins the sylvian fissure in only _____%. — 2%
   c. A sub-central sulcus is present in _____% of patients. — 98%
   d. The sylvian fissure terminates in the _____ _____. — supra-marginal gyrus
   e. The superior temporal sulcus is capped by the _____ _____. — angular gyrus

3. **Matching. Match the following Brodmann cortical areas and their functional significance:**

G7 p.84:128mm

Functional significance:
① primary motor cortex; ② Broca area (motor speech); ③ Wernicke area dominant hemisphere; ④ primary auditory area; ⑤ frontal eye fields; ⑥ primary somatosensory area; ⑦ premotor area; ⑧ primary visual cortex

Area:

a. Area 3, 1, 2   ⑥
b. Area 41, 42   ④
c. Area 4   ①
d. Area 6   ⑦
e. Area 44   ②
f. Area 17   ⑧
g. Area 40, 39   ③
h. Area 8   ⑤

4. **Complete the following regarding pars marginalis:**

G7 p.85:18mm

a. is the terminal part of the _____ gyrus   cingulate
b. is visible on axial view in > _____%   90%
c. is the _____ _____ of the midline paired grooves   most prominent
d. extends _____ into the hemispheres   deeper
e. on axial CT is located just posterior to the line _____ (the widest diameter)   9-3
f. it curves _____ in lower slices   posteriorly
g. it curves _____ in higher slices   anteriorly

5. **Complete the following regarding central sulcus:**

G7 p.85:95mm

a. Is visible in almost _____%   95%
b. Does it reach the midline?   no
c. Terminates in the _____ _____   para-central lobule

6. **True or False. The pterion is a region where each of the following bones comes together:**

G7 p.86:110mm

a. frontal   true
b. sphenoid (greater wing)   true
c. parietal   true
d. temporal   true
e. sphenoid (lesser wing)   false

7. **Matching. Match the bones/sutures that form the listed craniometric points.**
    Bone/suture:
    ① lambdoid suture; ② occipitomastoid suture; ③ parietomastoid suture; ④ frontal; ⑤ parietal; ⑥ temporal; ⑦ greater wing sphenoid
    Craniometric point:

G7 p.86:125mm

a. asterion   ①, ②, ③
b. pterion   ④, ⑤, ⑥, ⑦

8. **True or False. The name of the junction of lambdoid, occipitomastoid, and parietomastoid sutures is**

G7 p.86:140mm

a. pterion   false
b. asterion   true (Asterion is the junction of lambdoid, occipitomastoid suture, and parietomastoid suture.)

c. lambdoid   false
d. stephanion   false
e. glabella   false
f. opisthion   false

9. **The asterion junction overlies the**

G7 p.86:160mm

a. _____ sinus and the   transverse
b. _____ sinus.   sigmoid

10. **External landmark for the sylvian fissure is a line from the lateral canthus to a spot three quarters of the way posterior along an arc running over the convexity in the midline from the**

G7 p.87:135mm

a. _____ to the   nasion
b. _____.   inion

11. **True or False. In relation to external landmarks the angular gyrus is**

G7 p.87:145mm

a. one finger's breadth above the zygomatic arch   false

b. just above the pinna   true (The angular gyrus is just above the pinna and important as part of the Wernicke area in the dominant hemisphere.)

c. a thumb's breadth behind the frontal process of the zygomatic bone   false

d. at the junction of the lambdoid and sagittal suture   false

5

12. True or False. The motor strip of the motor cortex lies   G7 p.87:165mm

a.	at the level of the coronal suture	false
b.	within 2 cm of the coronal suture	false
c.	3 to 4 cm posterior to the coronal suture	false
d.	4 to 5.4 cm posterior to the coronal suture	true
e.	2 cm posterior to the mid-position of the inion-nasion arc	true
f.	5 cm straight up from the external auditory meatus	true

13. True or False. In the non-hydrocephalic adult the lateral ventricles lie   G7 p.88:87mm

a.	2 to 3 cm below the outer skull surface	false
b.	3 to 4 cm below the outer skull surface	false
c.	4 to 5 cm below the outer skull surface	true
d.	5 to 6 cm below the outer skull surface	false

14. True or False. In the non-hydrocephalic adult the anterior horns extend   G7 p.88:108mm

a.	1 to 2 cm anterior to the coronal suture	true
b.	2 to 3 cm anterior to the coronal suture	false
c.	3 to 4 cm anterior to the coronal suture	false

15. True or False. In the non-hydrocephalic adult the anterior horns extend   G7 p.88:130mm

a.	1 to 2 cm anterior to the foramen of Monro	false
b.	2.5 cm anterior to the foramen of Monro	true
c.	3 to 4 cm anterior to the foramen of Monro	false

16. True or False. The fastigium is located at   G7 p.88:145mm

a.	the midpoint of the Twinings line	false
b.	the floor of the fourth ventricle	false
c.	the apex of the fourth ventricle within the cerebellum	true (The fastigium is the apex of the fourth ventricle in the cerebellum.)
d.	1 to 2 cm anterior to the coronal suture	false

17. List the surface landmarks of the following cervical levels.   G7 p.89:35mm
Hint: htcc

a.	C3-4 _____ _____	hyoid bone
b.	C4-5 _____ _____	thyroid cartilage
c.	C5-6 _____ _____	cricothyroid membrane
d.	C6-7 _____ _____	cricoid cartilage

18. **Matching. Match the following surface landmarks and cervical levels:**   G7 p.89:35mm
Surface landmark:
① level of thyroid cartilage; ② cricoid cartilage; ③ angle of mandible; ④ cricothyroid membrane; ⑤ carotid tubercle; ⑥ 1 cm above thyroid cartilage (hyoid bone)
Cervical level:
a. C1-2   ③
b. C3-4   ⑥
c. C4-5   ①
d. C5-6   ④
e. C6   ⑤
f. C6-7   ②

5

■ Cranial Foramina and Their Contents

19. **Matching. Match the foramen with contents (choices may be used more than once).**   G7 p.89:75mm
Contents:
① nothing; ② middle meningeal artery; ③ VII facial; ④ V2; ⑤ V3; ⑥ V1; ⑦ IX, X XI
Foramen:
a. superior orbital fissure   ⑥
b. inferior orbital fissure   ④
c. foramen lacerum   ①
d. foramen rotundum   ④
e. foramen ovale   ⑤
f. foramen spinosum   ②
g. stylomastoid foramen   ③
h. jugular foramen   ⑦

20. **List the cranial nerves and the three branches of one found within the superior orbital fissure (SOF).**   G7 p.89:85mm
a. o_____   CN III oculomotor
b. t_____   IV trochlear
c. n_____   nasociliary nerve
d. f_____   frontal nerve ophthalmic division: all three branches
e. l_____   lacrimal nerve
f. a_____   VI abducens nerve

21. **Additional structures found in the SOF include the**   G7 p.89:85mm
a. s_____ o_____ v _____   superior ophthalmic vein
b. r_____ m_____ a _____   recurrent meningeal artery
c. which arises from the l_____ artery   lacrimal
d. o_____ b_____ of the   orbital branch of the middle
   m_____ m_____ a_____   meningeal artery
e. s_____ p_____ of the ICA   sympathetic plexus of the ICA

22. **Another name for the transverse crest is _____ _____.**

crista falciformis

G7 p.89:182mm

23. **Another name for the vertical crest is _____ _____.**

Bill's bar

G7 p.89:187mm

24. **Draw and label the nerves in the right porus acusticus.**

G7 p.90:22mm

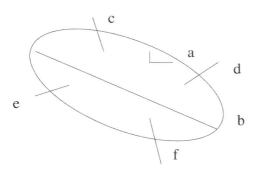

a. Bill's bar
b. transverse crest crista falciformis
c. cranial nerve VII
d. SV—superior vestibular
e. VIII
f. IV—inferior vestibular

Fig. 5.1

25. **Label the diagram of the right internal auditory canal.**

G7 p.90:22mm

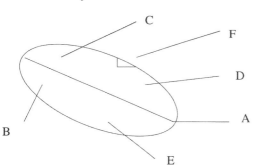

a. transverse crest
b. acoustic portion of CN VIII
c. cranial nerve VII in facial canal
d. superior vestibular nerve
e. inferior vestibular nerve
f. Bill's bar—vertical crest

Fig. 5.2

26. **Matching. Match the nerves of the IAC with the areas that they serve.**

G7 p.90:23mm

Nerves:
① facial n.; ② nervus intermedius;
③ acoustic portion of VIII n.; ④ superior branch of vestibular n.; ⑤ inferior branch of vestibular n.
Areas served:

a. Facial muscles   ①
b. Hair follicles   ②
c. Taste buds   ②
d. Hearing   ③
e. Utricle   ④
f. Superior semi-circular canal   ④
g. Lateral semi-circular canal   ④
h. Saccule   ⑤

5

■ Occipitoatlantoaxial-complex Anatomy

27. **Matching. Match the ligaments of the occipito-atlantoaxial complex with the statements below.**
    G7 p.91:32mm

    Ligaments:
    ① apical; ② alar; ③ cruciate;
    ④ ascending portion; ⑤ descending portion; ⑥ transverse portion;
    ⑦ posterior longitudinal; ⑧ tectorial;
    ⑨ anterior longitudinal; ⑩ anterior atlanto occipital

    Statements:
    a. Attaches the odontoid to the foramen magnum   ①
    b. Attaches the odontoid to the occipital condyle   ②
    c. Attaches the odontoid to the lateral mass of C1   ②
    d. Attaches C1 to the clivus and to C2   ③
    e. Attaches odontoid to clivus   ④
    f. Attaches C1 to C2   ⑤
    g. Traps the odontoid against the atlas   ⑥
    h. Extends cephalad to become the tectorial   ⑦
    i. The cephalad extension of the PLL   ⑧
    j. Extends cephalad to become the anterior atlanto-occipital   ⑨
    k. The cephalad extension of the anterior longitudinal   ⑩

28. **The most important spinal ligaments in maintaining atlanto-occipital stability are the**
    G7 p.92:95mm

    a. _____ membrane and the   tectorial
    b. _____ ligaments.   alar

■ Spinal Cord Anatomy

29. **The very large ascending tract closest to the dentate ligament is the _____.**
    lateral spinothalamic tract (LST) for pain and temperature from the opposite side of the body
    G7 p.93:120mm

30. **How is the lateral spinothalamic tract (LST) somatotopically organized?**
    G7 p.93:120mm

    a. Cervical is _____.   medial
    b. Sacral is _____.   lateral

31. **Which descending motor tract facilitates**
    G7 p.92:158mm

    a. extensor tone?   vestibulospinal tract
    b. flexor tone?   rubrospinal tract

32. **Matching. Match sensory function and anatomy.** G7 p.93:175mm
    Sensory function:
    ① pain and temperature: body; ② fine touch, deep pressure and proprioception: body; ③ light (crude) touch: body
    Anatomy:
    a. Receptors
        i.   Free nerve ending   ①
        ii. Meissner and pacinian corpuscles   ②-③
    b. First order neurons
        i.   Small   ①
        ii. Heavily myelinated   ②-③
        iii. Finely myelinated   ①
        iv. Large   ②
    c. Soma in dorsal root ganglion   ①-②-③
    d. Enter cord at
        i.   Zone of Lissauer   ①
        ii. Ipsilateral posterior columns   ②-③
    e. Synapse in
        i.   Rexed layer II   ①
        ii. Rexed layer III and IV   ②
        iii. Rexed layer VI and VII   ③
    f. Second order neurons
        i.   Cross obliquely in anterior white commissure   ①-③
        ii. Form the internal arcuate fibers   ②
    g. And enter the
        i.   Lateral spino-thalamic tract   ①
        ii. Medial lemniscus   ②
        iii. Anterior spino-thalamic tract   ③
    h. Second order neurons synapse on the ventral posterior lateral nucleus of the Thalamus   ①-②-③
    i. Third order neurons pass through IC to post-central gyrus   ①-②-③

33. **The major blood supply of the spinal cord vasculature** G7 p.95:60mm
    a. to the anterior cord arises from
        i.   the vertebral artery and enters at _____   C3
        ii. the deep cervical artery and enters at _____   C6
        iii. the costo cervical trunk and enters at _____   C8
        iv. thoracic levels _____ or _____   T4 or T5
        v.   and from the a_____ of A_____   artery of Adamkiewicz
    b. to the posterior spinal cord arises from: _____ to _____ radicular branches   10 to 23
    c. The "watershed zone" is at the _____ or _____ region   T4 or T5

5

34. List the body area with the appropriate root. G7 p.95:70mm

a. Nipple, root:_____   T4
b. Umbilicus, root:_____   T10
c. Inguinal crease, root:_____   T12
d. Anterior thigh, root:_____   L2-L3
e. Posterior thigh, root:_____   S1
f. Lateral calf, root:_____   L5
g. Medial calf, root:_____   L4
h. Posterior calf, root:_____   S1
i. Big toe, root:_____   L5
j. Little toe, root:_____   S1
k. Sole of foot, root:_____   S1
l. Lateral shoulder, root:_____   C5
m. Lateral forearm   C6
n. Thumb   C6
o. Middle finger   C7
p. Little finger   C8
q. Medial forearm   T1

35. Complete the following regarding upper extremity vs trunk dermatomes. Trunk sensory level is reported at T3 on a trauma patient. G7 p.95:70mm

a. This is a little _____ the clavicle.   below
b. You must check the _____ dermatomes.   arm
c. Dermatomes _____ to _____ are not represented on the trunk.   C5 to T2

36. Characterize spinal cord vasculature. The artery of Adamkiewicz serves the spinal cord from G7 p.96:35mm

a. T_____ distally and from the   T8
b. _____ side in   left
c. _____% of the population.   80%

37. The artery of Adamkiewicz is also known as G7 p.96:35mm

a. a_____   arteria
    r_____   radicularis
    a_____   anterior
    m_____   magna
b. Which side does it arise from?   L 80%, R 20%
c. What levels does it arise from 100% inclusive?   T9 and T12 75%
    T9 and L2 85%
    T5 and T8 15%
    T5 and L2 100%
d. What is its appearance on angiography?   characteristic hairpin shape

38. An artery that has a hairpin shape on angiography is named the _____.   artery of Adamkiewicz G7 p.96:52mm

5

■ Cerebrovascular Anatomy

39. **The artery that feeds a tentorial meningioma is named after**
    a. _____ and
    b. _____.

    Bernasconi
    Cassinari

    G7 p.99:118mm

40. **The artery that has a bayonet-type kink is the _____ _____.**

    ophthalmic artery

    G7 p. 99:118mm

41. **Circle of Willis is intact in _____%.**

    18%

    G7 p. 97:55mm

42. **Hypoplasia of at least one of the posterior communicating arteries occurs in _____%.**

    22 to 32%

    G7 p.97:55mm

43. **Absent or hypoplastic A1 occurs in _____%.**

    25%

    G7 p.97:55mm

5

44. **What are the seven segments of the internal carotid artery?**
    Hint: *can Peter laugh can Charlie only clap*
    a. c_____
    b. p_____
    c. l_____
    d. c_____
    e. c_____
    f. o_____
    g. c_____

    cervical
    petrous
    lacerum
    cavernous
    clinoid
    ophthalmic
    communicating

    G7 p.98:20mm

45. **What portion of the PCA traverses the ambient cistern?**

    P2

    G7 p.98:95mm

46. **What choroidal artery arises from it?**

    medial posterior choroidal artery

    G7 p.98:103mm

47. **Which cistern is traversed by the P3 segment of the PCA?**

    quadrigeminal cistern

    G7 p.98:102mm

48. **Name the segments of the carotid artery and their main branches.**
    a. C1 c_____

    b. C2 p_____
    c. C3 l_____
    d. C4 c_____
       i.   m_____ t_____
       ii. a_____ m_____ a_____
    e. C5 c_____
    f. C6 o_____
       i.   o_____
       ii. s_____ h_____
       iii. p_____ c_____
       iv. a_____ c_____

    cervical-carotid sheath
    IJV × PGSN × vagus posterior medial to external carotid
    petrous
    lacerum
    cavernous
    meningohypophyseal trunk
    anterior meningeal artery
    clinoidal
    ophthalmic
    ophthalmic
    superior hypophyseal
    posterior communicating
    anterior choroidal

    G7 p.99:45mm

g. C7 c_____ d_____ i_____   communicating divides into
    i.   A_____   ACA
    ii. M_____   MCA

49. What are the branches of the meningohypophyseal trunk?   G7 p.99:107mm
G6p.79:100mm

Hint: dit

a. d_____ m_____   dorsal meningeal
b. i_____ h_____   inferior hypophyseal
c. t_____ a_____   tentorial artery of Bernasconi and Cassinari

50. Complete the following concerning anterior circulation: G7 p.99:125mm

a. Occlusion of which artery results in Sheehan syndrome?   inferior hypophyseal artery
b. It serves _____ _____ _____ _____.   posterior lobe of pituitary
c. It is a branch of the _____ artery,   meningohypophyseal
d. which is a branch off the _____ _____segment of carotid.   cavernous C4
e. Occlusion causes pituitary infarct in _____ patients.   postpartum

51. The ophthalmic artery   G7 p.99:145mm

a. arises from the _____ segment of the ICA.   sixth
b. Is distal or inside cavernous sinus?   distal 89%, intracavernous 8%
c. Has what shape on lateral angiogram?   a bayonet-type kink

52. The sixth segment of the carotid artery   G7 p.99:150mm

a. is known as the _____   ophthalmic
b. begins at the _____ dural ring   distal
c. ends just proximal to _____-_____   P-comm
d. has its branches
    i.   o_____ artery and the   ophthalmic
    ii. s_____ h_____ artery   superior hypophyseal

53. What vessel supplies the inferior half of the posterior limb of the internal capsule?   anterior choroidal artery   G7 p.100:23mm

54. Complete the following about the anterior choroidal artery: G7 p.100:30mm

a. The anterior choroidal artery serves six sites. (Hint: gogoup)
    i.   g_____ p_____   globus pallidus
    ii.   o_____ t_____   optic tract
    iii. g_____ of i_____ c_____   genu of internal capsule
    iv.   o_____ r_____   optic radiations
    v.   u_____   uncus
    vi.   p_____ l_____   posterior limb of internal capsule

5

b. Occlusion may produce: hemiplegia, hemihypesthesia,
   Hint: 3 H   homonymous hemianopsia

   _____, _____, _____
   _____

c. MRI shows infarct in the _____.   posterior limb of the internal
   capsule

55. **What artery enters the supracornual**   plexal segment of the   G7 p.100:30mm
    recess of the temporal horn to supply   anterior choroidal artery
    the choroid plexus?

56. **Complete the following regarding**   G7 p.100:35mm
    P-comm and the anterior choroidal
    artery (ACH):
 a. They are _____ mm apart.   2
 b. The origin of the _____-_____ is   P-comm
    proximal.
 c. Is the Ach smaller or larger than the P-   smaller
    comm?
 d. Which artery has the hump of the plexal   Ach
    point?

57. **True or False. The carotid siphon**   G7 p.100:53mm
 a. is only that part of the carotid that   false
    passes within the cavernous sinus.
 b. If an aneurysm ruptures on the siphon   false
    there is no SAH.

58. **The carotid siphon**   G7 p.100:53mm
 a. begins at the posterior bend of the   cavernous
    _____ carotid and
 b. ends at the ICA _____.   bifurcation
 c. It includes the
    i.   ca_____   cavernous
    ii. op_____   ophthalmic
    iii. co_____.   communicating

59. **Complete the following about**   G7 p.102:168mm
    vertebral artery segments:
 a. The first segment enters the _____   sixth
    foramen transversarium.
 b. The second ascends _____ within the   vertically
    foramina transversaria.
 c. The second turns _____ as it exits the   laterally
    axis.
 d. The third curves _____ and   posteriorly and medially
    _____.
 e. The fourth pierces the _____.   dura

60. **The vertebral artery joins the other**   G7 p.103:20mm
    side at the level of the
 a. _____ _____ to form the   lower pons (pontomedullary
    junction)
 b. _____ _____.   basilar artery

61. The junction of the vertebral arteries is called the _____ _____.

vertebral confluens

G7 p.103:20mm

62. What are the six branches arising from the vertebral artery?
Hint: *A postman puts postcards away.*
   a. a_____ m_____
   b. p_____ m_____
   c. m_____
   d. p_____ s_____
   e. P_____
   f. a_____ s_____

anterior meningeal
posterior meningeal
medullary (bulbar)
posterior spinal
PICA
anterior spinal

G7 p.103:105mm

63. Complete the following statements about the PICA:
   a. PICA arises _____ mm distal to the point where VA becomes intradural.

   10

   b. PICA has an extradural origin in _____ to _____%.

   5 to 8%

   c. It includes five segments named
      i.   a_____ m_____
      ii. l_____ m_____
      iii. t_____-m_____ has _____ loop
      iv. t_____-v_____-t_____ has _____ loop
      v.   c_____ s_____
   d. and has three branches named
      i.   c_____
      ii. t_____-h_____
      iii. i_____ v_____

anterior medullary
lateral medullary
tonsillo-medullary, caudal

telo-velo-tonsillar, cranial (supratonsillar)
cortical segments

choroidal
tonsillo-hemispheric
inferior vermian

G7 p.103:120mm

64. The cranial loop on angio of the PICA is the _____ artery.

supratonsillar (telo-velo-tonsillar)

G7 p.103:165mm

65. The choroidal point
   a. is the point where the _____ artery
   b. arises from the _____ artery
   c. which is a branch of the _____
   d. enters into the _____ _____
   e. to serve the _____ _____

choroidal
supratonsillar
PICA
fourth ventricle
choroid plexus

G7 p.103:173mm

66. The copular point
   a. is the point where the _____ _____ artery
   b. arises from the _____.

inferior vermian

PICA

G7 p.103:65mm

67. Name the three segments of the posterior cerebral artery.
   a. c_____

   b. a_____
   c. q_____

crural (peduncular) segment (P1)
ambient segment (P2)
quadrigeminal segment (P3)

G7 p.104:65mm

5

68. Medial posterior choroidal artery arises from the   G7 p.104:84mm

a. _____ segment of PCA.   crural

b. It is also called _____.   P1

69. Lateral posterior choroidal artery arises from the   G7 p.104:92mm

a. _____ segment of the PCA.   ambient

b. It is also called _____.   P2

70. The third segment of PCA is named   quadrigeminal   G7 p.104:117mm
the _____ segment.

71. Name the branches of the external   G6 p.104:30mm
carotid from proximal to distal.
Hint: salfops m

a. s_____ _____   superior thyroid

b. a_____ _____   ascending pharyngeal

c. l_____   lingual

d. f_____   facial

e. o_____   occipital

f. p_____ _____   posterior auricular

g. s_____ _____   superficial temporal

h. m_____   maxillary

72. In relation to ICA, the ECA lies   G6 p.79:45mm

a. _____ and   anterior

b. _____ to ICA.   lateral

73. Which internal jugular vein is usually   the right   G7 p.104:140mm
dominant?

74. Which transverse sinus is usually   the right   G7 p.104:147mm
dominant?

75. Which vertebral artery is usually   the left by 60%   G7 p.102:156mm
dominant?

76. Name the major contributors to the   G7 p.105:25mm
great cerebral vein of Galen.

a. p_____ c_____ v_____   precentral cerebellar vein

b. b_____ v_____ of R_____   basal veins of Rosenthal

c. i_____ c_____ v_____   internal cerebral veins

77. The joining of the septal vein and the   venous angle   G7 p.105:35mm
thalamostriate vein with the internal
cerebral vein forms an angiographic
landmark called the _____
_____ at the foramen of Monro.

78. True or False. The cavernous sinus is   G7 p.105:140mm

a. a large venous space with multiple   false
trabeculations

b. a plexus of veins   true

5

79. **Draw the right and left cavernous sinus coronal view. On your drawing, label the following:**   G7 p.106:15mm

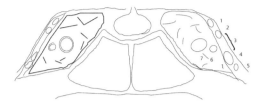

1. oculomotor (III)
2. trochlear (IV)
3. Parkinson triangle
4. ophthalmic (V1)
5. maxillary (V2)
6. abducent (VI)
7. carotid

Fig. 5.3

80. **Name six major contents of the cavernous sinus.**   G7 p.106:15mm

a. _____   CN III
b. _____   CN IV
c. _____   CN V1
d. _____   CN V2
e. _____   CN VI
f. _____   internal carotid artery

81. **Complete the following regarding the cavernous sinus:**

a. Which nerve in the cavernous sinus does not also pass through the superior orbital fissure?   V2 maxillary division of trigeminal   G7 p.106:30mm

b. Which foramen of the skull does that nerve pass through?   foramen rotundum   G7 p.106:30mm

c. Which nerve is not attached to the wall?   VI is not attached to lateral wall (abducens)   G7 p.106:85mm

82. **With regard to the cavernous sinus, the triangular space of Parkinson is bounded by what structures?**   G7 p.106:90mm

a. on its superior border _____   III and IV
b. on its inferior border _____   trigeminal V1 and V2

83. **Complete the following regarding persistent fetal anastomosis:**   G7 p.107:28mm

a. How many are there?   4
b. They result from a failure to _____.   involute
c. Name them.
   i.   t_____   trigeminal
   ii. o_____   otic
   iii. h_____   hypoglossal
   iv. p_____   proatlantal

84. **The most common persistent fetal anastomosis is the _____.**   trigeminal   G7 p.107:60mm

85. **First to involute in persistent fetal anastomsosis is the _____.**   otic   G7 p.107:125mm

■ Internal Capsule

86. Name the vascular supply for the following components of the internal capsule: G7 p.107:165mm

a.	anterior limb	lateral striate branches of MCA
b.	posterior limb	lateral striate branches of MCA
c.	ventral posterior limb	anterior choroidal
d.	genu	direct branches of ICA
e.	optic radiations	anterior choroidal

87. Name four thalamic peduncles and where their radiations go.   G7 p.108:75mm

a.	a_____, f_____ l_____	anterior, frontal lobe
b.	s_____, p_____ g_____	superior, postcentral gyrus
c.	p_____, o_____ p_____ a_____	posterior, occipital parietal areas
d.	i_____, a_____ a_____	inferior, auditory area

88. Draw the internal capsule and label which blood vessel serves which area.   G7 p.108:15mm
Hint: MIMA

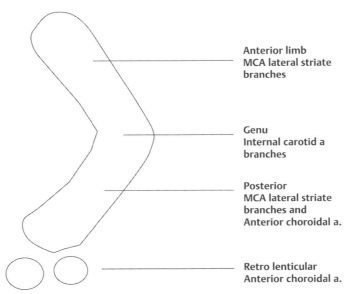

Anterior limb
MCA lateral striate branches

Genu
Internal carotid a branches

Posterior
MCA lateral striate branches and
Anterior choroidal a.

Retro lenticular
Anterior choroidal a.

Fig. 5.4

89. **Matching. Match the area in internal capsule with its function.**
Area in internal capsule:

G7 p.108:20mm

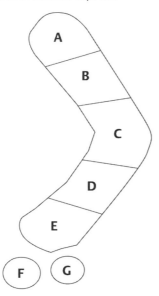

Fig. 5.5

Function:
1. Movement of face _____
2. Movement of foot _____
3. Vision _____
4. Hearing _____

C—genu
D—posterior limb
F—lateral geniculate
G—medial geniculate

■ Miscellaneous

90. **The Obersteiner-Redlich zone is**

G7 p.108:130mm

a. also known as the _____ _____ _____.   root entry zone

b. It is where the central _____ and peripheral _____ transition.   myelin, myelin

c. It is the zone where _____ tend to grow.   neoplasms

d. It is located on CN VIII, _____ from the brain stem.   8 to 12 mm

91. **The dentate ligament**

G7 p.108:150mm

a. separates _____   dorsal
b. from _____ roots in the spinal nerves.   ventral

92. **Which cranial nerve lies dorsal to the dentate ligament?**   CN XI spinal accessory   G7 p.108:155mm

■ Neurophysiology

93. Answer the following concerning the blood-brain barrier (BBB):   G7 p.109:60mm

a. What chemical opens the BBB?   mannitol
b. What chemical closes the BBB?   steroids
c. Which sites have no BBB?   pituitary   G7 p.109:70mm
   Hint: pppcta   pineal
                                       preoptic recess
                                       choroid plexus
                                       tuber cinereum
                                       area postrema
d. What pathology injures BBB?   hepatic encephalopathy
   Hint: histt   infections
                                       stroke
                                       trauma
                                       tumor

94. Complete the following statements about cerebral edema: G7 p.109:75mm

a. Cytotoxic
   i.   occurs with h_____ i_____   head injury
   ii. occurs with h_____   hematoma
   iii. shape is c_____   circular
   iv. occurs with C_____   CVA
   v.   BBB is c_____   closed
b. Vasogenic
   i.   shape is _____   V-shaped (like fingers of white matter edema)
   ii. occurs with t_____   tumors
   iii. occurs with m_____   metastasis
   iv. treat with s_____   steroids
   v.   with contrast it _____ and _____   enhances on CT and MR
   vi. BBB is o_____   open

95. Matching. Match the type of edema with the characteristics.   G7 p.109:80mm
Type of edema:
① cytotoxic edema; ② vasogenic edema
Hint: cytotoxic—early letters of alphabet
vasogenic—later letters of alphabet
Characteristics:

a. BBB open   ②
b. BBB closed   ①
c. Head injury   ①
d. Tumor   ②
e. Enhances   ②
f. Does not enhance   ①
g. Not appropriate to use steroids   ①
h. Appropriate to use steroids   ②
i. Circular shape on MR   ①
j. V-shaped finger like extensions on MR ②
k. Occurs with hematoma   ①
l. Occurs with CVA   ①

5

96. True or False. Cytotoxic edema has: G7 p.109:89mm
a. a disrupted BBB   false
b. expansion of the extracellular space   false
c. enhancement when contrast injected   false
d. no protein extravasation   true

97. Study Sheet.   G7 p.109:100mm
a. Cytotoxic:
b. Closed BBB
c. Head injury
d. Hematoma
e. Circular shape
f. CVA
g. Cells swell then shrink
h. Vasogenic:
i. Open BBB
j. Tumors
k. Metastasis
l. Steroids
m. Protein extravasates
n. Enhances on CT and MRI
o. Wide extracellular space
p. Stable cells

98. In pituitary embryology, posterior pituitary   G7 p.109:110mm
a. derives from the _____ evagination   downward
b. of _____ _____ cells   neural crest
   (neuroectoderm)
c. from the _____   floor
d. of the _____ ventricle.   third

99. The anterior pituitary   G7 p.109:120mm
a. develops from the _____   evagination
b. of _____ _____   epithelial ectoderm
c. of the _____,   oropharynx
d. known as _____ _____.   Rathke's pouch

100. Complete the following regarding neuroendocrinology: G7 p.109:150mm
a. The pituitary releases _____ hormones   8
b. from the anterior pituitary gland: 6
   _____ hormones.
c. Name them.
   Hint: pcpgtg
   i.   p_____   propriomelanocortin
   ii. c_____   corticotropin
   iii. p_____   prolactin
   iv. g_____ _____   growth hormone
   v.   t_____   thyrotropin
   vi. g_____   gonadotropin
d. and from the posterior pituitary
   i.   a_____   antidiuretic
   ii. o_____   oxytocin

101. The pituitary hormones that are
      released from the posterior pituitary
      are synthesized

G7 p109 :165mm

a. in _____   neurons
b. in the _____.   hypothalamus
c. Are these cells glands?   no
d. The hormones are conveyed by   axons
    _____
e. within the _____ _____   pituitary stalk
f. to the _____ pituitary gland   posterior
g. where they are_____.   released

■ Regional Brain Syndromes

102. **Matching. Match region with deficit.**
      Region:
      ① Pre-frontal lobes; ② frontal lobe;
      ③ parietal lobe—dominant; ④ parietal—
      non dominant; ⑤ occipital lobe;
      ⑥ cerebellum; ⑦ brain stem; ⑧ pineal;
      ⑨ olfactory groove
      Deficit:

G7 p.112:30mm

5

a. Apathy abulia   ②
b. Disorganized thoughts   ①
c. Contralateral neglect   ③ or ④
d. Language disorders   ③
e. Anosognosia   ④
f. Dressing apraxia   ④
g. Homonymous hemianopsia   ⑤
h. Truncal ataxia   ⑥
i. Ipsilateral ataxia   ⑥
j. Paralysis of upward gaze   ⑧
k. Poor planning   ①
l. Unilateral anosmia   ⑨

103. **Frontal eye fields for contra lateral
      gaze are**

G7 p.112:55mm

a. located in the _____ frontal lobe   posterior
b. in Broadmann area _____.   8
c. With a destructive lesion there, the   toward
    patient's eyes look _____ the lesion.   Hint: *destructive=toward*
d. With an irritative lesion there, the   away from
    patient's eyes look _____ _____   Hint: *irrigitative=away*
    the lesion.
e. Usually the lesions are _____.   destructive

104. **True or False. Regarding Foster-Kennedy syndrome:**

G7 p.114:125mm

a. usually from olfactory groove or medial third sphenoid wing tumor — true

b. contralateral anosmia — false (Ipsilateral not contralateral anosmia is part of the classic triad.)

c. ipsilateral central scotoma — true

d. contralateral papilledema — true

e. contralateral optic atrophy — false (ipsilateral optic atrophy)

f. usually meningioma — true

105. **True or False. Regarding Weber syndrome:**

G7 p. X:X mm

a. Weber syndrome includes CN III palsy with contralateral hemiparesis. — true

b. Weber syndrome includes CN VII palsy with contralateral hemiparesis. — false

c. Weber syndrome includes CN III palsy with ipsilateral hemiparesis. — false

d. Weber syndrome includes CN VI and VII palsy with contralateral hemiparesis. — false

e. Weber syndrome includes

G7 p.114:105

   i. Cranial nerve III palsy — false

   ii. Contralateral hemiparesis — false

   iii. Arm hyperkinesis — false

   iv. Ataxia — false

   v. Intention tremor — false

106. **True or False. Benedict syndrome is due to disruption of**

G7 p.114:115mm

a. cerebral peduncle — true

b. issuing fibers of CN III — true

c. red nucleus — true

107. **True or False. Millard-Gubler syndrome is due to disruption of**

G7 p.114:130mm

a. nucleus of VII — true

b. nucleus of VI — true

c. cortico spinal tract — true

108. **True or False. Regarding Parinaud syndrome:**

G7 p. 114:135mm

a. Parinaud syndrome includes downgaze palsy. — false

b. Parinaud syndrome includes lid retraction. — true

c. Parinaud syndrome includes nystagmus retractorius. — true

d. When Parinaud syndrome is combined with downgaze palsy it is known as the syndrome of the _____ _____. — sylvian aqueduct

5

109. **True or False. The following are** G7 p.115:70mm
contents of the jugular foramen:

a. transverse sinus   false

b. CN IX, X, and XI   true

c. CN X, XI, and XII   false

d. sigmoid sinus   true

e. petrosal sinus   true

f. branches from the ascending pharyngeal   true
artery

g. branches from the occipital artery   true

110. **Matching. Match the following** G7 p.115:110mm
numbered descriptions with the
lettered syndromes. Also indicate the
nerves involved and the results of the
lesion.
Description:
① Vernet; ② Collet-Sicard; ③ Villaret
Syndrome:

a. Which jugular foramen syndrome is *most*   ① involves CN,IX, X, XI taste,
likely due to an intracranial lesion?   vocal cords and SCM (sterno
cleido mastoid muscle)

b. Extracranial lesion?   ② above plus XII tongue

c. Retropharyngeal lesion?   ③ above plus Horner

111. **True or False. A jugular foramen** G7 p.115:155 mm
syndrome that spares CN IX is

a. Vernet   false

b. Collet-Sicard   false

c. Villaret   false

d. Tapia   true (Tapia X, XII vocal cords
and tongue)

112. **True or False. The following jugular** G7 p.115:180mm
foramen syndrome also results in a
Horner syndrome:

a. Vernet   false

b. Collet-Sicard   false

c. Jackson   false

d. Villaret   true

113. **True or False. Gerstmann syndrome** G7 p.113:70mm
includes

a. agraphia without alexia   true

b. left-right confusion   true

c. digit agnosia   true

d. tactile agnosia   false

e. acalculia   true

114. **True or False. Gerstmann syndrome**   true   G7 p.113:70mm
patients can read.

115. **True or False. Gerstmann syndrome**   false   G7 p.113:70mm
patients can write.

5

116. **True or False. Cortical sensory syndrome includes**   G7 p.113:110mm

a. loss of position sense — true
b. inability to localize tactile stimuli — true
c. astereognosis — true
d. loss of pain and temperature sense — false (Pain and temperature as well as vibration sense are preserved.)

117. **True or False. Anton Babinski syndrome includes**   G7 p.113:155mm

a. anosognosia — true
b. apathy — true
c. ipsilateral extinction to double-sided stimulation — false (contralateral extinction to double-sided stimulation)
d. dressing apraxia — true

118. **True or False. Wernicke aphasia includes**   G7 p.114:27mm

a. fluent aphasia — true
b. lesion is in Brodmann areas 41 and 42 — false (The lesion is in Brodmann 39 and 40.)
c. speech devoid of meaning — true
d. normal intonation — true

119. **True or False. Broca aphasia includes**   G7 p.114:40mm

a. dysarthria — true
b. lesion is in area 44 — true
c. an "apraxia" of motor sequencing — true
d. similar to conduction aphasia — false (Broca is a motor aphasia—faltering dysarthric speech. Conduction aphasia is fluent speech with paraphasias.)

120. **Alexia without agraphia**   G7 p.114:78mm

a. means that the patient can _____ — write
b. but cannot _____. — read
c. Surprisingly, such patients can usually do what with numbers? — read and name them
d. Lesion is located in the _____ lobe. — parietooccipital
e. On which side? — dominant (left) side
f. Serves to disconnect _____ _____ and — angular gyrus
g. _____ _____ — occipital lobes
h. also known as _____ _____ _____. — pure word blindness
i. This is contrasted with what syndrome? — Gerstmann
j. Where patient can _____ — read
k. but can't _____ — write
l. also known as _____ _____ _____. — agraphia without alexia

121. Matching. Match the numbered syndromes with the lettered phrases. G7 p.114:78mm
Syndrome:
① Gerstmann; ② Pure word blindness
Phase:
a. alexia without agraphia   ②
b. agraphia without alexia   ①
c. where patient can't read   ②
d. where patient can't write   ①

■ Babinski Sign

122. Fill in the blanks to complete the details of the Babinski reflex. G7 p.116:35mm
Hint: pcrstlpt
a. lateral _____ stimulation   plantar
b. originates as a _____ _____   cutaneous reflex
c. and stimulates the _____   receptors
d. in the _____ dermatome   S1
e. that travel via the _____ _____ tibial nerve
f. to the spinal cord segments number _____ (_____ limb)   L4-S2, afferent
g. The efferent limb travels via the _____ nerve (_____ limb)   peroneal, efferent
h. to the _____ _____   toe extensors

123. Summarize the Babinski sign. G7 p.116:65mm
a. receptor _____   S1 dermatome
b. afferent limb _____   tibial nerve
c. cord _____   L4-S2
d. efferent limb _____   peroneal nerve

124. Fill in the blanks to complete the details of eliciting the plantar reflex. G7 p.116:92mm
a. Stimulate the _____ _____ surface   lateral plantar
b. and the _____ _____   transverse arch
c. in a _____ movement   single
d. that lasts _____ seconds.   5 to 6
e. Response consists of _____ of the _____ _____.   extension of the great toe
f. _____ of the small toes is   Fanning
g. _____ clinically important. not

125. True or False. The Chaddock maneuver is described as G7 p. 116:108mm
a. scratching the lateral foot   true
b. pinching the Achilles tendon   false
c. sliding knuckles down shin   false
d. momentarily squeezing lower gastrocnemius   false

126. **Complete the following concerning Hoffman sign:**   G7 p.116:128mm
   a. H (from Hoffman) is the _____ letter   eighth
      of the alphabet.
   b. If unilaterally present Hoffman sign   C8
      indicates a lesion above _____.

■ Bladder Neurophysiology

127. **Complete the following concerning bladder physiology:**   G7 p.116:170mm
   a. The primary coordinating center for
      bladder function is in the
      i.   n_____ l_____ c_____   nucleus locus coeruleus
      ii. of the p_____.   pons
   b. This center coordinates
      i.   b_____ c_____ (d_____)   bladder contraction
           with   (detrusor)
      ii. s_____ r_____ (e_____   sphincter relaxation (external
           s_____).   sphincter)

128. **Voluntary cortical control**   G7 p.116:182mm
   a. inhibits the p_____ c_____.   pontine center—nucleus locus
                                                    coeruleus
   b. It originates in the
      i.   a_____ f_____ l_____   anteromedial frontal lobes
      ii. and g_____ of the c_____   genu of the corpus callosum
           c_____ and
   c. travels via the p_____ t_____   pyramidal tract
   d. to inhibit
      i.   c_____ of the   contraction of the
      ii. d_____ and contraction   detrusor and contraction
      iii. of the e_____ s_____.   external sphincter

129. **Immaturity, infarct, or cortical lesions cause**   G7 p.117:17mm
   a. inability to s_____   suppress
   b. the m_____ r_____   micturition reflex
   c. and results in i_____.   incontinence

130. **The efferents to the bladder**   G7 p.117:28mm
   a. travel in the _____ portion   dorsal
   b. of the _____ _____.   lateral columns

131. **Parasympathetic control**   G7 p.117:48mm
   a. detrusor _____   contracts
   b. internal sphincter _____   relaxes
   c. travels via the p_____ s_____   pelvic splanchnic
      nerves

132. **Somatic nerve**   G7 p.117:48mm
   a. external sphincter _____   contracts
   b. maintains c_____   continence
   c. travels via p_____ nerve   pudendal

133. **Sympathetic nerve**   G7 p.117:48mm
a. provides bladder neck _____ and   closure
b. travels via the i_____ h_____   inferior hypogastric
    plexus.

134. **True or False. The detrusor muscle of**   G7 p.117:53mm
the bladder contracts and the internal
sphincter relaxes under
a. PNS stimulation   true (parasympathetic
    nervous system stimulation)
b. somatic nerve stimulation   false
c. sympathetic nervous system stimulation   false
d. all of the above   false

135. **True or False. The following can cause**   G7 p.117:125mm
detrusor hyperreflexia:
a. CVA   true
b. spinal cord tumor   true
c. chronic bladder catheterization   false (Detrusor hyperreflexia
    can result from interruption
    of efferents anywhere from
    cortex to sacral cord.)
d. multiple sclerosis   true
e. Parkinson disease   true

136. **True or False. Interruption of the**   G7 p.117:142mm
efferents results in
a. atonic bladder   false—root lesion
b. overflow incontinence   false —root lesion
c. uncontrollable voiding   true
d. reflex bladder empting   true
e. voiding triggered by critical volume   true
f. produced by myelopathy   true
g. produced by head injury   true
h. produced by certain drugs   false—detrusor areflexia
i. produced by diabetes mellitus   false—automatic neuropathy

137. **True or False. Patients with multiple**   G7 p.118:127mm
sclerosis develop voiding symptoms
from demyelination primarily
involving the
a. posterior and lateral columns of lumbar   false
    spinal cord
b. lateral column of cervical spine   false
c. posterior column of lumbar spine   false
d. lateral column of lumbar spine   false
e. posterior and lateral columns of cervical   true (posterior and lateral
    spinal cord   columns of cervical spinal
    cord)

138. **True or False. Causes of urinary**   G7 p.118:145mm
retention are
a. urethral stricture   true
b. prostatic enlargement   true
c. detrusor areflexia   true
d. herpes zoster   true

5

6

Neuroradiology

■ Contrast Agents in Neuroradiology

1. **Characteristics of iodinated contrast agents**   G7 p.122:60mm
    a. may delay excretion of _____,   metformin
    b. which is an _____ _____ agent   oral hypoglycemic
    c. used in _____ _____ _____   diabtes type II
    d. It can produce
        i.   l_____ a_____   lactic acidosis
        ii. and r_____ f_____.   renal failure
    e. It should be held for _____ hours   48
        before and after administration of
        contrast agent.

2. **The primary approved agent for**   iohexol, Omnipaque   G7 p. 122:90mm
    intrathecal use is _____, trade
    name _____.

3. **Use Omnipaque cautiously in patients**   G7 p.123:70mm
    who have
    a. s_____ h_____   seizure history
    b. c_____-v_____ d_____   cardio-vascular disease
    c. c_____ a_____   chronic alcoholism
    d. m_____ s_____   multiple sclerosis
    e. and stop _____ medications   neuroleptic   G7 p.123:52mm
    f. at least _____ hours before procedure   48

4. **Complete the following for an**   G7 p.124:85mm
    iodinated contrast allergy prep:
    a. prednisone
        i.   pretest timing in hours   20 to 24 hours, 8 to 12 hours,
                                                         2 hours
        ii. dose in mg   50
        iii. route   PO
    b. Benadryl
        i.   pretest timing in hours   1
        ii. dose in mg   50
        iii. route   IM
    c. cimetidine
        i.   pretest timing in hours   1
        ii. dose in mg   300
        iii. route   PO or IV

■ Radiation Safety for Neurosurgeons

5. Characterize radiation safety.   G7 p.126:165mm

a. Rem is the absorbed dose in rads   Q
   multiplied by _____.

b. Q "is the quality factor"; the Q of x-ray is   1
   _____.

c. 1 rem causes _____ cases of cancer   300
   in every 1 million people.

d. Spine x-rays with obliques is _____   5   G7 p.127:18mm
   rem.

e. Cerebral angiogram is _____ rem.   10 to 20

f. Cerebral embolization is _____ rem.   34

6. Complete the following regarding   G7 p.127:80 mm
occupational radiation exposure:

a. It is advised to keep below _____   2
   rem per year,

b. averaged over a _____ year period.   5

7. Provide the precautions advised.   G7 p.127:110mm

a. Increase the _____ from the   distance
   radiation source.

b. Exposure is proportional to the _____   inverse square
   _____ of the distance.

c. Stay at least _____ feet away,   6,10
   preferably _____ feet away.

d. Double the distance and get _____ of   1/4
   the radiation.

e. What is better: lead "doors" or lead   doors
   aprons?

■ CAT Scan

8. For measurement on a CT scan   G7 p.128:46mm

a. The eyeball is _____ mm through its   25
   equator.

b. Give Hounsfield units for
   i.   air   -1000
   ii.   water   0
   iii. bone   +1000
   iv.   blood clot   75-80
   v.   calcium   100-300
   vi.   disc material   55-70
   vii. thecal sac   20-30

c. Effect of anemia on an acute subdural   isodense
   hematoma (SDH) in a patient with less
   than 23% HCT will look _____.

■ Sylvian Point

9. **True or False. The sylvian point is**   G5 p.559:10mm
   a. the apex of the insula   true
   b. usually 5 to 10 mm from the inner table   false (30 to 43 mm from inner
      of the skull   table)
   c. at or within 1 cm below the midpoint of   true
      a vertical line from the superior inner
      table to the orbital apex
   d. the point where the anterior choroidal   false (That is called the plexal
      artery enters the temporal horn of the   point.)
      lateral ventricle

■ Cerebral Angiography

10. **Answer the following concerning**   G7 p.134:145mm
    cerebral angiography:
    a. What is the overall risk, in %, of a   0.1%
       complication resulting in a permanent
       neurological deficit with angiography?
    b. What is the risk, in %, of neuropathy from   0.2%
       femoral angiogram?

11. **Complete the following about**   G7 p.134:145mm
    angiography (cerebral):
    a. The complication rate in
       i.   uncomplicated angiography is   0.1%
            approximately _____%.
       ii. asymptomatic carotid stenosis is   1.2%
            _____%.
    b. The most common of the persistent   persistent primitive
       carotid basilar anastomoses is _____   trigeminal artery
       _____ _____ _____.
    c. This occurs in _____% of angiograms.   0.6%
    d. The sylvian point marks the apex of the   insula
       _____.

12. **Characterize venous structures.**   G7 p.134:160mm
    a. Deep lesions cause changes in _____   venous
       structures.
    b. Superficial lesions cause changes in   arterial
       _____ structures.
    c. Malignant lesion (i.e., GBM) show an   draining vein
       early _____ _____.
    d. Meningiomas show draining veins   late
       _____.
    e. Meningiomas come _____ and stay   early, late
       _____.

6

13. The recurrent artery of Heubner arises from the

a. _____ segment of the

b. _____ _____ artery (80%)

c. and supplies the:

i.   a _____

ii. p _____

iii. c _____

A1

anterior cerebral

(Controversial item: Rhoton's Anatomy, page 119 column B 45 mm, recurrent branch most commonly arises from A^2—78% A^1—14% A^1–A^2 junction 8%)

anterior limb: internal capsule

putamen

caudate head

G7 p.134:145mm

14. What is the name of the artery that is the continuation of the anterior cerebral artery?

pericallosal artery

G7 p.101:15mm

15. Complete the following statements about neuroradiology:

a. The _____ _____ artery enters

b. the temporal horn via the _____ fissure.

c. This is called the p_____ p_____.

d. It is _____ mm to _____ mm from origin of that vessel.

e. What is unique about this point on the angiogram?

anterior choroidal

choroidal

plexal point

18 to 26 mm

It makes a distinct kink as seen on the lateral angiogram.

G7 p.101:70mm

16. True or False. From proximal to distal, the branches of the anterior cerebral artery are

a. medial orbitofrontal, frontopolar, callosomarginal, pericallosal — true

b. frontopolar, callosomarginal, medial orbitofrontal, pericallosal — false

c. frontopolar, medial orbitofrontal, pericallosal, callosomarginal — false

d. medial orbitofrontal, frontopolar, pericallosal, callosomarginal — false

G7 p.101:90mm

17. True or False. The sylvian triangle on a lateral ICA angiogram is formed by

a. superior insular line, angular artery, line between MCA origin, and most anterior ascending branch — true

b. superior insular line, line from bregma to torcula, line between posterior temporal branch, and lateral orbitofrontal branch — false

c. superior insular line, clinoparietal line, limbus sphenoidale — false

d. clinoparietal line, angular artery, line from bregma to torcula — false

G5 p.560:135mm

6

18. **True or False. The following are MCA branches:** G7 p.101:175mm
    a. lateral orbitofrontal — true
    b. ascending frontal — true
    c. medial orbitofrontal — false (The medial orbitofrontal is a branch of the anterior cerebral artery.)
    d. anterior temporal — true
    e. posterior parietal — true

19. **Complete the following about angiography (cerebral):** G7 p.105:86mm
    a. The foramen of Monro lies at the junction of what three veins?
       i. i_____ c_____ — internal cerebral
       ii. t_____ — thalamostriate
       iii. s_____ — septal
    b. This site is known as the _____ _____. — venous angle

20. **True or False. The following veins will drain into the straight sinus in the normal venous anatomy:** G7 p.105:130mm
    a. vein of Galen — true
    b. basal cerebral vein of Rosenthal — true (via the vein of Galen)
    c. inferior sagittal sinus — true
    d. vein of Labbé — false (It empties into the transverse sinus.)

21. **True or False. In the setting of a brain stem mass seen on a lateral vertebrobasilar angiogram, the displacement of the choroidal and colliculocentral points should be** G5 p.562:143mm
    a. both displaced anteriorly — false (They would both be displaced anteriorly by a cerebellar mass but posteriorly by a brain stem mass.)
    b. choroidal anteriorly, colliculocentral posteriorly — false (They outline the fourth ventricle and would move with it.)
    c. choroidal posteriorly, colliculocentral anteriorly — false (They outline the fourth ventricle and would move with it.)
    d. both displaced posteriorly — true (Both would be displaced posteriorly by a brain stem mass.)
    e. no displacement — false

6

22. **Complete the following about cerebral angiography:**

    G5 p.562:135mm

    a. True or False. On a lateral vertebrobasilar angiogram, the most sensitive indicator of the anterior border of the pons is the
       i. pontomesencephalic vein — true
       ii. basilar artery — false (Basilar artery may be off to one side.)
       iii. choroidal point — false (junction of posterior medullary loop and supratonsillar loop)
       iv. copular point — false (on the inferior vermian vein)

       G5 p.562:130mm

    b. Twinings line runs between
       i. t_____ — tuberculum
       ii. t_____ — torcula

■ Magnetic Resonance Imaging (MRI)

6

23. **Matching. Match the best completion for each of the following:**
    ① short TE, short TR; ② short TE, long TR; ③ long TE, short TR; ④ long TE, long TR

    G7 p.129:49mm

    a. T1-weighted MRI has: — ①
    b. T2-weighted image has: — ④

24. **Complete the following about magnetic resonance imaging (MRI):**

    G7 p.129:110mm

    a. List the three materials that appear white on T1-weighted imaging (T1WI) MRI. — fat, melanin, and subacute blood
    b. What color is pathology on T1WI? — low signal on T1 (dark)
    c. What color is pathology on T2WI? — high signal on T2 (white)

25. **Matching. Match the phrases with the appropriate signal.**
    ① high signal (bright); ② low signal (dark); ③ intermediate signal

    G7 p.129:145mm

    a. Fat on T1 is _____ — ①
    b. Fat on T2 is _____ — ②
    c. 7- to 14-day-old blood on T2-weighted MRI is: — ①
    d. 7- to 14-day-old blood on T1-weighted MRI is: — ①

    On T1 both fat and 7- to 14-day-old blood are high signal (white).
    On T2 fat drops out (i.e., is dark); blood remains white.

26. Complete the following about MRI: G7 p.129:170mm
 a. The best sequence for CVA is _____,   FLAIR
 b. which stands for _____-_____   fluid-attenuated inversion
    _____ _____.   recovery
 c. Cerebrospinal fluid (CSF) is _____.   black
 d. Most lesions appear _____ in this   bright
    sequence.
 e. Most lesions are more _____.   conspicuous

27. The best MRI sequence for
 a. SAH is _____   FLAIR   G7 p.130:15mm
 b. blood is _____ _____   gradient echo   G7 p.130:82mm

28. Gradient echo   G7 p.130:60mm
 a. aka _____ _____   T2 star
 b. aka _____   grass
 c. CSF and flowing blood appear _____   white
 d. In cervical spine produces a _____   myelographic
    effect
 e. Improves delineation of _____   bone spurs
    _____
 f. Also shows small old _____   hemorrhage
 g. It is the most sensitive MRI sequence for   blood
    _____.

29. Complete the following about MRI: G7 p.130:92mm
 a. True or False. An MRI sequence that
    summates T1 and T2 signals and causes
    fat to be suppressed is called the
    _____ sequence.
    i.   grass   false
    ii. stir   true
    iii. echo train   false
    iv. spin density   false
 b. STIR stands for _____ _____   short tau inversion recovery
    _____ _____.   (summates T1 and T2
    images)
 c. Use it to _____.   see tissues that enhance in
    areas of fat

30. If a MRI contrast is given to patients   nephrogenic systemic fibrosis   G7 p.130:125mm
 with severe renal failure, a rare
 condition called n_____ s_____
 f_____ may occur.

31. Name two contraindications to MRI.   G7 p.131:20mm

a. patients who contain _____ or _____

> ferro metals or cobalt (i.e., cardiac pacemaker, implanted neurostimulators, cochlear implants, ferromagnetic aneurysm clips, foreign bodies with a large component of iron or cobalt, metallic fragments in the eye, placement of stent, coil, or filter within past 6 weeks)

b. relative contraindication to MRI is _____

> claustrophobia

32. Complete the following regarding programmable valves and MRI: G7 p.131:80mm

a. Can such patients have MRI studies?   yes

b. You may need to check the _____ _____ after the MRI.   pressure setting

6

33. Hemorrhage on MRI. Related to time. T1   G7 p.132:15mm

Hint: George Washington Bridge

a. acute   g_____   gray

b. subacute   w_____   white

c. chronic   b_____   black

34. Hemorrhage on MRI. Related to time. T2   G7 p.132:15mm

Hint: layers of Oreo cookie

a. acute   b_____   black

b. subacute   w_____   white

c. chronic   b_____   black

35. Hemorrhage on MRI. Related to time.   G7 p.132:15mm

Hint: i - baby, i - di, bi - di, ba - by, da - da

a. hyper-acute

    i.   T1: i_____   isodense

    ii. T2: b_____   bright

b. acute

    i.   T1: i_____   isodense

    ii. T2: d_____   dark

c. subacute early

    i.   T1: b_____   bright

    ii. T2: d_____   dark

d. subacute late

    i.   T1: b_____   bright

    ii. T2: b_____   bright

e. chronic

    i.   T1: d_____   dark

    ii. T2: d_____   dark

36. Age of hemorrhage   G7 p.132:15mm
   a. hyper acute _____   <24 hours
   b. acute _____   1 to 3 days
   c. subacute early _____   3 to 7 days
   d. subacute late _____   7 to 14 days
   e. chronic _____   >14 days

37. Complete the following regarding   G7 p.132:20mm
   hemorrhage and the condition of
   hemoglobin:
   a. hyperacute o_____   oxy
   b. acute d_____   deoxy
   c. subacute early m_____   met
   d. subacute late m_____   met
   e. chronic h_____   hemosiderin

38. Complete the following regarding   G7 p.132:20mm
   hemorrhage and the location of   Also see
   hemoglobin: G7 p.1125:50mm
   a. hyperacute I_____   intracellular
   b. acute I_____   intracellular
   c. subacute early I_____   intracellular
   d. subacute late E_____   extracellular
   e. chronic I_____   intracellular

39. Complete the following regarding   G7 p.132:103mm
   diffusion weighted images (DWI):
   a. Its primary use is to detect
      i. i_____   ischemia
      ii. and a_____ p_____. active plaques
   b. It first generates on _____ map. ADC
   c. On DWI freely diffusible water is   dark
      _____.
   d. Restricted diffusion is _____.   bright
   e. Which is abnormal?   restricted diffusion

40. Characterize DWI.   G7 p.132:135mm
   a. Restricted perfusion usually indicates   cell death
      _____ _____.
   b. DWI abnormally will be present for   1 month
      _____.
   c. DWI abnormalities can light up within   minutes
      _____ of ischemia.

41. The most sensitive study for ischemia **PWI**   G7 p.133:13mm
   of the brain is the _____.

42. DWI and PWI mismatch identifies   G7 p.133:42mm
   penumbra.
   Hint: DWI death PWI
   a. Which modality shows irreversible cell   DWI
      injury (death)?
   b. Which modality shows reversible cell   PWI
      injury (penumbra)?

43. The important peaks in MRS are
G7 p.133:105mm
Hint: li-la-Na-crea-chol

a.	li_____	lipid
b.	la_____	lactate
c.	N a_____	N acetyl aspartate
d.	crea_____	creatine
e.	chol_____	choline

44. The significance of important peaks in MRS are
G7 p.133:105mm

a.	hypoxia	lactate
b.	a couplet peak	lactate
c.	nerve and axons	NAA
d.	a reference for choline	creatinine
e.	membrane synthesis	choline
f.	increased in tumor	choline
g.	increased in developing brain	choline
h.	reduced in CVA	choline

45. The test that may help distinguish hemangiopericytoma
G7 p.134:20mm

a.	from meningioma is the _____;	MRS
b.	specifically the presence of a large _____ peak.	inositol

46. The test that may help a surgeon avoid critical white matter
G7 p.134:118mm

a.	tracts during brain surgery is _____,	DTI
b.	which stands for d_____ t_____ i_____.	difffusor tensor imaging

■ Plain Films

47. Complete the following about plain films:
G7 p.135:115mm

a.	The basion is at the tip of the _____.	clivus
b.	The opisthion is at the anterior lip of the _____ _____.	occipital bone

G7 p.135:118mm

48. A lateral C-spine x-ray has four contour lines with two marking the borders of the spinal canal.
G7 p.135:160mm
Hint: apsp

a.	front of vertebral body called _____ _____ _____	anterior marginal line
b.	back of vertebral body called _____ _____ _____	posterior marginal line (marks anterior border of spinal canal)
c.	posterior margin of spinal canal called _____ _____	spinolaminar line
d.	posterior margin of spinous processes is called _____ _____ _____	posterior spinous line

6

49. Complete the following about spine films:

a. Cervical spine normal diameter is _____ mm.   17 ± 5 mm   G7 p.136:130mm

b. Stenosis is present when the anteroposterior diameter is less than _____ mm.   12 mm   G7 p.136:140mm

50. Complete the following about normal prevertebral soft tissue: G7 p.137:15mm

a. Anterior to C1: _____ mm   10

b. Anterior to C2, 3, 4: _____ mm   7

c. Anterior to C5-C6: _____ mm   22

51. Interspinous distances   G7 p.137:50mm

a. are abnormal if it is _____ times the adjacent levels on AP film   1.5

b. if present it represents: true or false
   i.   fracture   true
   ii. dislocation   true
   iii. ligament disruption   true

c. this is called _____ on lateral x-ray   fanning

52. C1 has how many ossification centers?   3   G7 p.137:84mm

53. C2 has how many ossification centers?   4   G7 p.137:140 mm

54. Matching. Match the following skull film findings with their characteristics: G7 p.138:115mm
① enlarged sella; ② J-shaped sella; ③ symmetrical ballooning; ④ erosion of posterior clinoids

a. craniopharyngioma   ④ erosion of posterior clinoids

b. pituitary adenoma   ① enlarged sella

c. optic glioma   ② J-shaped sella

d. empty sella   ③ symmetrical ballooning

55. True or False. On a skull x-ray, erosion of the posterior clinoids would most often be seen in the setting of   G7 p.138:115mm

a. craniopharyngioma   true

b. empty sella syndrome   false

c. pituitary adenoma   false

d. Hurler syndrome   false

e. optic glioma   false

6

56. **Complete the following regarding lumbosacral spine films:** G7 p.138:25mm

  a. The disc space with the greatest heigh is at _____   L45

  b. AP view. Look for "owl eyes."

     i. These correspond to the _____   pedicles

     ii. Can be eroded in _____ disease   metastatic

  c. Oblique views. Look for the neck of the scotty dog.

     i. It corresponds to the _____ _____   pars interarticularis

     ii. Discontinuity occurs in a _____   fracture

57. **True or False. The percentage of all patients over 20 years old who will have a calcified pineal gland visible on plain skull x-ray is** G5 p.570:55mm

  a. 0%   false

  b. 10%   false

  c. 20%   false

  d. 55%   true

  e. 90%   false

58. **True or False. The most common congenital anomaly of the craniocervical junction is** G7 p.139:140mm

  a. Chiari malformation   false

  b. basilar impression   true

  c. os odontoideum   false

  d. incomplete arch of C1   false

  e. C1-C2 subluxation   false

59. **True or False. Basilar invagination is seen in** G7 p.139:166mm

  a. hypoparathyroidism   false

  b. Paget disease   true

  c. osteogenesis imperfecta   true

  d. osteomalacia   true

  e. hyperparathyroidism   true

60. **True or False. In the evaluation of basilar invagination, in the normal patient, no part of the odontoid should be above the McRae line.**   true   G7 p.139:48mm

61. **True or False. A line used in the evaluation of the craniocervical junction is** G7 p.139:24mm

  a. McRae line   true

  b. Chamberlain line   true

  c. Wackenheim line   true

  d. Maginot line   false   G7 p.138:115mm

  e. Fischgold line   true

6

62. True or False. The most common G6 p.142:150mm
nondisc spinal lesion is:
a. synovial cyst   false
b. Tarlov cyst   false
c. astrocytoma   false
d. chordoma   false
e. metastatic tumor   true

■ Myelography

63. True or False. The risk of postlumbar G5 p.572:55mm
puncture headache is higher with
a. water-soluble contrast   false
b. non-water-soluble contrast   true

64. Matching. Match each of the following G5 p.571:145mm
two statements with answers 1, 2, 3,
or 4.
① 10%; ② 35%; ③ 65%; ④ 90%
a. In lumbar disc disease, what percentage   ②
of free fragments move inferiorly?
b. In lumbar disc disease, what percentage   ③
of free fragments move superiorly?

6

7

Operations and Procedures

■ Intraoperative Dyes

1. **Matching. Match the intraoperative dyes with their characteristics.**
   G7 p.144:70mm
   Dyes:
   ① indigo carmine; ② methylene blue;
   ③ fluorescein
   Characteristic:

   a. carries a small risk of seizures when administered intrathecally   ③

   b. is cytotoxic and should not be used at all   ②

   c. can be used to demonstrate arteriovenous malformation (AVM) vessels intraoperatively   ③

   d. used to identify cerebrospinal fluid (CSF) leaks and is considered safe   ①

■ Surgical Hemostasis

2. **Bone wax inhibits _____ formation.**   bone
   G7 p.146:82mm

3. **True or False. The following chemical hemostatic agent exerts its effect by promoting platelet aggregation:**
   G7 p.146:100mm

   a. Gelfoam (gelatin sponge)   false

   b. Oxycel (oxidized cellulose)   false

   c. Avitene (microfibrillar collagen)   true (Avitene, that is, microfibrillar collagen, provides platelet adhesion and aggregation. It loses its effectiveness with severe thrombocytopenia less than 10,000/mL.)

   d. thrombin   false

4. **Matching. Match the surgical hemostasis substance with its trade name.**

Trade name:
① Thrombostat; ② Gelfoam; ③ Oxycel;
④ Surgicel; ⑤ Avitene
Substance:

a. gelatin sponge   ②
b. oxidized cellulose   ③
c. regenerated cellulose   ④
d. microfibrillar collagen   ⑤
e. thrombin   ①

5. **Complete the following about surgical hemostasis:**

a. What may thrombin cause if placed on the brain?   significant edema
b. If the _____ has been _____.   the pia; disrupted

▪ Intraoperative Brain Swelling

6. **Complete the brain swelling intraoperative checklist.**

Hint: decompress

a. d_____ _____   drain CSF
b. e_____ _____   elevate head
c. c_____ (_____)   CO₂ (hypercarbia)
d. o_____ of _____ _____   obstruction of jugular veins
e. m_____   mannitol
f. p_____   pyperventilate
g. r_____ _____   remove bone
h. e_____ _____   excise brain (temporal or frontal lobes)
i. (s)
j. (s)

▪ Craniotomies

7. **Complete the following regarding the risks of craniotomy:**

a. increased neurological deficit _____%   10%
b. postop hemorrhage _____%   1%
c. infection _____%   2%
d. anesthetic complications _____%   0.2%

8. **Complete the following regarding anticonvulsants:**

a. True or False. Maintain their use if cortical incision is anticipated.   true (use Keppra)
b. Describe the method of loading.   500 mg PO or IV q 12 hours
c. For supratentorial craniotomy maintain for _____.   2 to 3 months

d.	For cortical incision maintain for _____.	2 to 3 months
e.	For aneurysm, AVM, or meningioma maintain for _____.	6 to 12 months
f.	For head injury (see Head Injury guidelines) use for _____.	1 week

9. **True or False. The following might be caused by pneumocephalus:**   G7 p.149:48mm

a.	lethargy	true
b.	confusion	true
c.	headache	true
d.	nausea	true
e.	vomiting	true
f.	seizures	true

10. **True or False. Simple pneumocephalus (the presence of air in the cranium not apparently under pressure) can cause neurologic symptoms postoperatively.**   true   G7 p.149:52mm

11. **Possible symptoms include l_____, c_____, h_____, n_____, v_____, and s_____.**   lethargy, confusion, severe headache, nausea, vomiting, and seizures (Obviously, other etiologies, including subclinical seizures, and metabolic causes should be ruled out.)   G7 p.149:52mm

12. **Symptoms usually improve over _____ days.**   1 to 3   G7 p.149:62mm

13. **If postoperative seizures occur, consider the following:**
Hint: abci   G7 p.149:100mm

a.	a_____ _____	anticonvulsant level—draw blood
b.	b_____	bolus—additional anticonvulsants
c.	c_____ _____	CAT scan—to identify if any cause
d.	i_____	intubate—to protect airway

■ Posterior Fossa Craniotomy

14. **True or False. The correct treatment for air embolism sustained during a craniotomy performed with the patient in a sitting position is**   G7 p.153:120mm

a.	to find and occlude site of entry or rapidly pack wound with sopping wet sponges	true
b.	bilateral or right-sided jugular venous compression	true

c.	ventilation with 100% O_2	true
d.	rotating the patient right side down	false (Patient should be turned left side down to trap air in the right atrium.)
e.	aspirating air from central venous pressure (CVP) catheter	true
f.	avoiding positive end-expiratory pressure (PEEP), which is ineffective and may worsen the risk of paradoxical air embolism	true

15. Complete the following about posterior fossa craniectomy and air embolism: G7 p.153:130mm

a. Effect of air in right atrium is
   i.   h_____   hypotension due to impaired venous return
   ii. a_____   arrhythmias
b. Paradoxical air embolism may occur if
   i.   p_____ f_____ o_____   patent foramen ovale
   ii. p_____ arteriovenous (AV) f_____   pulmonary AV fistula
c. Incidence in sitting position is _____%.   7 to 25%
d. Precautions require
   i.   D_____ _____ _____   Doppler precordial ultrasound
   ii. C_____ _____ _____ _____ _____   CVP catheter in right atrium
e. Earliest clue to occurrence is _____.   fall in end tidal pCO_2

16. How does air embolism cause problems?   G7 p.153:130mm

a. Air becomes trapped in the _____ _____,   right atrium
b. impairs _____ _____, and   venous return
c. produces _____.   hypotension

17. Outline the intraoperative treatment for air embolism during a craniotomy.   G7 p.153:145mm

   Hint: occlude
   i.   o_____   occlude entry site
   ii.   c_____   cover with wet laps
   iii. c_____   compress jugular veins
   iv.   l_____   left side down lower head
   v.   u_____   ventilate/increase volume
   vi.   d_____   discontinue nitrous
   vii. e_____   evacuate air

18. Earliest clues to occurrence include   G7 p.154:20mm

a. fall in _____ _____ _____   end tidal pCO_2
b. sound on Doppler is _____ _____   machinery sound
c. blood pressure _____   hypotension

19. **True or False. The following approach is most applicable for a vertebral endarterectomy:**   G7 p.155:22mm

a. midline suboccipital craniotomy — false

b. extreme lateral posterior fossa approach — false

c. paramedian suboccipital craniotomy — true (Paramedian suboccipital craniotomy gives decent access to the vertebral artery and to the posterior inferior cerebellar artery [PICA] and the vertebrobasilar junction.)

d. subtemporal craniotomy — false

20. **Consider the concept of "5-5-5."**   G7 p.155:90mm

a.

i. This relates to the _____ incision — skin

ii. for a linear _____ incision — paramedian

iii. for access to the _____. — CPA

b.

i. The first number relates to the mm medial to the _____ _____. — mastoid notch

ii. The second number relates to the _____ _____ the notch. — cm above

iii. The third number relates to the _____ _____ the notch. — cm below

21. **Matching. Match the incision with the objective.**   G7 p.155:90mm

Incision:

① 5-6-4, ② 5-5-5, ③ 5-4-6

Objective: approach for

a. the fifth nerve — ①

b. hemifacial spasm — ②

c. glossopharyngeal neuralgia — ③

d. microvascular trigeminal decompression — ①

e. vestibular schwannoma — ②

22. **Location of the inferior margin of the transverse sinus can be estimated**   G7 p.156:20mm

a. to be _____ f_____ _____ above the — two finger breadths

b. m_____ n_____. — mastoid notch

23. **Describe the Frazier burr hole.**   G7 p.156:90mm

a. It is used

i. p_____ — prophylactically

ii. to relive p_____ swelling — postoperative

iii. due to h_____ or — hydrocephalus

iv. e_____. — edema

b. It is located

i. _____ to _____ cm from the midline — 3 to 4

ii. _____ to _____ cm above the inion in adults — 6 to 7

iii. _____ to _____ cm above the inion in children — 3 to 4

7

24. **Complete the following regarding posterior fossa postop complications:**   G7 p.157:120mm
    a. Respiratory: prevent by _____   keeping patient intubated
    b. Hypertension: maintain SBP below   160 with nitroprusside
       _____ with _____
    c. Acute hydrocephalus: treat with   ventricular tap—external
       _____ _____   ventricular drain (EVD)
    d. Meningitis: prevent by prompt repair of cerebrospinal fluid (CSF) leak
       any _____ _____ _____

25. **Blood pressure above _____ is   160 mm Hg systolic   G7 p.157:148mm
    dangerous for the postoperative
    posterior fossa patient.**

26. **Complete the following regarding the   G7 p.157:160 mm
    posterior fossa:**
    a. Posterior fossa increased pressure is
       heralded by changes in
       i. b_____ p_____   blood pressure (increase)
       ii. r_____ p_____   respiratory pattern
    b. not by
       i.   p_____ i_____   pupillary inequality
       ii. m_____ s_____   level mental status
       iii. l_____ c_____   ICP changes

27. **Considerations for postoperative   G7 p.158:20mm
    posterior fossa emergency include**
    a. clinically
       i. blood pressure (BP) _____   high
       ii. respirations _____   labored
    b. recommended treatment
       i.   i_____   intubate
       ii. t_____ _____   tap ventricle
       iii. o_____ _____   open wound
    c. Should you
       i. obtain a computed tomographic   no
           (CT) scan first?
       ii. wait for operating room availability? no

28. **Indicate whether increased pressure in   G7 p.158:30mm
    the posterior fossa or supratentorial
    compartment produces a change in
    the following:**
    a. pupillary reflexes _____   supratentorial compartment
    b. level of consciousness _____   supratentorial compartment
    c. increase in intracranial pressure (ICP) supratentorial compartment
       _____
    d. changes in respiration _____   posterior fossa
    e. rise in blood pressure _____   posterior fossa

7

■ Pterional Craniotomy

29. **Matching. Match the head position with the location of the aneurysm.**
Head position:
① angled 30 degrees, ② angled 45 degrees, ③ angled 60 degrees
Location of aneurysm:

G7 p.159:70mm

a. ICA P-comm — ①
b. carotid terminus — ①
c. middle cerebral artery — ②
d. basilar bifurcation — ①
e. A-comm — ③

30. **Name the artery(ies) that cross the sylvian fissure.** — none cross   G7 p.161:92mm

■ Temporal Craniotomy

31. **True or False. A temporal craniotomy can allow access to the following structures:**   G7 p.162:120mm

a. foramen ovale — true
b. Meckel cave — true
c. labyrinthine and upper tympanic portion of the facial nerve — true

32. **A temporal lobectomy**   G7 p.163:115mm

a. can safely resect _____ cm in the dominant hemisphere — 4 to 5 (before injury to Wernicke area)
b. and _____ cm in the nondominant hemisphere. — 6 to 7 (before injury to optic radiations)

■ Frontal Craniotomy

33. **Complete the following regarding the superior sagittal sinus (SSS):**   G7 p.163:170mm

a. The risk in sacrifice of the SSS is _____ _____. — venous infarction
b. True or False. It almost always occurs with sacrifice of
  i.   the posterior third — true
  ii. the middle third — true
  iii. the anterior third — false

7

■ Skull Base Surgery

34. **The Dolenc approach is**   G6 p.609:95mm
   a. designed to remove the _____   anterior clinoid extradurally
       _____ _____
   b. and provide access to the _____   proximal carotid artery
       _____ _____.

■ Decompressive Craniectomy

35. **Indications for decompressive**   G7 p.165:55mm
       craniectomy are
   a.
       i.   m_____ m_____ cerebral   malignant middle
            artery occlusion
       ii. Primarily for the n_____ -   non-dominant
            d_____ hemisphere
   b. p_____ i_____ hypertension   persistent intracranial
   c. True or False. It is necessary to open the true   G7 p.165:110mm
       dura.
   d. Skull reimplantation can be considered   6 to 12   G7 p.165:140mm
       after _____ to _____ weeks
   e.   G7 p.165:147mm
       i.   A _____ opening is best   large
       ii. Approximately _____ by   12 by 12
            _____ cm or larger

■ Approaches to the Third Ventricle

36. **Study Chart.**   G7 p. 168:110mm
   a. t_____   transcortical
   b. t_____   transcallosal
       i.   a_____   anterior
       ii. p_____   posterior
   c. s_____   subfrontal
       i.   s_____   subchiasmatic
       ii. o_____   opticocarotid
       iii. l_____ t_____   lamina terminalis
       iv. t_____   transsphenoidal
   d. t_____   transsphenoidal
   e. s_____   subtemporal
   f. s_____   stereotactic

37. **What is the risk of postoperative**   5%   G7 p.168:125mm
       seizures after a transcortical approach
       to the anterior third ventricle (e.g., for
       a colloid cyst)?

38. What are the principles of tumor removal?

a. Veins must be preserved at all _____.   costs   G7 p.168:170mm

b. First remove the tumor from within the _____.   capsule   G7 p.168:180mm

c. If adhesions seem unyielding the most likely cause is i_____ i_____ evacuation.   incomplete intracapsular   G7 p.169:15mm

39. Complete the following: G7 p. 170:180mm

a. True or False. A disconnection syndrome (split-brain syndrome) is common with

   i.   posterior callosotomy through splenium   true (where more visual information crosses)

   ii. anterior callosotomy   false

   iii. callosotomy < 2.5 cm in length from a point 1 to 2 cm behind the tip of the genu.   false

b. Which of the above approaches avoids the disconnection syndrome best?   callosotomy < 2.5 cm in length from a point 1 to 2 cm behind the tip of the genu

40. Describe the transcallosal approach to the third ventricle.   G7 p.169:170mm

7

a. The superior sagittal sinus (SSS) is often to the _____ of the sagittal suture.   right

b. The cranial opening should be   G7 p.170:40mm

   i.   _____ anterior to the coronal suture   two third

   ii. and _____ behind it.   one third

c. The two cingulate gyri may be adherent in the midline and can be mistaken for the c_____ c_____.   corpus callosum   G7 p.170:130mm

d.

   i.   The corpus callosum has a distinct _____ color.   white

   ii. It is located beneath the paired _____ arteries.   pericallosal

e. The opening is usually made between the p_____ p_____ arteries.   paired pericallosal   G7 p.170:155mm

f. The trajectory of dissection is from the

   i.   c_____ s_____   coronal suture

   ii. the e_____ a_____ m_____.   external auditory meatus

   iii. The f_____ of M_____ lies along this line.   foramen of Monro

g.   G7 p.170:173mm

   i.   It is helpful to fenestrate the s_____ p_____   septum pellicidum

   ii. to prevent it from b_____ into the ventricle   bulging

   iii. especially in a case of c_____ c_____.   colloid cyst

41. **How can you tell which ventricle you are in?**   G7 p.171:38mm
    a. The foramen of Monro is located m_____.   medially
    b. If the choroid plexus goes to the left to enter the foramen of Monro you are in the _____ ventricle.   right
    c. If you see no choroid plexus and no veins you may be in a c_____ s_____ p_____.   cavum septum pellucidum   G7 p.171:80mm
    d. The safe way to enlarge the foramen of Monro is posteriorly between the _____ _____ and the _____.   choroid plexus; fornix   G7 p.171:115mm

42. **Complete the following about approaches to the third ventricle:**   G7 p.172:145mm
    a. The interhemispheric approach runs risk of injury to _____ _____ _____   bilateral cingulate gyrus
    b. which may produce _____ _____.   transient mutism
    c. The anterior transcallosal approach runs risk of injury to _____ _____   bilateral fornices
    d. which may produce problem with s_____-t_____ m_____ and n_____ l_____.   short-term memory and new learning   G7 p.172:135mm
    e. The transcortical approach is   G7 p.172:98mm
       i. made through the _____ _____ gyrus.   middle frontal
       ii. This is about the same spot used for e_____ v_____ d_____.   external ventricular drain
       iii. called _____ point.   Kocher

43. **Localizing levels in spine surgery. Most patients have _____ presacral vertebra.**   24   G7 p.173:175mm

44. **The aortic bifurcation is at the mid-body of _____.**   L3   G7 p.175:90mm

■ Transoral Approach to Anterior Craniocervical Junction

45. **Complete the following regarding transoral approach to anterior craniocervical junction:**   G7 p.176:125mm
    a. What percent of patients need posterior fusion after a transoral odontoidectomy?   75%
    b. The patient must be able to open the mouth at least _____ mm.   25   G7 p.177:115mm
    c.   G7 p.177:140mm
       i. The tubercle of the _____   atlas
       ii. can be palpated through the posterior _____   pharynx
       iii. in order to locate the _____.   midline
    d. If C1 sparing is not done the central _____ cm of the _____ is removed.   3; atlas   G7 p.177:168mm

7

e.   G7 p.177:175mm

   i.   There is about _____ to   20 to 25
        _____ mm working distance

   ii. between the _____ _____   two vertebral arteries
        _____ where

   iii. they enter the f_____ t_____   foramen transversarium
        at the inferior aspect of

   iv. the lateral masses of _____.   C2

46. **Complete the following regarding**   G7 p.178:110mm
     anterior access:

  a. To T3 use a s_____ s_____   sternal splitting
     approach.

  b. At T10 the attachment of the _____   diaphragm   G7 p.179:45mm
     increases the difficulty of this approach.

  c. The location of the bifurcation of the   L4-L5   G7 p.179:90mm
     vena cava is from just above to just
     below the _____ disc.

■ Surgical Fusion of the Cervical Spine

47. **What are the disadvantages of**   G7 p.179:140mm
     occipitocervical fusion?

  a. r_____ range of motion   reduces (movement at the
                                   occipitocervical junction)

  b. _____ is higher than _____   nonunion rate; C1-C2 fusion

48. **True or False. The following is an**   G7 p.179:150mm
     indication for occipitocervical fusion:

  a. congenital absence of C1 arch   true
  b. upward migration of the odontoid into   true
     the foramen magnum
  c. congenital anomalies of occipitocervical   true
     joints
  d. type II odontoid fracture   false

49. **Complete the following regarding**   G7 p.179:145mm
     occipitocervical fusion:

  a. Patient will lose about _____% of   30%
     neck flexion.

  b.   G7 p.180:80mm

   i.   Keel plate must be placed at the   thickest
       _____

   ii. region of the _____ occipital   midline
       bone.

   iii. It is advisable to _____ it pre-   measure
       operatively.

50. **True or False. After occipito-cervical**   G7 p.181:64mm
     fusion we use a halo for

  a. severe fractures   true
  b. elderly patients   true
  c. unreliable patients   true
  d. smokers   true
  e. 8 to 12 weeks   true

7

51. **True or False. The C1-C2 complex is**   G7 p.181:89mm
responsible for the following
percentage of axial rotation:

   a. 10%   false
   b. 15%   false
   c. 25%   false
   d. 50%   true
   e. 75%   false

52. **Complete the following regarding**   G7 p.181:89mm
anterior odontoid screw fixation:

   a. C1-C2 complex is responsible for   50%
       _____% of head rotation.
   b. Stability depends on the integrity of the   G7 p.181:101mm
      i.   o_____ p_____ and the   odontoid process
      ii. a_____ t_____ ligament   atlantoaxial transverse
   c. Indicated in patients who have a type   II, transverse   G7 p.181:130mm
      _____ odontoid fracture and an
      intact _____ ligament
   d. Contraindicated if there is a fracture   G7 p.181:140mm
      i.   of the _____ _____   vertebral body
      ii. and if the fracture is less than   6   G7 p.181:162mm
          _____ months old
   e.   G7 p.183:80mm
      i.   The immediate postop strength is   50%
          only _____%.
      ii. Therefore a brace is recommended   6
          for _____ weeks.
      iii. If the patient has osteoporosis use a   halo
          _____.

53. **Complete the following regarding**   G7 p.181:101mm
anterior odontoid screw fixation:

   a. The most important structure holding   transverse
      the odontoid in position against the
      anterior arch of C1 is the _____
      ligament,
   b. aka the _____ ligament.   atlantoaxial
   c. It is the horizontal limb of the _____   cruciate
      ligament.

54. **True or False. The following condition**   G7 p.181:130mm
is an indication for anterior odontoid
screw fixation:

   a. pathologic odontoid fracture   false
   b. type III odontoid fracture where the   false
      fracture line is in the caudal portion of
      body of C2
   c. type I odontoid fracture that is reducible   false
   d. type II irreducible odontoid fracture   false
   e. type II reducible odontoid fracture   true
   f. age of fracture is less than 6 months   true

55. What are indications for odontoid screw?   G7 p.181:131mm

a. Fracture must be _____   reducible
b. Type _____ fracture   II
c. Which ligament must be intact?   transverse

56. True or False. The following are contraindications for anterior odontoid screw fixation: G7 p.181:140mm

a. disruption of atlantal transverse ligament   true
b. disruption of apical ligament   false
c. fracture of C2 vertebral body   true
d. reducible odontoid type II fracture   false

57. Indications for odontoid screw fixation include   G7 p.181:160mm

a. type of fracture: _____   II odontoid
b. age of fracture: less than _____   6 months
   _____ old
c. ligament: t_____ l_____   transverse ligament intact
   i_____
d. judged by:
   i.   _____ and   MRI
   ii. _____ of _____   rule of Spence
e.
   i.   The immediate postop strength is   50%   G7 p.183:80mm
        only _____%
   ii. Therefore a brace is recommended   6
        for _____ weeks
   iii. If the patient has osteoporosis, use a   halo
        _____

58. Provide fusion rates with age of fracture.   G7 p.181:162mm

a. Fusion rates in fractures more than 18   25%
   months old: _____%
b. Fusion rates in fractures less than 6   90%
   months old: _____%

■ Atlantoaxial Fusion (C1-C2 Arthrodesis)

59. Characterize atlantoaxial fusion (C1-C2 arthrodesis).   G7 p.183:125mm

a. The patient will lose about _____% of   50%
   head rotation
b. Transarticular screws   G7 p.184:150mm
   i.   Danger is to the v_____   vertebral artery
        a_____
   ii. Provides i_____ s_____   immediate stabilization
   iii. Requires preop _____ to study   CT   G7 p.184:175mm
        vertebral arteries

7

60. **True or False. The following is an indication for atlantoaxial fusion:**
G7 p.183:140mm
a. type I odontoid fracture — false
b. disruption of alar ligament of dens — false
c. disruption of apical ligament of dens — false
d. vertebrobasilar insufficiency with head turning — true (Disruption of alar or apical ligament of dens does not render the spine unstable as long as the transverse ligament is intact.)

61. **Characterize bow hunter's sign.**
G7 p.183:82mm
a. What is bow hunter's sign? — vertebrobasilar insufficiency with head turning
b. What is the treatment for bow hunter's sign? — atlantoaxial fusion (C1-C2 arthrodesis)

62. **Characterize a C1-C2 fusion.**
G7 p.183:125mm Also G6 p.623:170mm
a. What mobility is lost?
   i. head rotation _____% — 50%
   ii. lateral mobility _____% — 35%
b. Which technique produces less loss of mobility?
   i. Brooks — All are the same in regard to loss of mobility.
   ii. Gallie — All are the same in regard to loss of mobility.
   iii. Sonntag — All are the same in regard to loss of mobility.

63. **Describe the fusion technique and differentiate.**
G7 p.184:75mm Also G6 p.624:120mm
a. Brooks fusion
   i. sublaminar to _____ — C1 and C2 sublaminar wiring
   ii. with _____ grafts — two-wedge bone
b. Gallie fusion
   i. sublaminar to _____ — C1 only
   ii. with _____ graft — "H" graft wired into place to C1 only
c. Sonntag fusion
   i. sublaminar to _____ — C1 only
   ii. with _____ graft — bicortical graft wedged between C1 and C2

64. **Characterize C1-C2 transarticular facet screw.**
G7 p.184:175mm
a. Special preop test needed is a thin cut CT scan from the
   i. _____ _____ — occipital condyles
   ii. through to C_____ — C3
   iii. to look for the location of the _____ _____. — vertebral arteries
b. A fusion rate of up to _____% has been reported. — 99%

7

65. **With postoperative immobilization:**   G6 p.625:25mm

a. The use of what apparatus is considered   halo brace
optimal immobilization of the cervical
spine?

b. It reduces cervical motion by _____%.   95%

c. It is mandatory for use in
   i.   r_____ _____   rheumatoid arthritis
   ii. o_____   osteopenia

d. The next best apparatus is the _____-   sternal-occipital-mandibular
_____-_____ _____ _____.   immobilizer (SOMI) brace

e. Use this apparatus for _____ weeks.   12 to 16

f. Follow with a _____ for _____   hard collar for 4 to 6
weeks.

g. Use _____-_____ _____ to   flexion-extension films
determine if this treatment was
satisfactory.

66. **Give the frequency of osseous fusions**   G6 p.625:60mm
for the listed techniques.

a. Brooks _____%   70 to 85%

b. Gallie _____%   70 to 85%

c. Sonntag _____%   97%

67. **True or False. The following is**   G6 p.625:80mm
associated with nonunion in
atlantoaxial fusion:

a. rheumatoid arthritis   true

b. cigarette smoking   true

c. osteoporosis   true

d. nonsteroidal antiinflammatory drugs   true
(NSAIDs)

68. **What are modifying correctible risk**   G6 p.625:100mm
factors for a C1-C2 arthrodesis?

a. c_____ s_____   cigarette smoking

b. m_____-o_____   malnutrition-osteoporosis

c. N_____   stopping suppressive drugs
(NSAID) 1 week before and
2 weeks after surgery

d. s_____   steroids

e. i_____   immunosuppressives

f. a_____ b_____   use autologous bone

69. **Complete the following:**   G6 p.625:105mm

a. How does smoking produce nonunion of   interferes with vascularization
fusions?   of healing bone grafts

b. What is the responsible chemical?   nicotine

c. Will it help if patients stop smoking by   no
using nicotine patches?

70. **Complete the following concerning an**   G7 p.183:85mm
anterior odontoid screw:

a. After placement what postop treatment   immobilization in cervical
is recommended?   brace

b. How long?   6 weeks

c. If patient has osteoporosis, use _____.   halo

7

71. Complete the following concerning a C1-C2 transarticular facet screw: G7 p.184:140mm

a. Indication—used in conjunction with _____ _____   Sonntag fusion

b. Benefit
    i. provides immediate _____   stabilization
    ii. avoids postoperative _____ _____   external orthosis

    iii. A major risk of the procedure is _____ _____ _____.   vertebral artery injury

72. Characterize atlantoaxial-axial fusion (C1-C2 arthrodesis).   G7 p.183:125mm

a. The patient will lose about _____% of head rotation.   50%

b. Transarticular screws   G7 p.184:150mm
    i. Danger is to the v_____ a_____   vertebral artery
    ii. Provides i_____ s_____   immediate stabilization
    iii. Requires preop _____ to study vertebral arteries   CT   G7 p.184:175mm

73. Complete the following regarding surgical fusion of lumbar and lumbosacral spine: G7 p.191:103mm

a. True or False. A lumbar fusion that includes L1
    i. Should not be terminated at L1   true
    ii. Should not be terminated at T12   true

b. Pedicle screws   G7 p.191:145mm
    i. Should be _____ to _____ % of pedicle   70 to 80%
    ii. Should be greater than _____ mm in the adult   5.5
    iii. The length should be _____ to _____% of the vertebral body   70 to 80%
    iv. typically _____ to _____ mm long   40 to 50

c. Medial angles for lumbar pedicle screws   G7 p.192:15mm
    i. L1 level—medial angle should be _____ degrees   5
    ii. L2 level—medial angle should be _____ degrees   10
    iii. L3 level—medial angle should be _____ degrees   15
    iv. L4 level—medial angle should be _____ degrees   20
    v. L5 level—medial angle should be _____ degrees   25
    vi. S1 level—medial angle should be _____ degrees   25
    vii. S2 level—medial angle should be _____ degrees   45

d. On AP view if screw tip
   i. Crosses the midline there is a _____ breech   medial
   ii. Does not pass medial to the medial edge of the pedicle there is likely a _____ breech   lateral

e. Posterior lumbar interbody fusion (Plif and Tlif)   G7 p.193:15mm
   i. Not appropriate if _____ height is preserved   disc
   ii. Usually supplemented with _____ _____   pedicle screws

f. Anterior lumbar interbody fusion   G7 p.195:18mm
   i. has a risk of _____ _____   retrograde ejaculation
   ii. of from _____ to _____%   2 to 45%

74. True or False or Unreliable. In assessing lumbar fusion the following tests can suggest success: G7 p.198:40mm

a. static x-rays   false
b. flexion—extension views   true
c. technetium 99 bone scan   false
d. good clinical outcome   unreliable
e. CT scan   true

75. Components necessary for bone graft fusion are   G7 p.198:100mm
Hint: IGC

a. Osteoinduction is _____ of mesenchymal cells.   recruitment
b. Osteogenesis is the process of forming _____ _____.   new bone
c. Osteoconduction structure adds _____ _____ and acts as a _____.   new vessels, scaffold

                                    Hint:
                                    *I*nduces mesenchymal cells to transform
                                    *G*enerates bone cells
                                    *C*onstructs bone scaffold

76. Allograft provides only osteo-_____.   conduction   G7 p.199:92mm

77. DBM   G7 p.199:92mm
a. aka as d_____ bone m_____   demineralized; matrix
b. has _____ and _____ properties   inductive and conductive

78. BMP   G7 p.199:145mm
a. aka bone m_____ p_____   morphogenic protein
b. has _____ properties   inductive
c. may cause e_____ b_____   ectopic bone
d. approved by FDA only for _____   Alif   G7 p.199:163mm

79. **Complete the following regarding graft procurement:**   G7 p.200:73mm

a. Anterior iliac bone graft
  i.   Obtain _____ to _____ cm   3 to 4
  ii. _____ to the anterior superior   lateral
       iliac crest
  iii. To avoid the l_____ f_____   lateral femoral cutaneous
       c_____ nerve
  iv. Also need to avoid injury to the   ilioinguinal and
       i_____ and i_____   iliohypogastric

b. Posterior iliac crest bone graft   G7 p.200:103mm
  i.   Obtain from the _____   medial
  ii. _____ to _____ cm of the   6 to 8
       iliac crest
  iii. To avoid the s_____ c_____   superior cluneal
       nerves
  iv. If injured, they cause b_____   buttock numbness or painful
       n_____ or p_____   neuromas
       n_____

c. The "dimple of Venus" lies directly   G7 p.200:133mm
  i.   above the s_____ joint.   sacro iliac
  ii. Incise a little _____ to it.   lateral
  iii. Avoid mistaking the s_____   sacrum
  iv. and the i_____ s_____.   iliac spine

■ Lumbar Punctures

80. **Complete the following regarding lumbar punctures:**   G7 p.201:175mm

a. For lumbar puncture (LP) the platelet $50{,}000/mm^3$
   count should be higher than _____.

b. In SAH, LP might increase the _____   transmural   G7 p.202:15mm
   pressure and precipitate aneurysmal
   rupture.

c. An LP in patients with spinal block may   14%   G7 p.202:25mm
   produce deterioration in as many as
   _____%.

81. **The spinal cord ends at the given location for what percentage of adults?**   G7 p.202:45mm

a. between T12 and L1   30%
b. between L1 and L2 middle thirds   51 to 68%
c. between L2 and L3   10%
d. between T12 and L2   94%

82. **The intercristal line**   G7 p.202:60mm

a. connects the superior border of the   iliac crests
   _____ _____

b. occurs in most adults between the   L4 and L5
   spinous processes of _____ and
   _____

83. Complete the following statements: G7 p.202:95mm

a. When an LP is performed, we must always advance the needle with _____ _____ in place.   the stylet

b. Otherwise we may introduce _____ _____,   epidermal cells

c. which could produce an iatrogenic _____ _____.   epidermoid tumor

84. Describe the Queckenstedt test and expected results.   G7 p.202:180mm

a. What do you compress?   the jugular vein

b. One or both?   one then the other, while measuring ICP

c. If no block what will happen with compression?   pressure should rise 10 to 20 cm from baseline

d. If no block what happens upon release of compression?   return to the original level within 10 seconds

e. If there is a block what will happen?   no rise in pressure from baseline

85. Complete the following about lumbar punctures: G7 p.203:85mm

a. Incidence of severe postpuncture headache is _____%.   0.1 to 0.5%

b. Severe means _____.   lasting longer than 7 days

86. Complete the following about lumbar punctures: G7 p.203:155mm

a. Can a sixth nerve (abducens nerve) palsy occur after lumbar puncture?   yes

b. If so when?   after 5 to 14 days

c. If it occurs when does it resolve?   4 to 6 weeks

87. True or False. Regarding fundus exam for papilledema: G7 p.204:25mm

a. It is a reliable test to assure safety of LP.   false

b. It is an unreliable test.   true

c. It takes 6 to 24 hours for papilledema to occur.   true

d. A better test of safety would be a C_____ s_____.   CT scan

88. True or False. If you suspect meningitis but cannot promptly get a CT scan   G7 p.204:85mm

a. you may do an LP without a CT scan   true (very small risk)

b. even if there is papilledema   true (risk is still low)

c. and if there are unequal pupils and/or hemiparesis   false (suggests an asymmetrical mass; do not do LP)

89. You suspect meningitis but cannot promptly get a CT scan. If the patient deteriorates during LP the anecdotal recommendation is to immediately _____ _____ _____.   replace the fluid   G7 p.204:85mm

7

90. **True or False. The following may reduce the frequency of post-LP headache:**   G7 p.204:135mm
    a. Use a small-size needle.   true
    b. Orient the bevel longitudinally.   true
    c. Position the patient flat in bed.   false (not shown to be truly beneficial)
    d. Remove only a little fluid.   false (not shown to be truly beneficial)
    e. Replace the stylet before removing the needle.   true
    f. Hydrate the patient after the LP.   false (not shown to be truly beneficial)

■ C1-C2 Punctures

91. **What condition makes lateral cervical puncture contraindicated?**   Chiari malformation   G7 p.205:125mm

■ Ventricular Catheterization

92. **True or False. Sites that may be used for ventricular catheterization are**   G7 p.207:80mm
    a. Keen point   true
    b. Dandy point   true (but may injure visual pathways)
    c. occipital-parietal region   true
    d. Kocher point   true

93. **Keen point**   G7 p207:168mm
    a. is about _____ cm superior to the PINNA   3
    b. is about _____ cm posterior to the PINNA   3
    c. places catheter into the _____   trigone

■ Ventriculostomy/ICP Monitors

94. **True or False. The site most commonly used for ICP monitoring is**   G7 p.207:180mm
    a. occipitoparietal region   false
    b. Frazier burr hole   false
    c. Keen point   false
    d. Dandy point   false
    e. Kocher point   true (2 to 3 cm from midline, approximate midpupil line; 1 cm anterior to coronal suture; aim toward ipsilateral inner-canthus and external auditory canal)

95. Another technique:
Hint: Easy as 1-2-3

G7 p.208:72mm

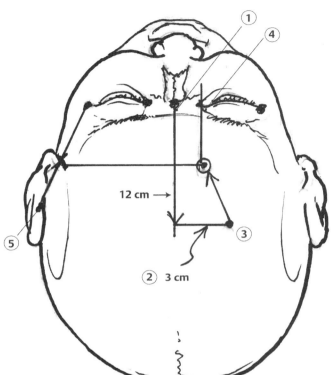

1. Nasion
2. Right
3. Kocher's point
4. medial canthus
5. auditory meatus

Fig. 7.1

Illustration by Tony Pazos

a. Measure 12 cm up the midline from the _____.   nasion

b. Measure 3 cm to the _____.   right

c. This is the approximate site of _____ point.   Kocher

d. Drill opening, puncture dura, aim catheter medially toward ipsilateral _____ _____   medial canthus

e. on a plane halfway between the contralateral lateral canthus and external _____ _____.   auditory meatus

(Thanks to Dr. Thomas Stilp, Chicago)

7

■ Ventricular Shunts

96. **List the layers to traverse in the placement of peritoneal catheter.**
Hint: samp³

G7 p.210:20mm

a. s_____ _____ — subcutaneous fat
b. a_____ _____ — anterior sheath
c. m_____ — muscle
d. p_____ _____ — posterior sheath
e. p_____ _____ — preperitoneal fat
f. p_____ — peritoneum

97. **Ventriculoatrial shunt should be revised when the catheter tip is above _____.**
T4

G7 p.211:110mm

98. **The needle to use in ommaya reservoir is a b_____ _____ or smaller gauge.**
butterfly 25

G7 p.212:160mm

99. **During third ventriculostomy**

G7 p.213:70mm

a. The opening is made
i. _____ to the mammillary bodies. — anterior
ii. This site is _____ to the basilar artery. — anterior
b. After puncturing the floor be certain that the m_____ of L_____ is also perforated. — membrane of Liliequist

G7 p.213:100mm

■ Sural Nerve Biopsy

100. **Nerve biopsy has a role in diagnosing the following:**
Hint: aCdHmv

G7 p.214:125mm

a. a_____ — amyloidosis
b. C_____-M_____-T_____ — Charcot-Marie-Tooth
c. d_____ a_____ — diabetic amyotrophy
d. H_____ d_____ — Hansen disease
e. m_____ l_____ — metachromatic leukodystrophy
f. v_____ — vasculitis

101. **Sural nerve biopsy**

G7 p.214:153mm

a. At the level of the ankle the sural nerve
i. lies between the _____ tendon — Achilles
ii. and the _____ malleolus. — lateral
b. A tourniquet distends the _____ _____ vein. — lesser saphenous
c. To biopsy only a portion of the fascicles open the _____ and tease out a few fascicles. — epineurium
d.

G7 p.215:115mm

i. Sensory loss is _____ — expected
ii. but may not last more than a _____ _____. — a few weeks

7

■ Nerve Blocks

102. **True or False. The following are risks of bilateral stellate ganglion block:**   G7 p.215:170mm
- a. glossopharyngeal nerve injury bilaterally — false
- b. respiratory compromise — true
- c. hypoglossal nerve injury bilaterally — false
- d. bilateral laryngeal nerve injury — true (Glossopharyngeal and hypoglossal nerves are higher in the cervical region.)

103. **The palpable landmark at C6 is called**   G7 p.216:23mm
- a. C_____ t_____ — Chassaignac's tubercle
- b. also known as a_____ t_____ of t_____ p_____ of C_____ — anterior tubercle; transverse process of C6
- c. also known as _____ _____ — carotid tubercle

104. **True or False. The following are signs of a successful stellate ganglion block:**   G7 p.216:40mm
- a. unilateral vocal cord paralysis — false
- b. hoarseness — false
- c. unilateral Horner syndrome — true
- d. upper extremity weakness from brachial plexus effect — false
- e. increased warmth of ipsilateral hand — true
- f. anhidrosis of the ipsilateral hand — true

105. **Complete the following concerning the intercostal nerve block:**   G7 p.216:115mm
- a. A good site for injection is the p_____ a_____ l_____. — posterior axillary line
- b. How many nerves need to be blocked to produce some anesthesia? — three
- c. Why so many? — overlap
- d. Order of structures from top down is _____ _____ _____ _____. (Hint: rvan) — rib, vein, artery, nerve

7

8

Developmental Anomalies

■ Arachnoid Cysts

1. **Characterize intracranial arachnoid**   G7 p.222:100mm
   cysts.
   a. Origin: c_____   congenital
   b. C_____ _____ _____ produce   cells of lining;
      _____.   CSF
   c. age: y_____ _____   young patients
   d. incidence per 1000 autopsies _____ 5
   e. symptoms of s_____, h_____   seizures, headache
   f. treatment: s_____, d_____,   shunt, drain,
      f_____   fenestrate
   g. path: s_____ a_____ m_____ split arachnoid membrane

2. **True or False. Acute deterioration in**   G7 p.223:65mm
   patients with known arachnoid cysts
   usually signifies
   a. rapid increase in cyst size   false
   b. postictal state   false
   c. rupture into subdural space   false
   d. rupture of bridging veins and cyst bleed true

3. **Complete the following about**   G7 p.222:177mm
   arachnoid cysts:
   a. The location of the only extradural type intra sellar
      of arachnoid cyst is in the _____ cyst.
   b. A retrocerebellar arachnoid cyst might Dandy-Walker
      mimic a _____-_____ syndrome.
   c. The most common location for an   sylvian fissure
      arachnoid cyst is the _____ _____.
   d. The next most common location is the cerebellopontine angle
      _____ _____.
   e. They are associated with ventriculo   64%   G7 p.224:45mm
      megaly in _____%.
   f. The best treatment is probably _____ shunting of cyst   G7 p.224:170mm
      of _____.

4. **Complete the following regarding intraspinal cysts:**   G7 p.224:70mm
   a. If you find one ventrally think _____   neurenteric cyst
      _____.
   b. If you find one dorsally think _____   arachnoid cyst
      _____.

■ Intracranial Lipomas

5. **Intracranial lipomas**   G7 p.225:130mm
   a. are usually found in the _____   midsagittal plane
      _____
   b. especially in the _____ _____.   corpus callosum
   c. They are frequently associated with   agenesis
      _____
   d. of the _____.   corpus callosum
   e. They may less frequently involve the
      i.   _____ _____   tuber cinereum
      ii. and the _____ _____.   quadrigeminal plate

6. **True or False. Characteristics of**   G7 p.225:145mm
   intracranial lipomas include
   a. Association with _____ abnormalities   congenital
   b. On CT they have a _____ density.   low
   c. Differential diagnosis is
      i.   d_____ c_____   dermoid cyst
      ii. t_____   teratoma
      iii. g_____   geminoma
   d. On MRI they have a _____ intensity   high (like fat)
      on T1.
   e. On MRI they have a _____ intensity   low
      on T2.

7. **Intracranial lipomas may present**   G7 p.225:178mm
   clinically with
   a. s_____   seizures
   b. h_____ d_____   hypothalamic dysfunction
   c. h_____   hydrocephalus
   d. m_____ r_____   mental retardation

■ Hypothalamic Hamartomas

8. **Hypothalamic hamartomas**   G7 p.226:50mm
   a. are frequent or rare?   rare
   b. are neoplastic or nonneoplastic?   nonneoplastic
   c. consist of a mass of _____ _____   neuronal tissue
   d. that arises from the
      i.   in_____ h_____ or   inferior hypothalamus
      ii. t_____ c_____   tuber cinereum

9. **Hypothalamic hamartomas clinically**   G7 p.226:98mm
   a. may present with a special type of   gelastic; laughing
      seizure called _____, which means
      _____ seizure

8

b.   may also have _____ attacks   rage

c.   G7 p.226:125mm

   i.   may also present with p_____   precocious puberty
      p_____
   ii.   due to release of g_____   gonadotropin releasing
      r_____ h_____   hormone
   iii. formed within the_____ cells   hamartoma

■ Neurenteric Cysts

10. Complete the following about   G7 p.227:100mm
neurenteric cysts:

a.   A neurenteric cyst is a central nervous   endothelium
system (CNS) cyst lined with _____

b.   resembling the _____ or _____   gastrointestinal or respiratory
tract.

c.   Regions affected are usually the   cervical or thoracic   G7 p.227:115mm
_____ or _____ areas.

d.   Histology is a cyst lined with c_____-   cuboidal-columnar epithelium
c_____ e_____

e.   with m_____-s_____ g_____   mucin-secreting goblet cells   G7 p.228:34mm
c_____.

8

■ Craniofacial Development

11. Complete the following about   G7 p.228:105mm
craniofacial development:

a.   The anterior fontanelle closes by age   2.5 years
_____.

b.   Head size is 90% of adult size at age   1 year
_____.

c.   The head stops enlarging by age   7 years   G7 p.228:130mm
_____.

d.   The skull is _____ at birth.   unilaminar
e.   Diploë appears by the _____ year   fourth
and
f.   reaches a maximum at age _____.   35 years
g.   Diploic veins form at age _____.   35 years
h.   Air cells in the mastoid occur in   sixth
_____ year.

12. True or false. Craniosynostosis   G7 p.228:172mm
a.   has been proven to occur after shunting.   false
b.   of one suture does not cause ↑ICP.   false—11 % have ↑ICP

13. Complete the following about   G7 p.229:157mm
craniofacial development:

a.   The most common craniosynostosis is   sagittal
_____.

b.   The male to female ratio is _____.   80:20
c.   The resulting skull shape is _____.   dolichocephalic/
scaphocephalic/boat shape

d. Surgery should be done within the age range of _____.

3 to 6 months

e. The strip craniectomy should be _____ cm wide.

3

14. Complete the following regarding coronal synostosis:

G7 p.230:28mm

a. Incidence of patients with craniosynostosis who have coronal synostosis is _____%.

18%

b. In which is it more common, males or females?

females

15. Coronal suture synostosis (CSS)

G7 p.230:35 mm

a. plus syndactyly is called _____ syndrome.

Apert

b. Unilateral CSS is called _____.

plagiocephaly

c. CSS plus hypoplasia of the face is called _____ disease.

Crouzon

d. Plagiocephaly has an unusual orbit appearance on x-ray called the _____ _____ _____.

harlequin eye sign

e. Plagiocephaly

i. Forehead on affected side is _____ or _____.

flattened or concave

ii. Supraorbital ridge has a _____ margin.

higher

16. Harlequin eye sign

G7 p.230:40mm

a. occurs in u_____ c_____ suture closure

unilateral coronal

b. seen on _____ _____ _____.

anteroposterior skull x-ray

c. The abnormal bony structure is the _____ _____

supraorbital margin

d. and is _____ than on the normal side.

higher

17. Complete the following about craniofacial development:

G7 p.230:80mm

a. What suture is closed to produce trigonocephaly?

metopic

b. It is usually associated with an abnormality of the _____ chromosome.

19 p

18. Characterize lambdoid synostosis.

G7 p.230:100mm

a. Male to female ratio is _____.

4:1

b. Side involved most frequently is _____.

right side

c. The frequency of involvement is _____% right.

70%

d. Does it have a ridge or an indentation to palpation?

not a ridge like the sagittal or coronal synostosis, but it has an indentation

8

19.   Considering lambdoid synostosis: G7 p.230:160mm

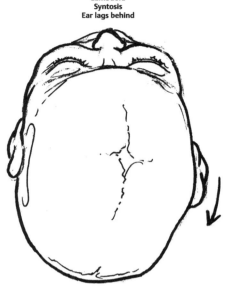

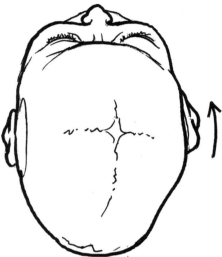

Lambdoid Syntosis Ear lags behind

Positional Flattening Ear pushed forward

Fig. 8.1   Illustration by Tony Pazos

8

a.   Differentiate from positional flattening by looking at the ears from the _____ _____ _____ _____.

top of the head

b.   In lambdoid synostosis you will see the ipsilateral ear _____ _____.

lags behind

c.   In positional flattening you will see the ipsilateral ear is _____ _____.

pushed forward (If flat side of occipital bone is same side as the posteriorly positioned ear it is a case of lambdoid synostosis; if not it is a case of positional flattening.)

20.   Answer the following concerning lambdoid synostosis treatment: G7 p.231:85mm

a.   True or False. All require surgery.

false (Only 15% won't respond to repositioning.)

b.   True or False. Surgery is indicated early (i.e., in 3 to 6 months).

false (One can observe for 3 to 6 months for improvement.)

c.   Ideal age for surgery is _____ to _____ months.

6 to 18

d.   Early surgery is indicated for s_____ d_____ and e_____ i_____ p_____.

severe disfigurement and elevated intracranial pressure

21. **Describe oxycephaly.**   G7 p.231:155mm
  a. Definition: _____ _____   tower skull
  b. Occurs if there is fusion of _____   multiple sutures
    _____
  c. Is there elevated ICP?   yes
  d. What is the status of the sinuses?   underdeveloped sinuses

22. **Complete the following about**   G7 p.232:60mm
    craniofacial development:
  a. Cranium bifidum is another name for   encephalocele or
    _____ or _____.   meningocele
  b. What type does not produce a visible   basal encephalocele
    soft tissue mass?
  c. Definition: an extension of _____   normal, confines   G7 p.232:75mm
    structures outside the normal _____
    of the skull
  d. A nasal polypoid mass in a newborn   encephalocele   G7 p.232:75mm
    should be considered an _____ until
    proven otherwise.

23. **Complete the following about**   G7 p.232:130mm
    encephalocele:
  a. Incidence of the basal form of   1.5%
    encephalocele is _____%.
  b. May exit the skull via a defect in
    i. c_____ p_____   cribriform plate
    ii. f_____ c_____   foramen cecum
    iii. s_____ o_____ f_____   superior orbital fissure
  c. Treatment is by a combined i_____   intracranial and transnasal
    and t_____ approach

■ Chiari Malformation

24. **Compare Chiari types I and II.**   G7 p.233:100mm
  a. medulla-caudal dislocation   Chiari I, no
                                                Chiari II, yes
  b. into cervical canal   Chiari I, tonsils
                                                Chiari II, vermis, medulla,
                                                fourth ventricle
  c. myelomeningocele   Chiari I, no
                                                Chiari II, yes
  d. hydrocephalus   Chiari I, no
                                                Chiari II, yes
  e. medullary kink   Chiari I, no
                                                Chiari II, 55%
  f. cervical nerves   Chiari I, normal
                                                Chiari II, upward
  g. age at presentation   Chiari I, adult
                                                Chiari II, infant
  h. symptoms   Chiari I, neck pain
                                                Chiari II, hydrocephalus,
                                                respiratory distress

8

25. Complete the following about Chiari malformation: G7 p.234:25mm

a. Chiari I has how many abnormalities?   1—with many names
b. List four names this abnormality has been called.
    i.   t_____ h_____   tonsillar herniation
    ii. c_____ d_____ of c_____   caudal displacement of cerebellum
    iii. p_____ e_____ of t_____   peglike elongation of tonsil
    iv. c_____ e_____   cerebellar ectopia

26. Chiari I   G7 p.234:25mm

a. has how many deformities?   1
b. is known by the following names
    i.   e_____   ectopia
    ii. e_____   elongation
    iii. d_____   displacement
    iv. h_____   herniation
c. symptoms
    i.   o_____ h_____   occipital headaches
    ii. c_____ p_____   cervical pain

27. What is the particular eye sign associated with Chiari I?   Downbeat nystagmus is considered a characteristic of this condition in 47%, but it can also occur in Chiari II.   G7 p.235:130mm

28. What percentage of Chiari I patients have hydrosyringomyelia?   20 to 30% of Chiari I patients have a syrinx.   G7 p.236:15mm

29. Characterize the location of tonsils and Chiari I.   G7 p.236:15mm

a. Normal range related to foramen magnum
    i.   high   8 mm above
    ii. low   5 mm below
    iii. mean   1 mm above
b. Chiari I range is
    i.   high   3 mm below
    ii. low   29 mm below
    iii. mean   13 mm below
c. Symptoms can occur with tonsils at _____ mm below.   2
d. Usual level considered cutoff for diagnosis is _____ mm below.   5

30. Possible better correlation with symptoms of tonsillar herniation is the degree of brain stem compression   G7 p.236:100mm

a. at the _____ _____   foramen magnum
b. as seen on the _____   axial
c. T_____ W1 MRI.   2

8

31. **The best results from surgery occur if treated within _____ years of onset of symptoms.**   2   G7 p.237:160mm

32. **Complete the following concerning Chiari I:**   G7 p.237:182 mm
    a. The most common postop complication is
       i. _____ _____   respiratory depression
       ii. in _____ %.   15%
    b. Occurs within how many days of surgery?   5
    c. Occurs mostly at what time of day?   night
    d. Death can occur from s_____ a_____.   sleep apnea
    e. Other risks of surgery include
       i. c_____ f_____ l_____   cerebrospinal fluid leak
       ii. injury to _____ _____ _____ _____   posterior inferior cerebellar artery (PICA)
       iii. h_____ of c_____ h_____   herniation of cerebellar hemispheres

33. **Complete the following concerning Chiari I:**   G7 p.238:30mm
    a. Operative results
       i. Main benefit may be to _____ progression   arrest
       ii. Best results in patients with _____ syndrome   cerebellar
       iii. which consists of   G7 p.238:55mm
            t_____ a_____   truncal ataxia
            l_____ a_____   limb ataxia
            n_____   nystagmus
            d_____   dysarthria
    b. Which responds better: pain or weakness?   pain   G7 p.238:55mm

34. **Factors that correlate with a worse outcome are**   G7 p.238:63mm
    a. a_____   atrophy
    b. s_____   scoliosis
    c. symptoms that are lasting more than _____ _____   2 years

35. **Which Chiari malformation is associated with myelomeningocele?**   Chiari II   G7 p.238:108mm

8

36. **Study Chart. Chiari II anatomical abnormalities: A to Z.**

G7 p.238:137mm

atlas assimilation
beaking of tectum
bony abnormalities
cerebellar folia poorly myelinated
cervical medullary junction compression
craniolacunia
corpus callosum agenesis
degenerated lower CN nuclei
enlarged massa intermedia
falx hypoplasia
fourth ventricle trapped
fusion of cervical vertebrae
gyri miniaturized
hydrocephalus
heterotopia
hydromyelia
Klippel-Feil deformity
low attachment of tentorium
massa intermedia enlarged
medulla oblongata
"z" bend microgyria
nuclei of lower CN degenerated
platybasia
peg of cerebellar tonsils
septum pellucidum absent
syringomyelia
tectum beaking (fusion)
tentorium low attachment
Z-shaped bend of medulla

37. **Considering Chiari II, presenting symptoms are due to dysfunction of**

G7 p.239:15mm

a. b_____ s_____   brain stem
b. l_____ c_____ n_____   lower cranial nerves

38. **Finding on presentation of Chiari II**
Hint: n2 chiari two

G7 p239 :30mm

a. n_____   nystagmus—down beat
b. n_____ _____   nasal regurgitation
c. c_____   cyanosis
d. h_____   hoarseness
e. i_____ _____ _____   impaired ventilatory drive
f. a_____ _____, _____   apneic spells, aspiration
g. r_____, _____ _____   regurgitation, respiratory arrest
h. i_____ _____   inspiratory stridor
i. t_____ _____ _____ _____ _____   tenth nerve (vagus) vocal cord paralysis
j. w_____ _____   weak arm—weak cry
k. o_____   opisthotonus

8

39. **Complete the following regarding Chiari II:**   G7 p.240:68mm

a. The most common cause of mortality is _____ _____.   respiratory arrest

b. The mortality at 6 years follow-up is _____%.   40%

c. Range of mortality
   i. Infants in poor condition (i.e., cardiopulmonary arrest, vocal cord paralysis, and/or arm weakness mortality) is _____%.   71%
   ii. There is gradual onset of symptoms in _____%.   23%
   iii. The worst prognostic factor for response to surgery is b_____ v_____ c_____ p_____.   bilateral vocal cord paralysis

■ Dandy-Walker Malformation

40. **Complete the following regarding Dandy-Walker malformation (DWM):**   G7 p.240:138mm

a. It is caused by a_____ of the f_____ of L_____ and M_____.   atresia of the foramina of Luschka and Magendie (old theory)

b. Results in
   i. agenesis of _____   vermis
   ii. large _____ _____ _____, which communicates with the   posterior fossa cyst
   iii. _____ _____, which becomes   fourth ventricle
   iv. _____.   enlarged

41. **To differentiate DWM from retrocerebellar arachnoid cyst observe for**   G7 p.241:28mm

a. v_____ a_____   vermian agenesis
b. cyst opens into f_____ v_____   fourth ventricle
c. enlarged p_____ f_____   posterior fossa
d. elevation of the t_____ H_____   torcular Herophili

42. **What is Dandy-Walker pathogenesis?**   G7 p.241:50mm

a. D_____   Dilation of fourth ventricle
b. A_____   Agenesis of vermis
c. N_____   Membrane of fourth ventricle
d. D_____   Dysembryo genesis
e. Y_____   Hydrocephalus

43. **DWM patients**   G7 p.241:60mm

a.
   i. Hydrocephalus is present in _____%   70 to 90%
   ii. and _____% of hydrocephalus patients have DWS.   2 to 4%

8

b. A common associated abnormality is   G7 p.241:92mm
    i.   _____ of the _____   agenesis of the corpus
          _____ in   callosum
    ii.   _____%.   17%
c. and c_____ a_____.   cardiac abnormalities
d. If treatment is necessary, you must shunt   cyst
    the ventricle, the cyst, or both?
e. If aqueductal stenosis you should shunt   ventricle
    _____ also.
f. But shunting the lateral ventricle alone   G7 p.241:122mm
    i.   is _____   contraindicated
    ii.   because it might cause _____   upward herniation
          _____.
g. To avoid _____ herniation   upward   G7 p.241:125mm
h. you must not shunt the _____ alone.   ventricle   G7 p.241:125mm

44. What is the prognosis in DWM?   G7 p.241:152mm
a. Seizures occur in _____%.   15%
b. Mortality occurs in _____ to   12 to 50%
    _____%.
c. Normal IQ is _____%.   50%

■ Aqueductal Stenosis

**45. True or False. Aqueductal stenosis is   false (Adults can present with   G7 p.241:179 mm
       seen only in children.**   symptoms as well.)

**46. What are the causes of aqueductal   G7 p.242:20mm
       stenosis?**
       Hint: aqectal
a. a_____   astrocytoma of brain stem
b. q_____   quadrigeminal plate mass
c. e_____   inflammation, infection
d. c_____   congenital atresia
e. t_____   tumors
f. a_____   arachnoid cysts
g. l_____   lipoma

**47. Complete the following concerning   G7 p.242:45mm
       aqueductal stenosis:**
a. It is associated with congenital   70%
    hydrocephalus in _____%.
b. MRI may show absence of
    i.   n_____ f_____ v _____   normal flow void
          in the
    ii.   a _____ of S_____.   aqueduct of Sylvius
c. MRI with contrast should be used to rule   tumor
    out _____.
d. Follow-up should be for at least   2 years
    _____
e. in order to rule out _____.   tumor   G7 p.243:22mm

48. **True or False. A patient with aqueductal stenosis of adulthood may have the following symptoms:**   G7 p.242:100mm
   a. headache   true
   b. visual disturbances   true
   c. decline of mental function   true
   d. gait disturbance   true
   e. papilledema (sign)   true
   f. ataxia   true
   g. urinary incontinence   true

49. **What are the treatment options for aqueductal stenosis?**   G7 p.242:175mm
   a. ventriculoperitoneal _____ _____   CSF shunting
   b. T_____ _____ _____   Torkildsen shunt in adults
      _____
   c. ETV = _____ _____ _____   endoscopic third ventriculostomy

■ Neural Tube Defects

50. **With neural tube defects there are classification systems. Give examples of**   G7 p.243:45 mm
   a. neurulation defects
      i.   a_____   anencephaly
      ii. m_____   myelomeningocele
   b. postneurulation defects
      i.   m_____   microcephaly
      ii. h_____   hydranencephaly
      iii. h_____   holoprosencephaly
      iv. l_____   lissencephaly
      v.   s_____   schizencephaly
   c. spinal defects
      i.   d_____   diastematomyelia
      ii. s_____   syringomyelia

51. **Complete the following about neural tube defects:**   G7 p.243:45mm
   a. Failure to fuse the anterior neuropore results in _____.   anencephaly
   b. Failure to fuse the posterior neuropore results in _____.   myelomeningocele
   c. The definition of microcephaly is head circumference _____ _____ _____ below the mean.   2 standard deviations
   d. In hydranencephaly the cortex is replaced by _____.   CSF
   e. Failure to cleave can result in _____.   holoprosencephaly

8

52. **Complete the following about neural tube defects:**   G7 p.243:45mm
   a. Give examples of neurulation defects.
      i.   a_____   anencephaly
      ii. c_____   craniorachischisis
      iii. m_____   myelomeningocele
   b. These defects are due to _____ of   nonclosure
      the neural tube.

53. **Complete the following about neural tube defects:**   G7 p.243:70mm
   a. Name five postneurulation defects.
      i.   h_____   hydranencephaly
      ii. l_____   lissencephaly (most severe)
      iii. h_____   holoprosencephaly
      iv. a_____ of _____ _____   agenesis of corpus callosum
      v.   d_____   diastematomyelia
   b. Which is the most severe?   lissencephaly

54. **Complete the following regarding lissencephaly:**   G7 p.243:120mm
   a. It is an example of an abnormality of   migration
      neuronal _____.
   b. It results in an abnormality of the   cortical
      _____ convolutions
   c. called _____.   agyria

55. **Name the key features of schizencephaly.**   G7 p.243:155mm
   a. _____ which communicates with   cleft; ventricle
      _____
   b. lined with _____ _____   gray matter
   c. Two types are
      i. o_____ l_____   open lipped
      ii. c_____ l_____   close lipped

56. **Complete the following about neural tube defects:**   G7 p.243:160mm
   a. In schizencephaly, the cleft wall is lined   gray matter
      with cortical _____ _____.
   b. In porencephaly, a cystic lesion is lined   connective or glial
      with _____ or _____ tissue.

57. **Hydranencephaly**   G7 p.244:49mm
   a. is a _____-neurolation defect.   post-
   b. Cranium is filled with _____.   CSF
   c. Is there a small or large head?   macrocrania
   d. Most common etiology is _____   bilateral ICA infarcts
      _____ _____.

58. **Angiography**   G7 p.244:137mm
   a. of anterior circulation shows _____   no flow
      _____.
   b. of posterior circulation shows _____.   normal

59. **Complete the following about neural tube defects:**   G7 p.244:150mm

a. What are the three types of holoprosencephaly? Please list in order of decreasing severity.

    i. a_____   alobar (single ventricle) most severe

    ii. s_____   semilobar

    iii. l_____   lobar (least severe)

b. They occur because of

    i. failure to _____   cleave

    ii. of the _____ _____.   telencephalic vesicle

60. **List the risk factors for neural tube defects.**   G7 p.245:120mm

a. B_____ i_____ B_{12} insufficiency

b. c_____   cocaine—maternal use

c. D_____   Depakene—use during pregnancy

d. f_____ a_____ i_____   folic acid insufficiency

e. f_____   fever in first trimester

f. h_____ e_____   heat exposure—maternal hot tub, sauna

g. o_____   obesity before and during pregnancy

h. v_____ a_____   valproic acid use during pregnancy

i. v_____   vitamins—prenatal up folic acid and B_{12}

61. **What are the tests for prenatal detection of neural tube defects?**   G7 p.245:160mm

a. serum _____ _____ (If high at 15 to 20 weeks be suspicious for neural tube defects.)   alfa fetoprotein (If high at 15 to 20 weeks be suspicious for neural tube defects.)

    i. u_____,   ultrasonography

    ii. which can detect what % of spina bifida cases?   90%

b. a_____   amniocentesis

62. **For prenatal detection of neural tube defects**   G7 p.245:168mm

a. test mother's serum for _____ _____.   alpha fetoprotein

b. Has a success rate for

    i. spina bifida open _____% and   91%

    ii. anencephaly _____%.   100%

    iii. Closed spinal dysraphism _____ _____ _____.   may be missed

c. An overestimate of gestational age will make us think that a high alpha fetoprotein level is _____.   normal

d. Real-time imaging is by _____.   ultrasonography

8

e. Identifies _____% of s _____   90% of spinal bifida
    b_____.

f. Obtaining fluid from the womb is called   amniocentesis
    _____.

g. It carries a risk of fetal loss of _____%. 6%

63. Characterize agenesis of the corpus   G7 p.246:70mm
    callosum.

a. On computed tomographic scan the
    typical appearance is as follows:
    i.   Third ventricle is _____.   expanded
    ii. Lateral ventricles are _____.   separated
    iii. Atria and occipital horns are   dilated
         _____.

b. Corpus callosum forms at age _____   2 weeks; rostral to caudal
    _____ after conception and forms
    from _____ to _____.

64. Complete the following concerning   G7 p.246:115mm
    the bundles of Probst:

a. They are aborted beginnings of the   corpus callosum
    _____ _____

b. bulging into the _____ _____.   lateral ventricles

65. Complete the following regarding   G7 p246 :155mm
    agenesis of the corpus callosum:

a. Does it always have clinical significance?   no, it may be an incidental
                                                    finding

b. Underlying cause may be an abnormality   chromosome
    of a _____.

66. List the features of spina bifida   G7 p.247:145mm
    occulta.
    Hint: bifidaocculta

a. b_____   bifida
b. i_____   incidental
c. f_____   foot deformity
d. i_____   innocuous
e. d_____   diastematomyelia
f. a_____   atrophy of leg
g. o_____   occurs in 20 to 30% of people
h. c_____   cutaneous stigmata
i. c_____   clinical importance often nil
j. u_____   urinary incontinence
k. l_____   lipoma, leg weakness
l. t_____   tethered cord
m. a_____   absent spinous process

67. Complete the following regarding   G7 p.248:28mm
    myelomeningocele:

a. The anterior neuropore closes at   25
    gestational age day _____.

b. The posterior neuropore closes at   28
    gestational age day _____.

8

68. **Complete the following concerning myelomeningocele (MM):**   G7 p.248:40mm

   a. Incidence if no previous child has a MM equals _____% or _____ per 1000.   0.2%, 2

   b. One previous MM child equals _____% or _____ per 1000.   2%, 20

   c. Two previous MM children equals _____% or_____ per 1000.   6%, 60

   d. Associated hydrocephalus equals incidence of _____%.   80%

   e. Associated Chiari II occurs in _____ children with MM.   most

69. **Answer the following about myelomeningocele:**   G7 p.248:40mm

   a. What is the incidence of meningocele or myelomeningocele?   1 to 2/1000 live births (0.2%)

   b. Does the risk increase in families with one affected child?   yes (The risk does increase to 2 to 3% in families with one previous myelomeningocele child.)

   c. Does the risk increase in families with two affected children?   yes (It further increases to 6 to 8% in families with two previous affected children.)

70. **True or False. All children born with myelomeningocele have an associated Chiari II malformation.**   false (Not all, but most, have Chiari II.)   G7 p.248:72mm

71. **True or False. Closure of myelomeningocele may result in the need for CSF shunting.**   true   G7 p.248:77mm

72. **Meningomyelocele patients develop allergy to _____.**   latex   G7 p.248:80mm

73. **True or False or Uncertain. Intrauterine closure of mm defect reduces**   G7 p.248:120mm

   a. Chiari II defect   true

   b. hydrocephalus   uncertain

   c. neurological dysfunction   false

74. **Complete the following concerning myelomeningocele:**   G7 p.248:140mm

   a. If ruptured start _____ (n_____ and g_____).   antibiotics (nafcillin and gentamicin)

   b. Perform surgery within _____ to _____ hours.   24 to 36 hours

   c. Better functional outcome occurs if children have spontaneous _____ of _____ _____.   movement of lower extremities

   d. Do multiple anomalies occur in myelomeningocele?   yes (average 2 to 2.5 additional anomalies in myelomeningocele)

8

75. Complete the following about myelomeningocele and early closure: G7 p.248:140mm

a. True or False. Results in improvement of neurological functions.

false (Early closure does not result in improvement of neurological function.)

b. True or False. Results in lower infection rate.

true (It does result in a lower infection rate.)

c. Myelomeningocele should be closed within 12, 24, or 36 hours?

24

76. Considering late problems in myelomeningocele repair, possible late problems include   G7 p.250:145 mm

a. brain _____

hydrocephalus— malfunctioning shunt

b. cervicomedullary junction _____

Chiari II compressing medulla

c. cord _____

syrinx

d. cauda _____

tethered cord

77. Characterize myelomeningocele outcome without treatment and with treatment.   G7 p.251:25mm

a. survive infancy without treatment _____% with treatment _____%

15 to 30%, 85%

b. normal IQ without treatment _____% with treatment ___%

70%, 80%

c. ambulatory without treatment _____% with treatment _____%

50%, 40 to 85%

d. continence without treatment _____ with treatment _____%

rare, 3 to 10%

78. For each of the following what are the facts to know concerning lipomeningocele?   G7 p.251:90mm

a. age for surgery

2 months is appropriate for surgery

b. band

thick fibrovascular band constricts

c. conus

is split

d. dura

is dehiscent

e. epidural fat versus

lipoma is distinct from epidural fat

f. placode

lipoma attached to neural placode

g. neuro exam

is normal 50%

h. sensory loss

most common neurological abnormality

i. stigmata

cutaneous

j. urologic exam

should be done preop

79. True or False. Lipomyelomeningocele is associated with tethered cord.

true   G7 p.251:90mm

80. **Study Chart.**

lipomeningocele
steps in surgical treatment:
untether the cord
Xomed
CUSA (Cavitron Ultrasonic
Surgical Aspirator)
recording from anal sphincter
free up sides from
attachment to dura
reduce bulk of fat using CUSA
in the midline
tie dura open to sides
place bovine pericardial graft
as dural substitute

G7 p.251:90mm
Courtesy of
Dr. David Frim

81. **True or False. The most common location of a dermal sinus tract is the**

G7 p.252:130mm

a. occipital region — false
b. cervical region — false
c. thoracic region — false
d. lumbosacral region — true

82. **What is the most likely cause of dermal sinus?**

G7 p.252:115 mm

a. Failure of the _____ ectoderm — cutaneous
b. to _____ — separate
c. from the _____-ectoderm — neuro
d. at the time of _____ — closure
e. of the _____ _____. — neural groove

83. **Dermal sinus items to know include**

G7 p.252:115mm

a. Location most common is the _____ area — lumbosacral
b. Results from _____ of _____ of _____ _____ — failure of separation of cutaneous ectoderm
c. from _____ _____ — neural ectoderm
d. appears as a _____ — dimple:
   i. hair? — with or without hairs
   ii. midline? — close to midline
   iii. skin stigmata? — yes
e. First manifestation is _____ dysfunction — bladder
f. Tract always courses _____ from lumbosacral area — cephalad

84. **True or False. An epidermoid cyst contains hair follicles and sweat glands.**

false (An epidermoid cyst contains stratified squamous epithelium with keratin from desquamated epithelium. A dermoid cyst is lined with dermis and contains sebum and hair.)

G7 p.252:145mm

8

85. **What is a major difference between epidermoid cyst and dermoid cyst?**
G7 p.251:145 mm
a. Epidermoid cyst is
  i. lined with s_____ s_____ e_____   stratified squamous epithelium
  ii. and contains only _____.   keratin (from desquamated epithelium)

b. Dermoid cyst is
  i. lined with _____   dermis
  ii. and contains _____ _____ such as   skin appendages
  iii. hair follicles?   yes
  iv. sebaceous glands?   yes

86. **True or False. A dermal sinus tract is a potential pathway for intradural infection such as meningitis or abscess.**   true
G7 p.251:155mm

87. **Radiologic evaluation of dermal sinus**
G7 p.253:48mm
a. If seen at births do _____   ultrasound
b. If first seen later do _____   MRI

88. **Given the above, indicate whether the dermal sinus tract should be excised at the given locations.**
G7 p.253:80mm
a. lumbar   yes
b. sacral   yes, though controversial
c. coccygeal   no

89. **Complete the following concerning the cranial dermal sinus:**
G7 p.253:140mm
a. The track extends _____.   caudally
b. If the dermal sinus tract enters the skull they do so _____ to the torcula.   caudal

---

■ Klippel-Feil Syndrome

90. **True or False. Klippel-Feil syndrome results from failure of**
G7 p.253:183mm
a. primary neurulation   false
b. secondary neurulation   false
c. dysjunction   false
d. segmentation   true (Klippel-Feil results from abnormal segmentation of the cervical somites between 3 and 8 weeks gestation.)

91. **Klippel-Feil syndrome**
G7 p.253:183mm
a. results from failure of _____ of _____ _____ at gestational age of _____.   segmentation of cervical somites; 3 to 8 weeks

b. Clinical triad
  i. Hairline is _____.   low
  ii. Neck is _____.   short
  iii. Motion is _____.   limited

8

c. Limitation of range of motion of the neck   3
occurs only if more than _____
segments are fused.

d. True or False. Other congenital   true
abnormalities may also be present.

e. True or False. Klippel-Feil causes   false (No symptoms ever
symptoms related to fused vertebrae.   attributed to the fused
                                        vertebrae.)

92. True or False. Anomalies seen in   G7 p.254:45mm
association with Klippel-Feil include

a. Sprengel deformity   true
b. webbing of the neck   true
c. basilar impression   true
d. unilateral absence of the kidney   true

93. Possible systemic congenital   G7 p.254:63mm
abnormalities include (be specific)

a. g _____   genitourinary—absence of
                                          one kidney

b. c _____   cardiopulmonary

■ Tethered Cord Syndrome

94. List six presenting signs and   G7 p.254:130mm
symptoms of tethered cord syndrome.

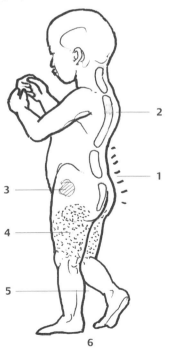

① cutaneous, 54%;
② scoliosis, 29%;
③ bladder, 40%;
④ sensations, 70%;
⑤ gait, 93%;
⑥ (+) pain, 37%

8

Fig. 8.2   Illustration by Tony Pazos

95. **True or False. In a patient with myelomeningocele with worsening scoliosis, spasticity, worsening gait, or deteriorating urodynamics, shunt evaluation is not part of the primary workup.**

false (In a myelomeningocele patient with worsening clinical symptoms, shunt evaluation and confirmation of normal intracranial pressure should be one of the first modalities of intervention.)

G7 p.255:15mm

96. **True or False.**

G7 p.255:33mm

a. Progressive scoliosis is not seen in conjunction with tethered cord syndrome.

false (Progressive scoliosis may be seen in up to 29% of patients with tethered cord syndrome.)

b. Early untethering may result in improvement in scoliosis

true

97. **True or False. The following is associated with adult tethered cord syndrome:**

G7 p.255:78mm

a. foot deformities

false (Foot deformities are associated with childhood tethered cord syndrome.)

b. pain — true
c. leg weakness — true
d. urological symptoms — true

98. **True or False. Urological symptoms are not common in the adult tethered cord syndrome.**

false (Urological symptoms are common in both pediatric and adult tethered cord syndrome.)

G7 p.255:95mm

99. **True or False. A tethered conus lies distal to L2 on radiographic evaluation.**

true

G7 p.255:130 mm

100. **Complete the following concerning tethered cord syndrome:**

G7 p.255:132mm

a. Name two criteria.
   i. conus below level _____   L2
   ii. thick filum greater than _____   2 mm diameter
b. A preop test that is strongly recommended is a_____.   cystometrogram

101. **Indicate the characteristics used to identify the filum.**

G7 p.255:180mm

a. The vessel on the surface is _____.   squiggly
b. The color of the filum is _____ _____ than nerve roots.   more white

102. **Complete the following outcome from tethered cord:**

G7 p.256:30mm

a. In meningomyelocele it is usually _____ to permanently untether.   impossible
b. Repeated untethering is advised till patient stops _____.   growing

8

c. Symptoms of retethering are especially   adolescent growth spurt
likely during the a_____ g_____
s_____.
d. Surgical release in an adult is
    i.   good for _____ and   pain
    ii. poor for _____ _____.   bladder function

■ Split Cord Malformation

103. **True or False. Diastematomyelia is**   false (Diastematomyelia is   G7 p.256:84mm
      associated with a nonrigid bony   associated with a rigid bony
      septum that separates two durally   septum that separates two
      ensheathed hemicords.   durally ensheathed
                                                 hemicords.)

104. **Complete the following concerning**   G7 p.247:95mm
      diastematomyelia:
      a. cutaneous stigmata h_____   tuft of hair hypertrichosis
      b. True or false. There are foot   true
          abnormalities
      c. specifically n_____ h_____-   neurogenic high-arched foot
          a_____ f_____.

■ Miscellaneous Developmental Anomalies

8

105. **True or False. In holoprosencephaly,**   true   G7 p.247:33mm
      there is absence of the septum
      pellucidum.

106. **Characteristic features of septo-optic**   G7 p.247:55mm
      dysplasia include
      Hint: h^3pvoplas$^3i^2$a
      a. h_____   hypopituitarism
      b. h_____   hydrocephalus
      c. h_____   hypersecretion of hormones
      d. p_____   pituitary infundibulum absent
      e. v_____   ventricles enlarged
      f. o_____   optic nerves absent (blind)
      g. p_____   panhypopituitarism
      h. l_____   little-dwarfism-Tiny Tim
      i. a_____   anterior midline structures
                               fail
      j. s_____   septum pellucidum absent
      k. s_____   schizencephaly
      l. s_____   sexual precocity
      m. i_____   isolated growth hormone
                               deficiency
      n. i_____   intelligence normal
      o. a_____   absence of midline
                               morphogenesis

**107.   True or False. Septo-optic dysplasia
frequently presents with symptoms of**   G7 p.247:55mm

a.   panhypopituitarism   true
b.   sexual precocity   true
c.   dwarfism   true
d.   blindness   true
e.   impaired intelligence   false (Most patients are of
                                                    normal intelligence.)

8

9

Neuroendovascular Intervention

■ Neuroendovascular Intervention

1. **True or False. The following conditions may be amenable to treatment by endovascular techniques:**
G7 p.262:50mm
   a. aneurysms — true
   b. AVMs — true
   c. carotid cavernous fistulas — true
   d. carotid stenosis — true
   e. tumor embolization — true

2. **The sheath may be removed when**
G7 p.263:55mm
   a. the aPTT is _____. — normal
   b. Normal aPTT is less than _____ seconds. — 36

3. **True or False. Stenting is useful for**
G7 p.263:145mm
   a. coiling of
      i. narrow-necked aneurysms — false
      ii. wide-necked aneurysms — true
      iii. ruptured aneurysms — false
   b. cerebroarterial dissections — true

4. **Complete the following regarding stenting:**
G7 p.263:145mm
   a. After stenting, _____ is prescribed — ASA
   b. for an _____ period of time. — indefinite
   c. _____ is prescribed for 6 weeks. — Plavix

9

10

Electrodiagnostics

■ Electroencephalogram (EEG)

1. What is the frequency of the following EEG rhythms?
Hint: dtab

G7 p.266:50mm

a.	delta	0 to 3 Hz
b.	theta	4 to 7 Hz
c.	alpha	8 to 13 Hz
d.	beta	>13 Hz

2. Matching. Match the following EEG patterns and their probable diagnostic pathology:

G7 p.266:80mm

Pathology:
① Creutzfeldt-Jakob disease; ② Hepatic encephalopathy-anoxia -hyponatremia; ③ SSPE—subacute sclerosing pan—encephalitis
EEG pattern:

a.	triphasic waves	②
b.	body jerks plus high-voltage periodicity with 4 to 15 seconds separation; no change with pain	③
c.	myoclonic jerks, bilateral sharp waves react to painful stimulation	①

3. True or False. Periodic lateralizing epileptiform discharges (PLEDs) may be produced by

G7 p.266:85mm

a.	herpes simplex encephalitis	true
b.	brain abscess	true
c.	embolic infarct	true
d.	brain tumor	true
e.	any acute focal cerebral insult	true

■ Evoked Potentials

4. **Complete the following statements about evoked potentials:** G7 p.267:72mm
   a. Evoked potentials offer limited usefulness because they are _____. delayed (and therefore less valuable in alerting surgeon to intraoperative injury)
   b. Criteria for significance
      i. increased latency of _____% 10%
      ii. decreased amplitude of _____% 50%

5. **Intraoperative SSEP may localize the primary sensory cortex by _____ _____ potential across the central sulcus.** phase reversal G7 p.267:82mm

6. **Evoked potentials during spine surgery** G7 p.267:82mm
   a. may remain unchanged by injury to the _____ cord anterior
   b. but are sensitive to injury to the _____ columns of the _____ cord posterior, dorsal

7. **True or False. Regarding transcranial (i.e., motor evoked) potentials:** G7 p.267:140mm
   a. Too painful to do on the awake patient true
   b. Feedback is prompt, almost immediate true
   c. Can't record continuously because of muscle contractions true
   d. Useful for cervical spine surgery true
   e. Useful for thoracic spine surgery true
   f. Useful for lumbar spine surgery false
   g. Have more special anesthetic requirements true

8. **Provide the SSEP deterioration plan.** G7 p.268:28mm
   Hint: r³s³tahe
   a. r_____ remove hardware
   b. r_____ reposition patient
   c. r_____ release traction
   d. s_____ sixty Hz
   e. s_____ steroids
   f. s_____ stop surgery
   g. t_____ temperature
   h. a_____ anemia
   i. h_____ hypotension
   j. e_____ electrode contact

10

9. **Name the location of the generators for the brain stem auditory evoked potentials (BSAER) test.**
   Hint: diplomu (Fig. 10.1)

G7 p.268:95mm

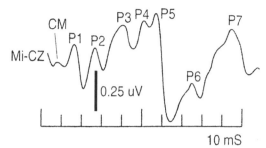

Fig. 10.1 (Reprinted with permission from Greenberg MS. Handbook of Neurosurgery, 6th ed. New York: Thieme; 2006:146. Copyright © 2006 Mark S. Greenberg. All rights reserved.)

a. P^1 d_____ e_____ n_____   distal eighth nerve
b. P^2 p_____ e_____ or c_____   proximal eighth or cochlear
   n_____   nucleus
c. P^3 l_____ p_____ /s_____   lower pons/superior olivary
   o_____ c_____   complex
d. P^4 m_____-u_____ p_____   mid-upper pons
e. P^5 u_____ p_____ or i_____   upper pons or inferior
   c_____   colliculus
f. d^1 _____ e_____ n_____   distal eighth nerve
g. p_____ e_____ n_____   proximal eighth nerve
h. lo_____   lower
i. m_____   middle
j. u_____ p_____   upper pons

10. **Name the parts of the EMG examination.**

G7 p.269:176mm

a. i_____ a_____   insertional activity
b. s_____ a_____   spontaneous activity
c. v_____ a_____   volitional activity

11. **How long following denervation of muscle after nerve injury do you start to see fibrillation potentials on electromyography (EMG)?**

G7 p.270:35mm

a. The earliest is _____, but   10 days
b. reliably not until _____.   3 to 4 weeks
c. Therefore don't order EMG until at least 4
   _____ weeks after injury.

12. **SNAP**

G7 p.270:99mm

a. aka _____ _____ action potential   sensory nerve
   ganglion
b. lies within the _____ _____.   neural foramen
c. Herniated disc is preganglion; therefore,   not affected
   SNAP is _____ _____.

10

13. H reflex G7 p.270:127mm
a. is practical only regarding the _____ 51
   root.
b. has similar information to the _____ ankle jerk
   _____.

14. True or False. Regarding EMG: G7 p.270:160mm
a. Is low yield for radiculopathy true
b. Best reserved for patients with weakness true
c. Pain without weakness, EMG has low true
   yield

15. True or False. Radiculopathy EMG is G7 p.270:170mm
a. Reliable if negative false—EMG is not sensitive for
   radiculopathy
b. Reliable if positive true—When positive it is very
   specific

16. True or False. Paraspinal mm testing is G7 p.271:70mm
    useful for lumbar disc disease.
a. Preop true
b. Postop false—muscles cut during
   surgery

10

11

Neurotoxicology

■ Ethanol

1. True or False. Primary effect of ethanol (ETOH) on the central nervous system (CNS) is
a. depression in neuronal excitability   true
b. depression in impulse conduction   true
c. depression in neurotransmitter release   true

G7 p.273:120mm

2. Complete the following concerning neurotoxicology:

a. Describe the Mellanby effect with respect to ETOH. The severity of intoxication is greater when blood alcohol level is _____.   rising

b. What is the effect of a blood alcohol level of
   i. 25 mg/dL?   mild intoxication, impaired cognition
   ii. 100 mg/dL?   vestibular/cerebellar dysfunction
   iii. 500 mg/dL?   usually fatal—respiratory depression

G7 p.273:140mm

3. Legal intoxication is a blood alcohol level of _____ mg/dL.   100 (80)

G7 p.273:155mm

4. As ETOH levels fall, hyperactivity may occur as compensation for the _____ effects of ETOH.   CNS depressant

G7 p.273:177mm

5. True or False. Regarding delirium tremens:

a. occurs within 4 days of ETOH withdrawal   true
b. agitation, confusion, autonomic instability   true
c. mortality 5 to 10% if untreated   true
d. benzodiazepine as first-line drug   true

G7 p.274:18mm

6. **True or False. Delirium tremens can be suppressed by**   G7 p.274:30mm

a. benzodiazepines   true
b. resumption of drinking   true
c. beta-adrenergic antagonists   true
d. A2 agonists   true

7. **What is the treatment for alcohol withdrawal syndrome?**   G7 p.274:55mm

a. Mainstay of treatment are the _____.   benzodiazepines
b. They reduce a _____ h_____   autonomic hyperactivity
c. and may prevent s_____   seizures
d. and/or _____ _____.   delirium tremens
e.   G7 p.274:55mm
   i. Also use _____   100mg/day
   ii. for _____ days   3 to 5
f.
   i. and _____ for seizures.   Dilantin   G7 p.274:172mm
   ii. Load with _____ mg/kg.   18

8. **True or False. Delirium tremens usually begins within _____ days of the onset of ETOH withdrawal.**   G7 p.275:20mm

a. 4   true
b. 5   false
c. 6   false
d. 7   false

9. **Complete the following about ethanol:**   G7 p.275:50mm

a. True or False. The classic triad of Wernicke encephalopathy is
   i. encephalopathy, ophthalmoplegia, and ataxia   true
   ii. apraxia, ophthalmoplegia, and encephalopathy   false
   iii. ophthalmoplegia, ataxia, and myelopathy   false
b. Eye signs occur in _____%.   96%
c. Gait disturbance occurs in _____%.   87%
d. Memory disturbance is called _____ _____ and occurs in _____%.   Korsakoff syndrome; 80%

10. **True or False. Wernicke encephalopathy is associated with**   G7 p.275:62mm

a. thiamine deficiency   true
b. vitamin B_{12} deficiency   false
c. folic acid deficiency   false
d. vitamin C deficiency   false

11

11.	**Complete the following about Wernicke encephalopathy (WE):**	G7 p.275:108mm
a.	Is there a unique MRI picture in WE?	yes
b.		
i.	There is a _____ signal	high
ii.	on _____ WI	T2
iii.	in the _____ thalamus	medial
iv.	the _____ of the fourth ventricle and	floor
v.	the p_____ gray	periaqueductal
vi.	of the _____.	midbrain
c.	What changes occur in the mammillary bodies?	atrophy

12.	**Complete the following about Wernicke encephalopathy (WE):**	G7 p.275:127mm
a.	What common treatment can precipitate acute WE?	IV glucose
b.	What should be given first: IV glucose or thiamine?	thiamine
c.	WE eye signs improve within _____.	days
d.	However residue of	
i.	K_____ s_____	Korsakoff syndrome
ii.	occurs in _____% in the form of	80%
iii.	h_____ n_____	horizontal nystagmus
iv.	and a _____.	amnesia

■ Opioids

13.	**True or False. Reversal of opioid toxicity is achieved with**	G7 p.276:20mm
a.	naloxone	true
b.	methadone	false
c.	Catapres	false
d.	Romazicon	false

14.	**Heroin, an opioid, causes small pupils called _____.**	miosis	G7 p.276:120mm

15.	**Complete the following about amphetamines:**	G7 p.277:36mm
a.	Toxicity is similar to _____.	cocaine
b.	Their use can result in CVA due to _____.	vasculitis

11

16. What are the features of carbon monoxide? G7 p.277:65mm

a. The largest source of poisoning in the United States is from _____.   CO
b. It harms by binding to _____.   Hb
c. It has an affinity for it _____ times that of O_2.   250
d. Cells need _____ mL O_2/100mL blood.   5
e. Blood normally contains _____ mL O_2/100mL.   20
f. The "cherry red" color of blood occurs in only _____%.   6%

17. In severe CO intoxication, CT scan may show G7 p.277:100mm

a. l_____ a_____ in the   low attenuation
b. g_____ p_____.   globus pallidus

18. True or False. Outcome G7 p.277:115mm

a. is more closely correlated with CO Hb levels   false
b. is more closely correlated with hypotension   true
c.
   i. _____% die   40%
   ii. _____% have persistent sequelae   30 to 40%
   iii. _____% make a full recovery   30 to 40%

11

12

Coma

◼ General

1. **Write out the Glasgow Coma Scale (GCS) and indicate the score assigned to each point on the scale.**   G7 p.279:50mm
    a. eyes
        i.   e_____   4 spontaneous
        ii. y_____   3 to speech
        iii. e_____   2 to pain
        iv. s_____   1 nil
    b. verbal
        i.   v_____   5 oriented
        ii. o_____   4 confused
        iii. i_____   3 inappropriate
        iv. c_____   2 incoherent
        v.   e_____   1 nil
    c. motor
        i.   m_____   6 obeys
        ii. o_____   5 localized
        iii. v_____   4 withdrawal
        iv. i_____   3 decorticate
        v.   n_____   2 decerebrate
        vi. g_____   1 nil

2. **True or False. A patient with a GCS score E2 V1 M2 (GCS 5) is in a coma.**   false (Whereas 90% of patients with GCS ≤ 8 are in a coma, coma is defined as inability to obey commands, speak, or *open the eyes* even to pain.)   G7 p.279:70mm

3. **Define coma.**   A GCS less than 8 is a generally accepted operational definition of coma.   G7 p.279:105mm

4. **List the three locations of brain lesions that produce coma.**   G7 p.279:155mm
    a. u_____ p_____ and m_____   upper pons and midbrain
    b. d_____   diencephalic
    c. b_____ c_____ h_____   bilateral cerebral hemisphere

12

5. **Disinhibition by removal of the corticospinal pathways above the midbrain typically results in _____ posturing.**   decorticate   G7 p.279:180mm

6. **Complete the following about coma in general:**   G7 p.279:182mm
    a. Decorticate lesion is at _____.   midbrain
    b. Decerebrate lesion is at _____.   intercollicular level between vestibular nuclei and red nucleus
    c. Locked-in syndrome lesion is at _____.   ventral pons

7. **Complete the following about coma in general:**   G7 p.280:15 mm
    a. In decorticate posturing
        i. The upper extremities are in _____.   flexion
        ii. The lower extremities are in _____.   extension
    b. In decerebrate posturing
        i. The upper extremities are in _____.   extension
        ii. The lower extremities are in _____.   extension

8. **Decorticate and decerebrate posturing have what lower extremity movements in common?**   G7 p.280:20 mm
    a. e_____   extension
    b. i_____ _____   internal rotation
    c. p_____ _____   plantar flexion

9. **A patient is brought to the emergency room in a coma after being found down. Pupils are equal and reactive. Painful stimulus elicits no movement. No signs of trauma are evident. Studies show Na$^+$ 130, K$^+$ 4.9, C 1—100, HCO$_3$ 2—15, BUN 30, Cr 1.2, Glu 440. The *likely* cause of coma is _____ _____.**   diabetic ketoacidosis   G7 p.280:62mm

10. **What stroke syndromes can lead to coma?**   G7 p.280:110 mm
    a. b_____ c_____ i_____   bilateral cortical infarcts
    b. b_____ d_____ i_____   bilateral diencephalic infarcts (i.e., top of basilar)
    c. b_____ s_____   brain stem

11. **A patient in coma eventually arouses with apathy, memory loss, and vertical gaze paresis. The most likely etiology for the coma was _____ _____ _____.**   bilateral diencephalic infarcts   G7 p.280:128mm

12

12. **Indicate the effect of midline shift on level of consciousness.**   G7 p.281:155mm
   a. 0 to 3 mm _____   alert
   b. 3 to 4 mm _____   drowsy
   c. 6 to 8.5 mm _____   stuporous
   d. 8 to 13 mm _____   comatose

13. **The three categories of disorders in the differential diagnosis of pseudocoma are**   G7 p.281:20 mm
   a. l_____-i_____ s_____ and   locked-in syndrome and
      v_____ p_____ i_____   ventral pontine infarction
                                            (EEG normal)
   b. p_____ d_____, c_____, and   psychiatric disorders,
      c_____ r_____   catatonia, and conversion
                                            reaction
   c. n_____ w_____ and m_____   neuromuscular weakness and
      g_____, G_____-B_____   myasthenia gravis, Guillain-
      s_____   Barré syndrome

■ Approach to the Comatose Patient

14. **A patient presents with coma. Your first move is to assess and secure the _____.**   airway   G7 p.281:60mm

15. **Complete the following about approach to the comatose patient:**   G7 p.281:103mm
   a. What percent of patients with Wernicke encephalopathy present with coma?   3%
   b. You would initially treat those patients with _____.   thiamine

16. **True or False. The following breathing pattern is most likely to be observed in a comatose child with fulminant hepatic failure after acetylsalicylic acid (ASA) use during a viral infection:**   G7 p.282:65mm
   a. Cheyne-Stokes   true (Seen with diencephalic lesions or, as in this case, bihemispheric dysfunction. The child has a toxic/metabolic encephalopathy as a result of hepatic failure due to Reyes syndrome.)
   b. hyperventilation   false
   c. cluster   false
   d. apneustic   false
   e. atoxic   false

17. **What is the significance of equal, reactive pupils in a comatose patient?**   indicates toxic metabolic cause   G7 p.282:133mm

12

18. **What is the most useful single sign in distinguishing metabolic from structural coma?**   the light reflex (Equal and reactive pupils indicate toxic/metabolic cause with few exceptions.)   G7 p.282:138mm

19. **The *only* metabolic causes of fixed/dilated pupils are**   G7 p.282:141mm
    a. a_____ e_____   anoxic encephalopathy
    b. g_____ t_____   glutethimide toxicity
    c. a_____ u_____   anticholinergic use (i.e., atropine)
    d. b_____ t_____ p_____   botulinum toxin poisoning

20. **True or False. The following is a metabolic cause of fixed, dilated pupils:**   G7 p.282:141mm
    a. atropine   true
    b. glutethimide toxicity   true
    c. hyperammonemia   false
    d. anoxic encephalopathy   true
    e. botulinum toxin poisoning   true

21. **In a third nerve palsy**   G7 p.282:165mm
    a. the pupil is _____   dilated
    b. and the eye looks _____ and _____.   down and out

22. **True or False. The following ocular findings can be seen in comatose patients with pontine lesions:**   G7 p.282:176mm
    a. pinpoint pupils   true
    b. periodic alternating gaze   false (Periodic alternating gaze usually indicates bilateral cerebral dysfunction.)
    c. ocular bobbing   true
    d. bilateral conjugate deviation to cold calorics   false

23. **In frontal lobe lesions patient looks toward**   G7 p.283:30mm
    a. the _____ side   moving
        i.   in destructive lesions that is _____   away from hemiparesis, toward the moving extremities
        ii. in irritative lesions (seizures) that is _____   away from seizure focus, toward the jerking extremities
    b. lesion is in the f_____ c_____ for c_____ g_____   frontal center for contralateral gaze

24. **In a pontine lesion the eyes deviate toward the _____ side.**   nonmoving   G7 p.283:30mm

12

25. **True or False. The eyes "look toward the side of the destructive lesion" in all destructive supratentorial lesions causing bilateral conjugate gaze deviation.**

false (Whereas the above is true for lesions affecting the frontal gaze center, medial thalamic hemorrhage can result in gaze deviation away from the lesion, "wrong way gaze," i.e., toward the nonmoving side.)

G7 p.283:45mm

26. **Name three causes of bilateral downward gaze deviation in a comatose patient.**
   a. t_____ l_____   thalamic lesion
   b. m_____ p_____ l_____   midbrain pretectal lesion
   c. b_____   barbiturates

G7 p.283:55mm

27. **Complete the following concerning internuclear ophthalmoplegia:**
   a. Lesion is in the _____ _____ _____.   medial longitudinal fasciculus
   b. Fibers are interrupted that go to the _____ _____ _____ _____.   contralateral third nerve nucleus
   c. Results in
      i.   loss of _____   adduction
      ii.   of the _____ eye   ipsilateral
      iii. on _____ _____ _____   spontaneous eye movement
      iv.   or in response to _____ _____   reflex movement (doll's, calorics)
      v.   and convergence _____   is not impaired

G7 p.283:105mm

28. **True or False. The ciliospinal reflex is indicative of**
   a. parasympathetic pathways   false
   b. spinothalamic pathways   false
   c. integrity of the periaqueductal gray   false
   d. sympathetic pathways   true

G7 p.284:80mm

---

12 ■ **Herniation Syndromes**

29. **True or False. Subfalcine herniation is of concern because:**
   a. Anterior cerebral artery territory infarcts may occur.   true
   b. Transtentorial herniation may occur.   true
   c. There is no obvious concern.   false

G7 p.284:137mm

30. **True or False. Decreased consciousness occurs early in uncal herniation.**   false (It occurs late in uncal herniation, early in central herniation.)

G7 p.285:15mm

31. **True or False. Uncal herniation syndrome rarely gives rise to decorticate posturing.**   true

G7 p.285:20mm

32. Upward cerebellar herniation   G7 p.285:95mm
  a. can occlude the _____,   SCAs
  b. resulting in _____ infarction.   cerebellar

33. Central herniation   G7 p.285:142mm
  a. can occlude the _____,   PCA
  b. resulting in _____ _____.   cortical blindness
  c. It can shear basilar artery _____ and   perforators, Duret   G7 p.285:150mm
     cause D_____ hemorrhages.

34. True or False. This stage of central   G7 p.285:170mm
   herniation is reversible.
  a. medullary stage   false
  b. diencephalic stage   true
  c. lower pons   false
  d. upper pons   false

35. List the distinguishing features of the   G7 p.286:15mm
   pupils and respiratory pattern for the
   following injuries:
  a. injury at the diencephalon
     i. pupils _____   react to light
     ii. respiratory pattern is _____   Cheyne-Stokes
  b. injury at the midbrain
     i. pupils _____   midposition
     ii. respiratory pattern is _____   hyperventilation
  c. injury at the pons
     i. pupils _____-_____   pin-point
     ii. respiratory pattern is _____   apneustic
  d. injury at the medulla oblongata
     i. pupils are _____   dilated, fixed (markedly open)
     ii. respiratory pattern is _____   ataxic

36. True or False. Internuclear   false (at the upper pons   G7 p.286:65mm
   ophthalmoplegia is prominent at the   stage)
   "lower pons" stage of central
   herniation.

37. Matching. Use the numbered options   G7 p.286:75mm
   to complete the following statements:
   ① Parasympathetics are lost;
   ② Sympathetics are lost; ③ Both are
   lost.
  a. Why does injury to the pons result in pin-   ②
     point pupils?
  b. Why does injury of herniation result in   ③ (i.e., bilateral third nerve
     dilated fixed pupils?   palsy)

38. Matching. Use the numbered options   G7 p.286:128mm
   to complete the following questions:
   ① 3%; ② 9%; ③ 15%; ④ 18%
   What percentage of patients who had
   symptoms of central herniation had:
  a. good outcome?   ②
  b. functional outcome?   ④

12

39. **True or False. Regarding uncal herniation:**   G7 p.286:168mm
   a. The earliest consistent sign is
      i.   impaired consciousness   false
      ii. unilateral dilated pupil   true

40. **What shape is the suprasellar cistern?**   pentagonal   G7 p.287:20 mm

41. **True or False. Unilateral dilated pupil in early third nerve stage of uncal herniation is seen in the following percentage of patients ipsilateral to the lesion:**   G7 p.287:52mm
   a. 65%   false
   b. 75%   false
   c. 85%   true
   d. 95%   false

■ Hypoxic Coma

42. **Complete the following statements concerning anoxia. Pathological lesions seen in**   G7 p.287:140mm
   a. cortex
      i.   _____ cortical layer   third
      ii. _____ horn   Ammon
   b. basal ganglia
      i.   g_____ p_____   globus pallidus
      ii. c_____   caudate
      iii. p_____   putamen
   c. cerebellum
      i.   P_____ cells   Purkinje
      ii. d_____ nucleus   dentate
      iii. i_____ o_____   inferior olive
   d. What tissue is more sensitive to anoxia— gray or white matter?   gray (It has a greater requirement of O_2.)
   e. Are steroids useful after cardiac arrest?   no   G7 p.288:170mm

12

13

Brain Death

■ Brain Death in Adults

1. The apnea test G7 p.289:158mm
a. assesses f_____ of m _____. function of medulla
b. To be a valid test of brain death, $PaCO_2$ must reach _____ mm Hg without respirations. 60 mm Hg
c. This usually takes _____ minutes. 6

2. Name five complicating conditions that must not be present to declare an adult brain dead. G7 p.290:134mm
Hint: hipps
a. h_____ hypothermia: core temperature less than 32.2°C (90°F)
b. i_____ intoxication (i.e., paralytics, barbiturates, benzodiazepines)
c. p_____ postresuscitation (i.e., could be in shock, or atropine may have been used in resuscitating, causing fixed, dilated pupils)
d. p_____ pentobarbital level > 10 µg/mL
e. s_____ shock (SBP less than 90)

■ Brain Death in Children

13

3. Are there different age-dependent observation periods to declare brain death? If so, what are they? yes G7 p.293:35mm
a. newborn to 7 days observe for 7 days
b. age 7 days to 2 months observe for 2 days; 2 exams, 2 electroencephalographs 48 hours apart
c. age 2 months to 12 months observe for a day; 2 exams, 2 electroencephalographs 24 hours apart
d. older than 12 months 12 hours observation

14

Cerebrospinal Fluid

■ General Information

1. **The volume (mL) of cerebrospinal fluid (CSF) in**   G7 p.297:80 mm
   a. a newborn is _____   5
   b. an adult is _____   150

2. **What is the intracranial:spinal ratio of distribution of CSF in adults?**   50:50   G7 p.297:80mm

3. **What percentage of CSF is produced in the lateral ventricles?**   80%   G7 p.297:80mm

4. **The amount of CSF volume produced per day for**   G7 p.297:84mm
   a. adults is _____   450 to 750 mL/d
   b. newborns is _____   25 mL/d

5. **What is the rate of CSF formation mL/min in adults?**   0.3 to 0.5   G7 p.297:84mm

6. **What is the CSF pressure in a patient in lateral decubitus position in the following age groups?**   G7 p.297:87mm
   a. newborn   9 to 12 cm H_2O
   b. 1 to 10 years old   < 15
   c. young adult   < 18 to 20
   d. adult   < 18 (7 to 15)

7. **Where is CSF produced other than in the choroid plexus?**   G7 p.297:95mm
   a. i_____ s_____   interstitial space
   b. e_____ l_____ of the v_____   ependymal lining of the ventricles
   c. d_____ of n_____ r_____ s_____ in s_____   dura of nerve root sleeves in spine

8. **Complete the following concerning CSF general information:** G7 p.297:115 mm

a. What is the rate of CSF production? 0.3 to 0.5 mL/min

b. That equals how many mL per day? 450 to 750

c. Normal CSF has

  i. _____ lymphocytes 0 to 5

  ii. _____ polymorphonuclear leucocytes (PMN) 0

  iii. _____ red blood cells (RBCs) 0

d. White blood cells (WBCs) above _____ is suspicious. 5 to 10

e. WBCs above _____ is definitely abnormal. 10 WBCs per cubic mm

f. Subtract _____ WBC for every _____ RBCs. 1; 700

g. Subtract _____ mg protein for every _____ RBCs. 1; 1000 G7 p.298:65mm

9. **Does intracranial pressure (ICP) have any effect on CSF formation?** no (The rate of formation is *independent* of CSF pressure *except* if the ICP is so high that it causes *reduction in cerebral blood flow [CBF].*) G7 p.297:120mm

10. **Complete the following concerning CSF general information:** G7 p.297:130mm

a. True or False. CSF absorption is a pressure-dependent phenomenon. true

b. Where does it take place?

  i. a_____ v_____ arachnoid villi → dural venous sinuses

  ii. c_____ p_____ choroid plexus

  iii. l_____ lymphatics

■ CSF Constituents

11. **True or False. The composition of CSF is exactly the same in the ventricles as in the lumbar subarachnoid space.** false (It differs slightly.) G7 p.297:153mm

12. **True or False. The following are normally found in CSF:** G7 p.297:170mm

a. lymphocytes true

b. mononuclear cells true

c. polymorphonuclear leucocytes false

d. RBCs false

14

13. **True or False. CSF osmolarity and plasma osmolarity are equal, with a ratio 1:1. What is the other constituent that is also equal among the following?**   G7 p.298:160mm

    a. Na   true
    b. K^+ false
    c. Cl^- false
    d. IgG   false

14. **True or False. CSF proteins**   G7 p.299:110mm

    a. are equal in adults and children — false (30 in adults and 20 in children)
    b. in prematures are ~60 mg/dL — false (in prematures 150 mg/dL)
    c. in newborn are ~40 mg/dL — false (about 80 in newborn)
    d. normally rise ~1 mg/dL/yr of age in adults — true

15. **How do you differentiate true leukocytosis from normal white blood cell count included in the traumatic tap?**   G7 p.298:30mm

    a. ratio of _____ to _____ — RBC to WBC
    b. normal is _____ — 700:1
    c. or subtract 1 WBC for every _____ _____ — 700 RBCs

16. **What conditions would affect the WBC:RBC ratio of 1:700?**   G7 p.298:30mm

    a. a_____ — anemia
    b. p_____ l_____ — peripheral leukocytosis

17. **In case of a traumatic tap, how could you estimate the original count in that CSF in a patient who has anemia or peripheral leukocytosis?** — use Fishman's formula WBC original CSF = WBC CSF – (WBCbld × RBCCSF) RBCbld. Note: WBC and RBC per mm^3 in peripheral blood   G7 p.298:30mm

18. **How would you estimate the correct protein in the CSF of a traumatic tap?**   G7 p.298:65mm

    a. Subtract _____ mg of protein — 1
    b. for every _____ RBCs/mm^3. — 1000

19. **Answer the following about subarachnoid hemorrhage:**   G7 p.300:35mm

    a. How long does it take for RBC to disappear? — 2 weeks
    b. How long does it take for xanthochromia to disappear? — many weeks

14

■ Artificial CSF

20. True or False. In the use of neuroendoscopy, endogenous CSF and "artificial CSF" should have which of the following characteristics in common?

G7 p.300:84mm

a. physiological temperature   true
b. membrane active ion concentrations true
c. osmolarity   true
d. pH   true

■ CSF Fistula

21. The Rosenmüller fossa is located just _____.

inferior to the cavernous sinus (Rosenmüller fossa is located *just inferior to the cavernous sinus* exposed by drilling the anterior clinoid in a paraclinoid aneurysm. Upper lateral pharyngeal recess. Limited above by the sphenoid and occipital bone. Communicates with the nasal cavities.)

G7 p.301:50mm

22. True or False. The following are characteristics of traumatic CSF fistula:

G7 p.301:77mm

a. They occur in 2 to 3% of all patients with head injury.   true
b. 60% are noted within days of trauma.   true
c. 95% occur within 3 months of trauma.   true
d. < 5% of cases of CSF rhinorrhea stop within 1 week.   false (70% of cases stop within 1 week.)
e. Adult:child ratio is 1:10.   false (adult:child ratio is 10:1)
f. Occurrence is common before age 2 years.   false (occurrence uncommon prior to 2 years of age)
g. Anosmia is common.   true (78% have anosmia.)
h. Most CSF otorrhea ceases in 5 to 10 days.   true

23. Complete the following concerning posttraumatic CSF fistula:

G7 p.301:78mm

a. Rhinorrhea stops within _____ week in _____%.   1; 70%
b. Otorrhea stops within _____ days in _____%.   5 to10; 80 to 85%

G7 p.301:93mm

24. True or False. Regarding CSF fistulas:

G7 p.301:117mm

a. Anosmia is common in traumatic leaks.   true (78% in traumatic leaks)
b. Anosmia is common in spontaneous leaks.   false (rare in spontaneous leaks; approximately 5%)

14

25. The infection rate for

G7 p.301:96mm

a. penetrating injuries and CSF fistulas is _____%.   50%

b. penetrating injuries without fistula is _____%.   4.6%

26. Study Chart.

G7 p.301:110mm

a. Regarding spontaneous CSF fistula: Hint: spontaneous fistula h

sense of smell preserved

pneumocephalus is not common

otitis media

neck stiffness

tumor-pituitary-meningioma

allergic rhinitis

meningitis

empty sella syndrome

otitis media may result in CSF leak

undeveloped floor of anterior fossa

sense of smell preserved

cribriform plate agenesis

sinusitis (paranasal sinusitis)

foot plate of stapes is dehiscent—CSF into eustachian tube

facial canal fistula into middle ear

insidious, ICP is high, intermittent

serous effusion

transsphenoidal surgery consequence

unable to hear due to Mundini dysplasia

labyrinthine anomalies

adenoma of pituitary

hydrocephalus

27. Complete the following concerning meningitis in CSF fistula:

G7 p.302:45mm

a. Posttraumatic CSF leak has an incidence of meningitis of _____%.   5 to 10%

b. Does CSF leakage after surgery have a *higher* or *lower* incidence of meningitis?   higher

c. If the leakage site is not identified before surgery failure to close CSF leaks is _____%.   30% (recurrent leak postop)

d. The most common pathogen is _____ and its percentage is _____%.   pneumococcus; 83%

28. **What are the characteristics of the fluid suggesting the presence of rhinorrhea or otorrhea resulting from a CSF fistula?**

G7 p.302:92mm

a. CSF fluid is _____.
   as *clear* as water (unless infected or blood present).

b. True or False. Fluid causes excoriation.
   false (Fluid doesn't cause excoriation of the nose.)

c. Fluid tastes _____.
   salty (in rhinorrhea).

d. Glucose is greater than _____ mg %.
   normal CSF glucose > 30 mg%

e. It contains a special chemical called _____.
   B2-transferrin (present in CSF)

f. The special sign when it drops on a sheet is called a _____.
   ring sign (An old but unreliable sign. Described as a ring of blood surrounded by a larger concentric ring of clear fluid [suggests the presence of CSF] seen when blood-tinged fluid allowed to drip onto linen [sheet or pillowcase].)

29. **Name five characteristics of fluid that suggest the presence of CSF fistula.**
   Hint: bcsfg

G7 p.302:100mm

   *B*2 transferrin
   *c*lear
   *s*alty taste
   *f*luid does not excoriate
   *g*lucose—high > 30 mg % vs. 5 mg % in tears and mucous

30. **True or False. The procedure of choice to localize the site of CSF fistula is**

G7 p.303:34mm

a. magnetic resonance imaging
   false

b. iohexol cisternography
   true

c. computed tomography with intravenous contrast
   false

d. plain x-ray
   false

14

15

Hydrocephalus

■ Hydrocephalus

1. Complete the following statements about hydrocephalus: G7 p.307:42mm

a. Incidence of congenital hydrocephalus is _____%. 0.2%

b. Size of normal temporal horns should be no wider than _____ mm. 2 mm

c. Width of brain (internal diameter) compared with largest width of frontal horns should normally be _____. 2 times or more

d. Therefore, a ratio of frontal horns to internal diameter of _____% suggests hydrocephalus. > 50%

2. True or False. Indicate if the following are considered "true" hydrocephalus: G7 p.307:82mm

a. hydrocephalus ex vacuo false

b. obstructive hydrocephalus true

c. communicating hydrocephalus true

3. True or False. The following are characteristics of hydranencephaly: G7 p.307:115mm

a. preneurulation defect false

b. cause may be from infection true

c. cause may be from bilateral internal carotid artery (ICA) infarcts true

d. electroencephalography (EEG) shows no cortical activity true

e. transillumination specific and very helpful false

4. Complete the following regarding hydranencephaly: G7 p.307:115mm

a. Hydranencephaly is defined as total or near total absence of the _____. cerebrum

b. It occurs before or after neurulation? postneurulation

c. The most common cause is _____ _____ _____. bilateral ICA infarcts

d. Other causes are
   i.   n_____ h_____   neonatal herpes
   ii. i_____   infection
   iii. t_____   toxoplasmosis
e. The best way to differentiate   EEG   G7 p.244:98mm
   hydranencephaly from maximal
   hydrocephalus is to perform an

   _____.

f. Other tests include
   i.   c_____ t_____   computed tomography (CT)
   ii. m_____ r_____ i_____ magnetic resonance imaging
                                      (MRI)
   iii. a_____   angiography

5. **What are key features regarding**   G7 p.307:140mm
   benign external hydrocephalus (also
   known as external hydrocephalus)?
a. Subarachnoid spaces are _____.   enlarged over frontal poles in
                                        first year of life
b. Ventricles are _____.   normal or minimally enlarged
c. They are distinguished from subdural cortical vein sign
   hematoma by the _____ _____

   _____.
d. It usually spontaneously _____ by   resolves; 2 years of age
   _____.

6. **Complete the following concerning**   G7 p.307:160mm
   external hydrocephalus:
a. It occurs in what age group?   infants in first year of life
b. What is the cortical vein sign?   MRI or CT shows veins
                                        extending from brain to inner
                                        table of skull
c. The cortical vein sign helps differentiate benign external
   _____ from _____.   hydrocephalus from subdural
                                        hematoma
d. Postulated cause of benign external defect in CSF reabsorption
   hydrocephalus (BEH) is _____.
e. BEH usually resolves by age _____.   2
f. Concern is caused by _____.   large head size

7. **"X" linked hydrocephalus**   G7 p.308:60mm
a. is a type of _____ hydrocephalus that inherited
b. occurs in _____% of patients with   2%
   hydrocephalus.
c. Gene is located on _____.   Xq28
d. It causes abnormality in _____   LICAM
   membrane receptor and   G7 p.308:110mm
e. produces classical syndromes including
   i.   c_____ c_____ h_____   corpus callosum hypoplasia
   ii. r_____   retardation
   iii. a_____ t_____   adducted thumbs
   iv. s_____ p_____   spastic paralysis
   v.   h_____   hydrocephalus

15

8. **Complete the following regarding radiographic finding of L1 syndrome:**   G7 p.308:140mm
   a. Large
      i.   p_____ h_____   posterior horn
      ii. m_____ i_____   massa intermedia
      iii. q_____ p_____   quadrigeminal plate
   b. Small (hypoplastic)
      i.   c_____ c_____   corpus callosum
      ii. c_____ v_____   cerebellar vermis
   c. Rippled
      i.   v_____ w_____   ventricular wall
   d. Which feature is pathognomonic?   rippled ventricular wall   G7 p.308:160mm
      r_____ v_____ w_____
   e. Available treatment for retardation?   none

9. **True or False. Shunt dependency is likely in hydrocephalus due to**   G7 p.309:53mm
   a. aqueductal stenosis   true
   b. spina bifida   true
   c. communicating hydrocephalus (i.e., secondary to arachnoidal adhesions)   false (shunt independence more likely to occur)

10. **True or False. With respect to a disconnected or nonfunctioning shunt:**   G7 p.309:57mm
    a. A disconnected shunt may continue to function by CSF flow through a subcutaneous fibrous tract.   true
    b. If in doubt, better to watch, not shunt.   false
    c. Patients with a nonfunctioning shunt should not be followed with serial CT scans but possibly with serial neuropsychological evaluations.   false

11. **True or False. When deemed "arrested" no further follow-up is needed.**   false, deterioration can still occur   G7 p.309:60mm

12. **True or False. With regard to "arrested hydrocephalus":**   G7 p.309:115mm
    a. It is interchangeable with the term "uncompensated hydrocephalus."   false
    b. Arrested hydrocephalus satisfies the following criteria in the absence of a cerebrospinal fluid (CSF) shunt   false
       i.   ventriculomegaly nonprogressive   true
       ii. normal head growth curve   true
       iii. continued psychomotor development   true

13. **Hydrocephalus-radiologic criteria:**   G7 p.310:60mm
    a. skull
       i.   inner table shows _____ _____ cranium   beaten copper
       ii. sella shows _____   erosion

15

b. ventricles
    i. Frontal horns ballooning look like   Mickey Mouse
        M_____ M_____.
    ii. Frontal horns' percent of brain width   50%
        is > _____%.
    iii. Temporal horns' width is   2 mm
        >_____mm.
    iv. Anteroposterior (AP) view shows   disproportion of ventricle size
        _____.   and cortical sulci
    v. Third ventricle on AP view shows   bowing laterally
        _____ _____.
    vi. Third ventricle on lateral view shows   bowing down into sella
        _____ _____ _____
        _____.

c. brain
    i. transependymal _____   edema
    ii. corpus callosum is _____   thin/atrophic
    iii. and shows _____   stretching
    iv. and _____ _____   upward bowing

14. Regarding the characteristics of the   G7 p.310:140 mm
    etiology of hydrocephalus:
a. True or False. There is excess production   true
    of CSF.
b. True or False. There is impaired   true
    absorption of CSF.
c. True or False. It is congenital without   true
    myelomeningocele.
d. Congenital with myelomeningocele   Chiari II
    usually occurs with _____.
e. Chiari I if a cause has _____   fourth ventricle outlet
    _____ _____ _____.   obstruction
f. Aqueductal stenosis presents symptoms   infancy
    in _____.
g. Secondary aqueductal stenosis is due to   intrauterine infection,
    _____ _____, _____, or   hemorrhage, or tumor
    _____.
h. Atresia of foramina of Luschka and   Dandy-Walker syndrome
    Magendie is called _____-_____
    _____.

15. Complete the following concerning   G7 p.311:10mm
    etiologies of hydrocephalus:
a. Chiari II is associated with _____.   myelomeningocele
b. Aqueductal stenosis usually manifests   infancy
    itself in which age group?
c. Of postop pediatric post-fossa tumor   20%   G7 p.311:117mm
    patients, _____% develop
    hydrocephalus and need a shunt.
d. This may be delayed for up to _____.   1 year
e. Dandy-Walker malformation occurs in   2.4%
    what percent of patients with
    hydrocephalus?

15

16. **Conditions that may mimic hydrocephalus are**   G7 p.311:130mm
    i.   h_____   hydranencephaly
    ii. a_____   atrophy
    iii. a_____ of c_____ c_____   agenesis of corpus callosum
    iv. s _____ o_____ d_____   septo optic dysplasia

17. **List signs and symptoms of hydrocephalus in young children.**   G7 p.312:45mm
    i.   h_____   hydrocephalus
    ii.   y_____   young children
    iii. d_____   diplopia on lateral gaze
                                          (abducens palsy)
    iv.   r_____   respiratory pattern irregular
    v.   o_____   outward protrusion of
                                          fontanelle
    vi.   c_____   cracked pot sound of
                                          Macewen
    vii. e_____   enlargement of cranium
                                          relative to face
    viii. p_____   poor head control, Parinaud
                                          syndrome
    ix.   h_____   hyperactive reflexes
    x.   a_____   abducens nerve palsy, apneic
                                          spells
    xi.   l_____   large head
    xii. u_____   upward gaze palsy
    xiii. s_____   scalp veins prominent
    xiv. s_____   setting sun sign
    xv.   s_____   splaying of cranial sutures
                                          (seen on plain skull x-rays)

18. **List the signs and symptoms of active hydrocephalus in older children/adults with rigid cranial vault.**   headache, nausea, vomiting   G7 p.312:45mm
    Hint: hcp   changes in gait, and urine
                                          control
                                          papilledema, upward gaze or
                                          abducens palsy

19. **Occipital frontal circumference (OFC) in the normal child should equal the distance from crown to _____.**   rump   G7 p.312:115mm

20. **For the indicated ages give the expected normal head circumference pattern.**   G7 p.313:15mm
    Hint: At 33 weeks the circumference is
    33 cm. In a child younger than 33 weeks
    the head circumference is greater in cm
    than the age of the child in weeks old.
    After 33 weeks head circumference
    growth slows so that at 40 weeks of age
    the head circumference is 36 cm.
    a. premature (ages in weeks)
        i.   28   29 cm
        ii. 29   30 cm

15

iii. 30	31 cm
iv. 31	31.5 cm
v. 32	32 cm
vi. 33	33 cm
vii. 34	33.5 cm
viii. 35	34 cm
ix. 36	34.5 cm
x. 37	35 cm
xi. 38	35 cm
xii. 39	35.4 cm
xiii. 40	36 cm

b. full term (ages in months)
Hint: Note the pattern; with each month head circumference increases by 1 cm.

i. 1	40 cm
ii. 2	42 cm
iii. 3	43 cm
iv. 4	44 cm
v. 5	45 cm
vi. 6	46 cm

c. What is the upper limit of head circumference for a baby?

i. 28 weeks gestational age	29 cm
ii. 33 weeks gestational age	33 cm
iii. 2 months old	42 cm
iv. 3 months old	43 cm
v. 4 months old	44 cm
vi. 6 months old	46 cm

■ Treatment of Hydrocephalus

21. **Answer the following about the treatment of hydrocephalus:**

a. True or False. Hydrocephalus is a medically treated condition.

false (mainly to be treated surgically)

G7 p.314:40mm

b. Diuretic therapy can include a_____ and f_____.

acetazolamide and furosemide

G7 p.314:68mm

c. Be sure to watch for the complication of _____ _____.

electrolyte imbalances

G7 p.314:95mm

d. Role of spinal taps in hydrocephalus is to t_____.

temporize (Hydrocephalus after intraventricular hemorrhage may be only transient, and serial taps [ventricular or lumbar] may temporize until resorption resumes, but lumbar taps can be performed only for communicating hydrocephalus.)

15

e.   Critical protein level of CSF is _____.   100 mg/dL (If reabsorption does not resume when protein content of CSF is < 100 mg/dL, then it is unlikely that spontaneous resorption will occur and a shunt will usually be necessary.)   G7 p.314:120mm

22.   Complete the following concerning spinal taps and hydrocephalus: G7 p.314:110mm
a.   Protein above _____ will not be absorbed.   100 mg/dL
b.   Protein below _____ may be absorbed.   100 mg/dL

23.   Complete the following concerning surgery and hydrocephalus: G7 p.314:110mm
a.   Third ventriculostomy when looking into ventricle
    i.   Where is thalamostriate vein?   lateral wall
    ii.   Where is septal vein?   medial wall
    iii.   Where is choroid plexus?   enters foramen of Monro
b.   Where is puncture of third ventricle to occur?   anterior to mammillary bodies
c.   Into the _____ cistern   interpeduncular
d.   Watch out for _____.   basilar artery
e.   Success rate is _____%,   approximately 50% (60 to 90% range) for aqueductal stenosis   G7 p.315:70mm
f.   but only 20% for _____ _____.   preexisting pathology

24.   Concerning shunts and hydrocephalus, what type of shunts do you know?   G7 p.315:140mm
    Hint: palmt
a.   v_____ s_____   ventriculoperitoneal shunt
b.   v_____ a_____   ventriculo-jugular vein–right cardiac atrial
c.   l_____   lumboperitoneal
d.   m_____ s_____   miscellaneous shunts– ventriculopleural
e.   T_____ s_____   Torkildsen shunt (ventricle– cisterna magna)

25.   What is shunt usage priority?   G7 p.315:145mm
    Hint: palmt
a.   most often used _____ _____   ventriculoperitoneal shunt
b.   abdominal abnormality _____   ventriculoatrial shunt
    _____

    surgery
    peritonitis
    morbid obesity

c. pseudotumor cerebri _____
_____

*l*umboperitoneal shunt–small ventricles

d. alternative _____ _____
e. acquired obstructive hydrocephalus
_____ _____

*m*iscellaneous shunts
*T*orkildsen shunt

26. **Which are the miscellaneous shunts?**
    Hint: gupc

    G7 p.316:22mm

    i.   g_____
    ii.   u_____

    iii. p_____
    iv.   c_____

    ventricle to *g*all bladder shunt
    ventricle to *u*reter or bladder shunt
    ventriculo*p*leural shunt
    *c*yst shunt (arachnoid cyst or subdural hygroma cavity to peritoneum)

27. **Name six possible shunt complications.**
    Hint: odesma

    G7 p.316:160mm

    i.   o_____
    ii.   d_____
    iii. e_____
    iv.   s_____

    v.   m_____
    vi.   a_____

    obstruction
    disconnection of shunt parts
    erosion through skin
    seizures–5.5% first year, 1.1% after 3 years
    metastases of tumor cells
    allergy to silicone

28. **What are ventriculoperitoneal shunt complications?**
    Hint: h^{2}alo^{3}mvps

    G7 p.316:125mm

    i.   h_____
    ii.   h_____
    iii. a_____
    iv.   l_____

    v.   o_____

    hernia–inguinal 17%
    hydrocele
    CSF ascites
    lengthen catheter with growth (preventable)
    obstruction by omentum or debris
    by peritoneal cyst (infection or talc from surgical gloves) severe peritoneal adhesions malposition of catheter tip collapsed ventricular wall choroid plexus

    vi.   o_____

    vii. o_____
    viii. m_____

    obstruction or strangulation of intestine
    overshunting
    migration of tip to:
    scrotum
    perforation of stomach, bladder, diaphragm

    ix.   v_____
    x.   p_____
    xi.   s_____

    volvulus
    peritonitis
    subdural hematoma

15

29. **What are ventriculoatrial shunt complications?**   G7 p.317:55mm
    Hint: liverssh

i. l_____	lengthening in children
ii. i_____	infection
iii. v_____	vascular
	perforation
	thrombophlebitis
	pulmonary microemboli
iv. e_____	shunt embolus
v. r_____	retrograde blood flow
vi. s_____	superior vena cava obstruction
vii. s_____	subdural hematoma
viii. h_____	hypertension (pulmonary)

30. **What are lumboperitoneal shunt complications?**   G7 p.317:70mm
    Hint: Carols

i. C_____	Chiari I malformation (70% made worse)
ii. a_____	arachnoiditis and adhesions
iii. r_____	radiculopathy (from tube-hard to control)
iv. o_____	overshunting (sixth and seventh cranial nerve dysfunction)
v. l_____	leakage of CSF
vi. s_____	scoliosis due to laminectomy (14% in children)

■ Shunt Problems

31. **When do you tap the shunt?**   G7 p.322:65mm
    a. to study CSF for

i. i_____	infection
ii. c_____	cytology
iii. b_____	blood

    b. or to assess function

i. measure p_____	pressure
ii. instill c_____	contrast

    c. inject m_____   medication

32. **When tapping a shunt, what is normal CSF pressure as measured from the ventricle?**   less than 15 cm of CSF in relaxed recumbent position   G7 p.322:130mm

33. **How often does the patient have to pump the shunt?**   Patient must not touch the pump unless instructed to do so.   G7 p.323:48mm

15

34. **What are acute symptoms of undershunting?**   G7 p.323:140mm
    Hint: salvadib h

   a. s_____   seizures
   b. a_____   ataxia
   c. l_____   lethargy
   d. v_____   vomiting
   e. a_____   apnea
   f. d_____   diplopia
   g. i_____   irritability
   h. b_____   bradycardia
   i. h_____   headache

35. **What are signs of acute increase in intracranial pressure?**   G7 p.323:165mm
    Hint: p^4b^2

   a. p_____   Parinaud syndrome
   b. p_____   palsy of abducens
   c. p_____   papilledema
   d. p_____   prominent scalp veins
   e. b_____   blindness or field cut
   f. b_____   bulging fontanelle

36. **What are complications of overshunting?**   G7 p.325:130 mm
    Hint: s^4i

   a. s_____   slit ventricles 12%
   b. s_____   subdural hematoma
   c. s_____   sylvian aqueduct occlusion
   d. s_____   skull changes—
                                  craniosynostosis or
                                  microcephaly
   e. i_____   intracranial hypotension

37. **Intracranial hypotension**   G7 p.326:23mm
   a. When patient is erect, column of CSF   siphon effect
       produces a s_____ e_____.
   b. Diagnose by documenting a drop in ICP   supine to erect
       when patient changes from _____ to
       _____ position.

38. **Slit ventricles can be diagnosed by frontal-occipital horn ratio of less than _____.**   0.2   G7 p.326:50mm

39. **Name categories of patients with slit ventricles.**   G7 p.326:80mm
    Hint: pahms

   a. p_____   pseudotumor cerebri
   b. a_____   asymptomatic slit ventricles
   c. h_____   intracranial hypotension
   d. m_____   migraine
   e. s_____   slit ventricle syndrome

15

40. Complete the following concerning hydrocephalus and subdural hematomas (SDs):   G7 p.327:105mm

   a. Cause of SD in patients with shunts is _____ of the brain and _____ _____ _____ _____ _____.

collapse; tearing of the bridging veins

   b. Risk factors

      i. b_____ a_____

      ii. l_____-s_____ h_____

      iii. n_____ v_____ p_____

brain atrophy
long-standing hydrocephalus
negative ventricular pressure

41. If subdural hematoma develops as a shunt complication the subdural is located on   G7 p.327:140mm

   a. the same side as the shunt _____%

32%

   b. opposite side of the shunt _____%

21%

   c. bilaterally _____%

47%

42. Treatment for subdural hematoma that occurs due to shunting for hydrocephalus could include   G7 p.328:25mm
Hint: bcdht

   a. b_____

burr holes

   b. c_____

craniotomy

   c. d_____

drainage–subdural peritoneal shunt

   d. h_____

higher pressure shunt

   e. t_____

tie off shunt

43. True or False. In VP shunt and laparoscopic surgery, abdominal insufflation can increase ICP.

true   G7 p.328:145mm

◼ Normal Pressure Hydrocephalus

44. What are the symptoms of normal pressure hydrocephalus?   G7 p.329:65mm
Hint: dig

   a. d_____

dementia (wacky)

   b. i_____

incontinence of urine (wet)

   c. g_____

gait disturbances (wobbly)

45. What is the etiology?   G7 p.329:85mm
Hint: mistapa

   a. m_____

meningitis

   b. i_____

idiopathic

   c. s_____

subarachnoid hemorrhage

   d. t_____

trauma

   e. a_____

aqueductal stenosis

   f. p_____

posterior fossa surgery

   g. A_____

Alzheimer disease

46. In clinical triad, which symptom precedes the others?

gait disturbance   G7 p.329:145mm

15

47. **Note the clinical features of NPH as expected (+) or not expected (−).**   G7 p.329:145mm
   a. Wide-based gait   +
   b. Shuffling steps   +
   c. Unsteadiness on turning   +
   d. Difficult initiating steps   +
   e. Feel glued to the floor   +
   f. Ataxia of limbs   −
   g. Slowness of thought   +
   h. Unwitting urinary incontinence   −
   i. Papilledema   −
   j. Seizure   −
   k. Headaches   −

48. **True or False. Concerning cisternography for normal pressure hydrocephalus (NPH), what finding predicts a 75% improvement with a shunt? Radionucleotide in the ventricle at**   G7 p.333:78mm
   a. 24 hours   false
   b. 48 hours   false
   c. 72 hours   true (late scan 48 to 72 hours)

49. **In NPH what is the sequence in which symptoms are likely to improve with shunting?**   G7 p.334:125mm
   Hint: igd
   a. i_____   incontinence
   b. g_____   gait
   c. d_____   dementia

■ Blindness and Hydrocephalus

50. **Blindness in hydrocephalus may be due to**   G7 p.335:30mm
   Hint: pop
   a. p_____   papilledema—chronic—optic atrophy
   b. o_____ _____ _____ optic chiasm compression dilation of third ventricle
   c. p_____ _____ _____ posterior cerebral artery _____   occlusion compressed at tentorial edge

51. **Blindness clinical criteria for localization are _____ _____ and _____ _____.**   G7 p.335:70mm   pregeniculate blindness and postgeniculate blindness
   a. Characteristics for pre-_____   pregeniculate blindness
      i. o_____ n_____ a_____—   optic nerve atrophy—severe s_____
      ii. p_____ r_____—p_____   pupillary reflexes—poor
      iii. due to p_____, h_____, a_____   pressure, hypotension, anemia

15

b. Characteristics for p_____   postgeniculate blindness
   b_____
   i.   o_____ n_____ a_____—   optic nerve atrophy—minimal
        m_____
   ii. p_____ r_____—n_____   pupillary reflexes—normal
   iii. due to _____ _____   hypoxia macular sparing in
        _____   PCA occlusion, no macular
                                                      sparing in trauma to occiput

**52. Cortical blindness may be associated   G7 p.335:82mm
      with**
   a. Anton syndrome = d_____ of   denial of visual deficit
      v_____ d_____
   b. Riddoch phenomenon = a_____ of   appreciation of moving
      m_____ o_____, but n_____   objects, but no appreciation
      a_____ of s_____ o_____   of stationary objects

■ Hydrocephalus and Pregnancy

**53. Patients with shunt for hydrocephalus   G7 p.336:65mm
      should prior to conception**
   a. have up-to-date _____ or _____   CT or MRI
   b. have assessment of any m_____   medications
   c. if prospective mother's hydrocephalus is   2 to 3%
      accompanied by a neural tube defect
      (NTD), her child could be born with an
      NTD incidence of _____ to
      _____%
   d. have genetic c_____   counseling
   e. start v_____   vitamins
   f. avoid excessive h_____   heat

**54. If shunt malfunctions during   G7 p.336:100mm
      pregnancy, you may**
   a. in the first two trimesters _____ the   revise
      VP shunt
   b. in the third trimester use a _____-   ventriculo-atrial,
      _____ or a _____-_____ shunt   ventriculo-pleural

55. During labor and delivery   G7 p.336:175mm
   a. Use p_____ a_____.   prophylactic antibiotics
   b. If patient is asymptomatic deliver via   vagina
      _____.
   c. If patient is symptomatic deliver via   cesarean
      _____.
   d. In light of increased cranial pressure   epidurals
      avoid _____.

15

16

Infections

■ General Information

1. Complete the following regarding antibiotics:

G7 p.342:127mm

a. An antibiotic good for neurosurgical prophylaxis is _____.

Ancef (cefazolin)

b. An antibiotic good for shunt surgery prophylaxis is _____.

Ancef (cefazolin)

c. The above are _____ cephalosporins.

first-generation

d. A third-generation cephalosporin good for treatment of Lyme disease is _____.

Rocephin (ceftriaxone)

G7 p.343:33mm

■ Prophylactic Antibiotics

2. Describe the administration of prophylactic antibiotics.

G7 p.342:127mm

a. Ancef—also known as _____

cefazolin

b. dose and route

1 to 2 g IV

c. when? _____ before surgery

60 minutes

d. and repeat every _____ hours for _____ hours

6; 24

e. if allergic to _____ use _____

penicillin; vancomycin

f. dose and route _____

1 g IV

g. and repeat every _____ hours for _____ hours

8; 24

■ Meningitis

3. List the differential diagnosis of chronic meningitis.

G5 p.213:40 mm

Hint: msfict

a. m_____ c _____

meningeal carcinomatosis

b. s_____

sarcoidosis

c. f_____

fungal

d. i_____

infection

e. c_____

cysticercosis

f. t_____

tuberculosis

4. **Describe the treatment for posttraumatic meningitis.**   G7 p.344:60mm
   a. for gram-negative   imipenem or cipro
   b. for gram-positive   vancomycin
   c. continue until _____   1 week after CSF sterilization
   d. Surgery may be needed to _____   repair fistula
      _____.

■ Shunt Infection

5. **What are the characteristics of shunt infection?**   G7 p.345:97mm
   a. Risk of early infection is _____%.   7% overall
   b. Risk of mortality is _____%.   10 to 15%
   c. Risk of late is _____% within   2.7 to 31% (typically 6%)   G7 p.345:179mm
      6 months.
   d. Organism is _____ _____.   *Staphylococcus epidermidis*

6. **What are the characteristics of shunt nephritis?**   G7 p.346:88mm
   a. v_____ s_____   ventriculovascular shunt
   b. c_____ l_____-l_____   chronic low-level infection
      i_____
   c. i_____ c_____ d_____ in   immune complex deposit in
      g_____   glomeruli
   d. p_____ and h_____   proteinuria and hematuria

7. **Gram-negative bacillus (GNB) shunt infection compared with gram-positive bacillus (GPB)**   G7 p.346:165mm
   a. morbidity   higher in GNB
   b. Gram stain   more than 90% + Gram stain
                                         (in contrast to GPB only 50%)
   c. protein   ↑ protein
   d. glucose   ↓ glucose
   e. neutrophils   ↑ neutrophils
   f. The reason we must identify GNB
      infection is because
      i. treatment _____ _____ than   is different
          for staph and
      ii. there is a higher _____ for GNB. morbidity

8. **What is the treatment for shunt infection?**   G7 p.347:60mm
   a. Remove _____.   shunt
   b. Insert _____ _____ _____.   external ventricular drain
                                         (EVD)
   c. Administer antibiotics of _____ plus   vancomycin plus rifampin   G7 p.347:105mm
      _____   (change to nafcillin if
                                         possible)
   d. for _____ days.   14—with CSF sterilization
   e. Add i_____ a_____   intrathecal antibiotics
   f. by clamping _____ for _____   EVD for 30
      minutes.

16

Wound Infections

9. **Describe laminectomy wound infection treatment.**

    G7 p.349:15mm

    a. B_____ — Betadine—if purulent—half strength follow with normal saline

    b. c_____ — culture

    c. d_____ — debride wound

    d. e_____ — empirically vancomycin plus third generation cephalosporin (ceftazidime)

    e. f_____ — fill (pack) with iodoform ¼ inch

    f. g_____ — gradually reduce packing trim by 1 inch each day

    g. h_____ — hospital—change pack every 8 hours

    h. h_____ — home—change pack twice a day

Osteomyelitis of the Skull

10. **Complete the following concerning Pott puffy tumor:**

    G7 p.349:130mm

    a. Treatment
        i.   f_____ r_____ — flap removal
        ii.   d_____ — debridement
        iii. antibiotics for _____ weeks. For first week use _____ — 6 to 12; IV
        iv.   c_____ — cranioplasty after 6 months
    b. Most common organism is _____ _____. — *Staphylococcus aureus*

Cerebral Abscess

11. **What are the risk factors for cerebral abscess?**

    G7 p.350:85mm

    Hint: Abcdefghi
        i.   A_____ — AIDS
        ii.   b_____ — bacterial sepsis
        iii. c_____ — cyanotic heart disease
        iv.   d_____ — dental abscess
        v.   e_____ — endocarditis
        vi.   f_____ — fistula (arteriovenous)
        vii. g_____ — gastrointestinal infection
        viii. h_____ — hematogenous spread
        ix.   i_____ — infection pulmonary

16

12. **Complete the following about cerebral abscess:** G7 p.351:75mm

a. What percentage of cerebral abscesses fail to grow organism on culture? 25%

b. The most common organism is _____. Streptococcus, 30 to 50%

c. The most common organisms in frontal-ethmoid sinusitis are _____ _____ and _____ _____. Streptococcus milleri and Streptococcus anginosus

d. The most common organism in traumatic causes is _____ _____. Staphylococcus aureus

e. The most common organism in transplant patients is _____ _____. Aspergillus fumigatus

f. The most common organism in infants is _____ _____. gram negative

g. The most common organisms in AIDS patients are _____ and _____. toxoplasmosis and Nocardia

h. The most common dental source is _____. actinomyces

i. The most common organisms following neurosurgical procedures are _____ _____ and _____. Staphylococcus epidermidis and aureus

13. **Indicate the value of the following diagnostic tests or treatment for brain abscess:** G7 p.352:40mm

a. lumbar puncture (LP) dubious value—may herniate

b. computed tomography (CT) excellent

c. leukocyte scan excellent

d. effect of steroids tests become less positive—can mislead

14. **Describe the four stages of cerebral abscess.** G7 p.352:120mm

a. stages
    i. stage 1 e_____ c_____ early cerebritis
    ii. stage 2 l_____ c_____ late cerebritis
    iii. stage 3 e_____ c_____ early capsule
    iv. stage 4 l_____ c_____ late capsule

b. number of days
    i. stage 1 1 to 3
    ii. stage 2 4 to 9
    iii. stage 3 10 to 13
    iv. stage 4 14

c. histologic characteristics
    i. stage 1 inflammation
    ii. stage 2 developing necrotic center
    iii. stage 3 neovascularity reticular network, necrotic center
    iv. stage 4 collagen capsule necrotic center gliosis around capsule

16

15. **Conservative management of cerebral abscess is appropriate**   G7 p.353:130mm
   a. if the abscess is less than _____ cm in diameter   3
   b. or it is in the _____ _____ phase.   early cerebritis (where surgery would not be appropriate)

16. **List the empiric antibiotics used for cerebral abscess.**   G7 p.354:60mm
   Hint: vcmc or r
   a. v_____   vancomycin
   b. c_____   cefotoxime
   c. m_____ or   metronidazole (Flagyl)
   d. c_____ or   chloramphenicol
   e. r_____   rifampin

17. **For how long should IV antibiotics be used in cerebral abscess?**   6 weeks   G7 p.354:135mm

18. **Complete the following regarding *Nocardia*:**   G7 p.356:40mm
   a. It arises from the _____.   soil
   b. What is the duration of treatment?   many months
   c. Is it a fungus?   no, it is a bacterium

■ Subdural Empyema

19. **Complete the following regarding subdural empyema:**   G7 p.357:20mm
   a. It spreads as a result of _____ _____.   direct extension
   b. The leading cause was previously c_____ o_____ m_____.   chronic otitis media
   c. The leading cause now is _____.   frontal sinusitis, 65 to 75%
   d. Is LP used for diagnosis?   no, rarely positive and it is hazardous
   e. Fatal cases are associated with v_____ i_____ of the b_____.   venous infarction of the brain

■ Viral Encephalitis

20. **Complete the following regarding herpes simplex:**   G7 p.358:150mm
   a. HSE stands for _____ _____ _____.   herpes simplex encephalitis
   b. It has a predilection for the t_____, o_____ l_____ and l_____ s_____.   temporal, orbitofrontal lobes and limbic system
   c. Definitive diagnosis requires b_____ b_____ and v_____ i_____.   brain biopsy and virus isolation
   d. Treat promptly with _____.   acyclovir

16

21. **HSE has the following characteristic:**   G7 p.359:70mm
    a. CSF: _____-_____   leukocytosis-monocytes
    b. EEG: p_____ l_____ e_____   periodic lateralizing
       d_____ on electroencephalography   epileptiform discharges
    c. CT e_____ in t_____ l_____   edema in temporal lobes
    d. Hemorrhage on _____ means   CT; poorer prognosis
       _____ _____.
    e. MRI shows t_____ s_____.   transsylvian sign
    f. Significance: if bilateral it is highly   HSE
       suggestive of _____.

22. **Transsylvian sign**   G7 p.359:105 mm
    a. indicates temporal lobe e_____   edema
    b. that extends across the s_____   sylvian fissure
       f_____.

23. **General treatment for intracranial**   G7 p.360:60mm
    pressure (ICP) elevation involves the
    following:
    a. e_____ h_____ of b_____   elevate head of bed
    b. m_____   mannitol
    c. h_____   hyperventilate

24. **Complete the following concerning**   G7 p.360:85mm
    acyclovir treatment:
    a. The dose is _____   30 mg/kg/day is divided every
                                                       8 hours
    b. for a duration of _____ days.   14 to21
    c. If you identify HSE before GCS drops you   limit mortality
       can l_____ m_____.

■ Creutzfeldt-Jakob Disease

25. **Complete the following about**   G7 p.361:30mm
    Creutzfeldt-Jakob disease:
    a. CJD stands for _____ _____   Creutzfeldt-Jakob disease
       _____.
    b. The prognosis is _____ _____.   invariably fatal
    c. The EEG shows _____.   characteristic bilateral sharp   G7 p.361:43mm
                                                       waves 0.5 to 2.0 per second
    d. Prion stands for _____ _____   proteinaceous infectious
       _____.   particles
    e. Diagnostic triad   G7 p.362:160mm
       Hint: dEm
       i.   d_____   dementia
       ii. E_____   EEG
       iii. m_____   myoclonus

26. **What is the biopsy procedure in**   G7 p.363:150mm
    suspected CJD?
    a. Use a _____ cranial saw   manual
    b. to avoid _____ of the infection.   aerosolization
    c. Avoid cutting the _____ with the saw.   dura
    d. Clearly _____ containers .   label
    e. Fix is _____% phenolized formalin.   15%

16

■ Neurologic Manifestations of AIDS

27. **Name four conditions in AIDS producing focal CNS lesions.**   G7 p.364:75mm

a. t_____   toxoplasmosis

b. l_____   lymphoma

c. p_____ m _____ l _____   progressive multifocal leukoencephalopathy (PML)

d. *C*_____   *Cryptococcus*

28. **Complete the following about the neurologic manifestations of AIDS:**   G7 p.364:95mm

a. What is the most common lesion causing mass effect in AIDS patients?   toxoplasmosis

b. Does this occur early or late in the course of HIV infection?   late

c. Central nervous system (CNS) lymphoma is associated with what virus?   Epstein-Barr virus

d. PML is associated with what virus?   polyoma or J-C virus (not to be confused with Creutzfeldt-Jakob)

29. **An imaging characteristic of toxoplasmosis in AIDS patients is**   G7 p.365:170mm

a. number   multiple

b. density   low

c. located   basal ganglia

d. enhancement   ring—"multiple enhancing lesions in the basal ganglia"

30. **Complete the chart by listing the CT and MRI findings in each of the following:**   G7 p. 365:171mm

a. toxoplasmosis
  i. number   more than 5
  ii. enhance   ring
  iii. location   basal ganglia
  iv. mass effect   moderate
  v. miscellaneous   edema

b. lymphoma
  i. number   less than 5
  ii. enhance   homogeneous
  iii. location   subependymal
  iv. mass effect   mild
  v. miscellaneous   may cross corpus callosum

c. PML
  i. number   multiple
  ii. enhance   no
  iii. location   white matter
  iv. mass effect   none
  v. miscellaneous   high on T2 and low on T1

16

31. **Complete the following about the neurologic manifestations of AIDS:** G7 p. 366:135mm
a. treatment for toxoplasmosis
   i. p_____   pyrimethamine
   ii. s_____   sulfadiazine
b. How promptly should we see improvement clinically and radiologically?   2 to 3 weeks G7 p. 367:68mm
c. If successful how long should toxoplasmosis be controlled?   for patient's lifetime if meds are continued
d. Biopsy should be considered if there is no response in _____ _____.   3 weeks (some say 7 to 10 days) G7 p. 367:82mm

32. **Complete the following about the neurologic manifestations of AIDS:** G7 p.366:160mm
a. Can toxoplasmosis be radiologically distinguished from
   i. lymphoma?   no
   ii. PML?   usually
b. Therefore check
   i. for toxo _____ _____ _____   serum toxo titers
   ii. for lymphoma _____ study for c_____, PCR a_____ of v_____ D_____   LP (if no mass effect); cytology; amplification of viral DNA

33. **Considerations for performing a biopsy of a brain lesion in a HIV+ patient** G7 p.367:15mm
a. if toxo titers are _____   negative
b. if no response to toxo meds in _____   3 weeks
c. True or False. Biopsy is equally valuable in lesions that enhance or don't enhance.   false (more valuable in enhancing lesions to differentiate toxoplasmosis from lymphoma) G7 p.367:113mm
d. technique for biopsy _____   stereotactic
e. What two areas should be sampled?   enhancing rim and the center
f. Positive biopsy can be expected in _____%.   96% G7 p.367:120mm

34. **Indicate the survival times for AIDS patients with the following conditions:** G7 p.367:160mm
a. CNS toxo _____   15 months
b. PML _____   15 months
c. lymphoma _____   3 months versus 1 month without treatment
d. lymphoma in nonimmunosuppressed patient _____   13.5 months

Lyme Disease—Neurologic Manifestations

35. Complete the following regarding Lyme disease: G7 p.368:30mm

a. It is caused by a _____.   spirochete transmitted by a tick

b. The hallmark skin lesion is called e_____ c_____ m_____.   erythema chronicum migrans

c. The clinical triad consists of
 i.   c_____ n_____   cranial neuritis
 ii. m_____   meningitis
 iii. r_____   radiculopathy

d. On clinical exam, don't be misled into diagnosing _____ _____.   Bell palsy (The seventh nerve weakness in Lyme disease is common.)

e. On CSF exam, don't be misled into diagnosing _____ _____.   multiple sclerosis (MS) (from the oligoclonal bands that also occur in Lyme disease)

f. What is the most common cause of bilateral Bell palsy?   Lyme disease cranial neuritis   G7 p.368:110mm

36. Complete the following about Lyme disease neurologic manifestations: G7 p.369:100mm

a. What two conditions share an uncommon CSF finding?   MS (multiple sclerosis) and Lyme disease

b. The CSF component they share is _____ _____.   oligoclonal bands

Parasitic Infections of the Central Nervous System

37. Cysticercosis is a disease caused by   G7 p.370:60mm

a. Which organism?   *Taenia solium*

b. At which life cycle stage?   larval stage

c. The life cycle stages (4) include the following:
 Hint: eael
 i.   e_____   embryo
 ii. a_____   adult
 iii. e_____   eggs
 iv. l_____   larva

d. The current best test is _____- _____ _____ _____.   enzyme-linked immunoelectrotransfer blot

38. Complete the following statements about parasitic infections of the CNS: G7 p.370:65mm

a. Cysticercosis is caused by
 i.   the p_____ t_____   pork tapeworm
 ii. *T_____ s_____*   *Taenia solium*

b. Echinococcus is caused by
 i.   the d_____ t_____   dog tapeworm
 ii. *E_____ g_____*   *Echinococcus granulosa*   G7 p.373:80mm

c. What is hydatid sand?   germinating parasitic scoleces   G7 p.373:120mm

16

d. Caution is advised during removal not to _____.   rupture the *Echinococcus* cyst and contaminate adjacent tissues   G7 p.373:135mm

39. Describe the life cycle of cysticercosis.   G7 p.370:85mm

a. Pig contains _____ _____ in its flesh.   encysted embryo

b. Humans eat undercooked _____ with _____ in it.   pork with embryo

c. Embryo matures to an _____.   adult

d. The _____ produces eggs.   adult

e. Eggs are released in the _____ of the human.   feces

f. The same or a different human _____ the _____.   ingests the eggs (from contaminated fingers, vegetables, or water)

g. Eggs in this host release _____   larvae

h. which burrow through the _____ _____ _____ to _____.   small bowel wall to circulation

i. Larva lands and develops a _____ _____   cyst wall

j. and becomes an _____ _____   encysted embryo

k. in _____ months.   4

40. Answer the following concerning neurocysticercosis: G7 p.371:107mm

a. What is the permanent host for the adult tapeworm?   human

b. What is the intermediate host?   human or animal (pig)

41. Answer the following concerning neurocysticercosis: G7 p.371:175mm

a. What is the significance of CT scan with

　　i. low-density cysts with eccentric punctate high-density spots in an enhancing ring?   living cysticerci

　　ii. above plus edema?   dying cysticerci

　　iii. intraparenchymal punctate calcifications?   dead parasites

b. What may soft tissue x-rays show?   calcifications in thigh or shoulder

c. What might MRI show?   intraventricular or cisternal cysts

42. Complete the following regarding CT in cysticercosis: G7 p.372:20mm

a. Ring-enhancing cysts suggest _____ _____.   living cysticerci

b. Intraparenchymal punctate calcifications suggest _____ _____.   dead parasites

c. Ring-enhancing cyst with edema suggests

　　i. _____ with   recently dead or dying parasite

　　ii. _____   inflammatory reaction

16

Fungal Infections of the CNS

43. **What organism can cause a cerebral abscess in an organ transplant patient?**

Aspergillus fumigatus

G7 p.374:80mm

44. **Name the most common fungal infection of the CNS diagnosed in the living patient.**

cryptococcosis

G7 p.374:100mm

Amoebic Infections of CNS

45. **Describe amoebic infections of the CNS.**

G7 p.375:120mm

   a. The only amoeba known to cause infection is _____ _____.

Naegleria fowleri

   b. Infection occurs 5 days after exposure in warm _____.

freshwater

   c. The amoeba gains entry to the CNS via the _____ _____.

olfactory mucosa

   d. 95% die within _____ _____

1 week

   e. due to _____.

↑ ICP

   f. Prescribe with _____ _____.

amphotericin B

Spine Infections

46. **Describe spinal epidural abscess.**

G7 p.367:140mm

   a. Most common site for spinal epidural abscess is the _____ at _____%.

thoracic level at 50%

   b. The next most common is

   i. _____ at _____%

lumbar at 35%

   ii. _____ at _____%

cervical at 15%

   c. Symptoms of epidural abscess are

   i. s_____ p_____

severe pain over the area

   ii. p_____ upon p_____

pain upon percussion

   iii. f_____

fever

47. **What is the pathophysiology of cord in spinal epidural abscess?**

G7 p.377:45mm

   a. compression by

   i. m_____ of a_____

mass of abscess

   ii. b_____ by c_____ of o_____ v_____ b_____

bone by collapse of osteomyelitic vertebral body

   b. infarction by v_____ t_____

venous thrombophlebitis

   c. direct spread to cord can cause _____

myelitis

16

48. Complete the following regarding causes of spinal epidural abscess: G7 p.377:100mm

a. hematogenous—most commonly from
  i. f_____   furuncle
  ii. IV _____ _____   drug abuse
b. direct extension from a p_____   psoas abscess
   a_____
c. spinal procedures
  i. d_____   discectomy (incidence of SEA 0.67%)
  ii. n_____   needles (catheters)
d. Underlying causes are
   Hint: idlra
  i.   i_____ c_____   immune compromised
  ii. d_____   diabetes
  iii. IV d_____ a_____   IV drug abuse
  iv. r_____ f_____   renal failure
  v.   a_____   alcoholism

49. Complete the following concerning psoas abscess: G7 p.377:160mm

a. Muscle extends from T_____ to L_____   T12 to L5
b. Psoas is the primary hip_____   flexor
c. Innervated by _____   L2, L3
d. Proximity to sources of _____   infection
e. Pain on _____ flexion   hip
f. CT shows _____ of psoas shadow   enlargement   G7 p.378:80mm
g. Inside the _____ wing   iliac

50. Cultures from spinal epidural abscess patients can be expected to show the following: G7 p.378:100mm

a. *Staphylococcus aureus* _____%   50%— the main organism
b. no growth _____%   30 to 50%
c. *Streptococcus* (frequency)   second-most-common organism
d. tuberculosis (TB) associated with _____ disease _____%   Potts disease; 25%
e. multiple organisms _____%   10%

51. Complete the following regarding spinal epidural abscess (SEA):   G7 p.378:175mm

a. If during the spinal tap you encounter pus, what should you do?   stop advancing needle and send pus for culture
b. The best test if you suspect SEA is _____.   MRI
c. Treatment includes
   Hint: eabc
  i.   e_____   evaluation
  ii. a_____   antibiotics
  iii. b_____   bracing—immobilization
  iv. c_____   compression relief if present

16

d. If no organism is known, start empiric antibiotics of
Hint: cvr

   i.   c_____   cephalosporin third-generation (cefotaxime)

   ii.   v_____   vancomycin
   iii.   r_____   rifampin

52. Complete the following regarding spinal infections: G7 p.380:35mm

a. The length of time IV antibiotics should be administered for spinal epidural abscess is _____.   3 to 4 weeks

b. The length of time IV antibiotics should be administered for vertebral osteomyelitis is _____.   6 to 8 weeks

c. Follow with _____.   serial sedimentation (ESR) rates

d. Mortality is _____%.   4 to 31%
e. Recovery of neurologic deficit is _____ _____.   very rare

f. An exception to the rule is _____ _____—_____% improve.   Potts disease—50% improve neurologically

■ Vertebral Osteomyelitis

53. Complete the following regarding spine infections: G7 p.380:85mm

a. vertebral osteomyelitis risk factors
Hint: d^{3}e

   i.   d_____   drug abusers
   ii.   d_____   dialysis patients
   iii.   d_____   diabetes
   iv.   e_____   elderly

b. What condition in renal patients can mimic infection on MRI?   destructive spondyloarthropathy   G7 p.1233:30mm

c. Sources of infection are never found in _____%.   37% (consider urinary tract infection [UTI], respiratory tract, teeth)

d. Neurologic deficits occur in _____% of Pott's disease patients.   10 to 47%

54. Answer the following about spine infections: G7 p.382:105mm

a. How long does it take for plain x-rays to demonstrate changes in osteomyelitis?   2 to 8 weeks

b. What % of cases can be successfully managed nonoperatively?   90%

55. True or False. Regarding treatment of vertebral osteomyelitis: G7 p.383:73mm

a. Instrumented fusion is contraindicated.   false
b. It is permitted even in pyogenic infections.   true

16

■ Discitis

56. One differentiates spine destruction from G7 p.384:45mm

a. infection: i_____ d_____   involves the disc
b. metastases: m_____ d_____   miss the disc and involve the
                                         vertebral body

57. What is the MRI triad of infection? Enhancement of G7 p.384:120mm

a. a_____ p_____ p_____   annulus posterior portion
b. b_____ m_____   bone marrow
c. d_____ s_____   disc space

58. What is the CT triad of infection? G7 p.384:160mm

a. e_____ p_____ f_____   end plate fragmentation
b. p_____ s_____   paravertebral swelling
c. p_____ a_____   paravertebral abscess

59. Complete the following regarding discitis: G7 p.385:70mm

a. Cultures are positive
   i. from disc space in _____%.   60%
   ii. from blood in _____%.   50%
b. The usual pathogen is _____.   *Staphylococcus aureus*
c. Special staining is required to detect   TB in all cases
   _____.

60. Complete the following about discitis: G7 p.386:100mm

a. In children discitis manifests itself by the   walk or stand or sit
   child refusing to _____ or _____
   or _____.
b. Postop discitis is suggested when the   G7 p.387:90mm
   i. Erythrocyte sedimentation rate   20 mm/hour
       (ESR) is raised in infection to above
       _____ and does not come down.
   ii. CRP reactive protein above   10; 2
       _____ mg/L at _____ weeks
       postop.
c. Interval between surgery and   G7 p.387:135mm
   radiological changes in discitis
   i. plain x-rays _____ weeks   12 (1 to 8 months range)
   ii. polytomography _____ weeks   3 to 8

61. The empiric antibiotic treatment for postop discitis is G7 p.388:30mm

a. v_____   vancomycin
b. r_____   rifampin
c. C_____   Ceftizox

16

17

Seizures

Seizures

1. **Name the two major categories of seizures.**

   G7 p.394:60mm

   a. g_____   generalized
   b. p_____   partial

2. **List the six major types of primary generalized seizures.**
   Hint: magcat

   G7 p.394:60mm

   a. m_____   myoclonic
   b. a_____   atonic (drop attacks)
   c. g_____   generalized (grand mal)
   d. c_____   clonic
   e. a_____   absence (petit mal)
   f. t_____   tonic

3. **What are the major differences between primary generalized and partial seizures?**

   G7 p.394:60mm

   a. primary generalized
      i. areas involved   bilateral and symmetrical
      ii. percent of seizures   40% of all seizures
      iii. consciousness   loss of consciousness at onset
      iv. significance   does not suggest structural lesion

   b. partial
      i. areas involved   one hemisphere
      ii. percent of seizures   57% of all seizures
      iii. consciousness   no loss of consciousness at onset
      iv. significance   suggests structural lesion

4. Matching. Match the type of seizure with its listed characteristic(s). More than one may apply.   G7 p.394:70mm

Characteristic:
① 3% of seizures; ② 40% of seizures; ③ 57% of seizures; ④ consciousness lost from onset; ⑤ tonic clonic motor activity; ⑥ involves both hemispheres; ⑦ no postictal confusion; ⑧ spike and wave exactly 3/s; ⑨ represents a structural lesion

Seizure:
a. generalized   ②, ④, ⑤, ⑥
b. partial   ③, ⑨
c. unclassified   ①
d. absence   ⑦, ⑧

5. The main difference is that simple partial seizures have   G7 p.394:120mm

a. _____ _____ of _____   no loss of consciousness
   and complex partial seizures have
b. _____ of _____.   loss of consciousness

6. Briefly describe the following characteristics of absence seizures: G7 p.395:70mm

a. motor involvement _____   absent
b. postictal state _____   absent
c. loss of consciousness _____   absent
d. characteristic electroencephalography   abnormal EEG 3/s spike and
   (EEG) of _____   wave
e. effect of hyperventilation _____ induces seizures

7. Briefly describe the following characteristics of uncinate seizures: G7 p.395:100mm

a. arise from _____-_____   uncus-hippocampus
b. produce hallucinations of _____ odor
c. kakosmia is perception of _____ bad odors
   where none exist

8. Complete the following about seizures: G7 p.395:120mm

a. What is the most common cause of   mesial temporal sclerosis
   intractable temporal lobe epilepsy?
b. due to _____   loss of cells in hippocampus
c. treated by _____   medication till refractory then
                                       surgery

9. Name the rare syndrome with the following features: childhood onset, drop attacks, treatment by valproic acid, and surgery by corpus callosotomy.   Lennox-Gastaut syndrome   G7 p.396:45mm

10. **Describe Todd paralysis.**   G7 p.396:60mm
    a. occurs after _____   seizure
    b. causes _____   weakness
    c. resolves with _____   time
    d. another name for it is _____   postictal paralysis

11. **Name factors that lower seizure**   G7 p.396:90mm
    threshold.
    Hint: seizure history
    i.   s_____   stroke
    ii.   e_____   elevated temperature, fever
    iii. i_____   infection, intoxication
    iv.   z_____   "zzzzs" lost (sleep
                                   deprivation, fatigue)
    v.   u_____   uremia
    vi.   r_____   repeated seizures (kindling)
    vii. e_____   electrolyte imbalance pH,
                                   Mg++, low NA, high Ca++
    viii. h_____   hyperventilation,
                                   hyponatremia, hypoglycemia,
                                   hypercalcemia
    ix.   i_____   ischemia
    x.   s_____   stimulation (photic)
    xi.   t_____   trauma, tumor
    xii. o_____   opioids
    xiii. r_____   removal or withdrawal of
                                   alcohol or antiseizure meds
                                   suddenly
    xiv. y_____   youth (birth asphysia,
                                   congenital central nervous
                                   system [CNS] abnormalities)

■ Special Types of Seizures

12. **Complete the following about special**   G7 p.396:150mm
    types of seizures:
    a. Incidence of new-onset seizures per   44 per 100,000
       100,000 person years is _____.
    b. % that recur   27%
    c. If all studies are normal can you release   no
       the patient from your care?
    d. What should you do?   repeat CT or MRI
    e. For how long?   6 months and again in 1 or   G7 p.397:140mm
                                               2 years

13. **What are the two categories of**   G7 p.398:48mm
    posttraumatic seizures?
    a. _____ within _____ days   early within 7 days after
                                               trauma
    b. _____ beyond _____ days   late beyond 7 days after
                                               trauma

17

14. Complete the following about special types of seizures: G7 p.398:55mm

a. True or False. Anticonvulsants prevent early posttraumatic seizures and reduce the frequency of late posttraumatic seizures.

false (Anticonvulsants have been shown to reduce the risk of *early* posttraumatic seizures, up to 1 week, but they do not reduce the frequency of *late* posttraumatic seizures.)

b. Therefore, you should stop antiepileptic drugs (AEDs) after _____.

1 week

15. Incidence of seizures in early posttrauma period (1 to 7 days) is   G7 p.398:70mm

a. _____% in severe head injuries   30%

b. _____% in mild to moderate head injuries   1%

16. Incidence of late seizures (greater than 7 days) is _____% over a 2-year period.   10 to 13%   G7 p.398:90mm

17. True or False. The incidence of posttraumatic seizures is higher with closed head injuries than with penetrating head injuries.

false (The incidence is higher with penetrating head injuries; occurs in 50% of cases followed 15 years.)   G7 p.398:120mm

18. Answer the following concerning posttraumatic seizures: G7 p.398:140mm

a. Is there any treatment that reduces the

   i. frequency of late posttraumatic seizures?   no

   ii. frequency of early posttraumatic seizures?   yes

   iii. by how much?   75%

b. What may reduce the frequency?   antiseizure medication

   i. To be used for how long?   1 week

   ii. Are there any exceptions to that length of time?   yes

   iii. What are they?   penetrating wound, craniotomy, prior seizures

c. What do we mean when we say late posttraumatic seizure (PTS)?   1 week after the trauma

19. What occurs with long-term Dilantin use?   adverse cognitive effects   G7 p.398:150mm

20. True or False. Antiepileptic drugs have been shown to   G7 p.398:160mm

a. impede epileptogenesis   false

b. reduce the incidence of late posttraumatic seizures   false

c. improve outcome by reducing posttraumatic seizures   false

d. reduce seizure recurrence after epilepsy has developed   true

e. all of the above   false

17

21. **True or False. Indications for AEDs after trauma include**   G7 p.399:15mm
    a. alcohol abuse   true
    b. computed tomographic (CT) scan shows blood in brain   true
    c. Glasgow Coma Scale (GCS) score below 10   true
    d. seizure after injury   true

22. **Using AEDs after head trauma can result in _____ in early posttraumatic seizures.**   reduction   G7 p.399:15mm

23. **True or False. In appropriate patients, antiepileptic drugs should be tapered off after**   G7 p.399:50mm
    a. 24 hours   false
    b. 48 hours   false
    c. 7 days   true
    d. 14 days   false
    e. 6 months   false

24. **True or False. Physicians should continue antiepileptic drugs longer than 1 week in patients with**   G7 p.399:55mm
    a. penetrating brain injury   true
    b. development of late posttraumatic seizures   true
    c. prior seizure history   true
    d. undergoing craniotomy   true

25. **True or False. Ethanol withdrawal seizures are seen in 33% of habitual drinkers within _____ of stopping or reducing ethanol intake.**   G7 p.399:95mm
    a. 1 to 2 hours   false
    b. 3 to 5 days   false
    c. 7 to 30 hours   true
    d. 1 to 2 weeks   false

26. **Answer the following about alcohol withdrawal patients:**   G7 p.399:105mm
    a. What occurs first: delirium tremens (DTs) or seizures?   seizures
    b. Risk of onset of seizures lasts for _____.   48 hours (2 days)
    c. Risk of onset of DTs lasts for _____.   96 hours (4 days)   G7 p.274:30mm
    d. Risk persists for _____ days.   1 to 3 days   G7 p.275:20mm
    e. Are AEDs recommended?
       i.   for prophylaxis?   yes, as prophylaxis only
       ii. for treatment?   no (Because seizure is usually single, brief, and self-limited, AEDs are not indicated once seizure has occurred.)

27. **True or False. Patients with ethanol withdrawal seizures should receive long-term antiepileptic drugs if they have**

G7 p.399:175mm

a. history of prior ethanol withdrawal seizures — true

b. recurrent seizures — true

c. history of prior seizure disorder unrelated to ethanol — true

d. risk factors for seizures (e.g., subdural hematoma) — true

■ Nonepileptic Seizures

28. **Answer the following about nonepileptic seizures (NES):**

G7 p.400:32mm

a. aka pse_____ — pseudoseizures

b. aka psy_____ — psychogenic

c. True or False

  i. They are real events. — true

  ii. They may not be under voluntary control. — true

  iii. They are helped by AEDs. — false

  iv. Up to 50% of these patients also have legitimate seizures at times. — true

29. **What are the features suggestive of nonepileptic seizures (NES)?**

G7 p.401:75mm

a. This feature is 90% specific for NES: _____ of the _____ — arching; back

b. Another feature that is very specific is w_____ — weeping

c. Forced eye _____ — closing

d. Bilateral shaking with preserved _____ — awareness

e. Variable _____ _____ — seizure types

f. Clonic UE or LE movements that are _____ _____ _____ — out of phase

g. Pelvic _____ — thrust

h. Altered by _____ — distraction

30. **A feature strongly suggestive of epileptic seizure is l_____ t_____ l_____.** — lateral tongue laceration

G7 p.401:160mm

17

31. **True or False. Nonepileptic seizures (NES) can be detected with the following:**   G7 p.401:135mm

    a. out of phase (arrhythmic) motor activity   true
    b. lack of vocalization at start of seizure   true
    c. lack of postictal confusion or lethargy   true
    d. absence of urinary incontinence   false (Absence of urinary incontinence may be the case in both epileptic seizures and NES and therefore can't be used to differentiate.)
    e. suggestible or inducible seizures   true

32. **True or False. Which serum hormone may be used to confirm a true seizure versus nonepileptic seizures (psychogenic seizures)?**   G7 p.401:165mm

    a. TSH   false
    b. ACTH   false
    c. Cortisol   false
    d. GH   false
    e. prolactin   true

33. **To use this test, blood must be drawn promptly because peak levels of the hormone are reached in _____ .**   20 minutes   G7 p.401:165mm

34. **True or False. The most common type of seizure is**   G7 p.402:85mm

    a. ethanol withdrawal   false
    b. tumor induced   false
    c. posttraumatic   false
    d. febrile   true
    e. epileptic   false

35. **True or False. Antiepileptic drugs that prevent afebrile seizures after a febrile seizure include**   G7 p.402:115mm

    a. phenobarbital   false
    b. phenytoin   false
    c. valproic acid   false
    d. carbamazepine   false
    e. none of the above   true (Diazepam may be helpful during period of fever.)

■ Status Epilepticus

36. **True or False. Status epilepticus is defined as more than 5 minutes of**   G7 p.402:178mm

    a. continuous seizures   true
    b. multiple seizures without fully recovering consciousness   true
    c. persistent seizure despite 1st and 2nd line AED   true

17

37. Complete the following about status epilepticus (SE):   G7 p.403:170mm
a. The mean duration of status is _____ hours.   1.5
b. The mortality from SE is _____ %.   1 to 2%
c. The mortality from underlying acute event is _____ %.   10 to 12%
d. Irreversible changes from repetitive electrical discharges begin to appear in neurons as early as _____ minutes.   20
e. Cell death may occur after _____ minutes.   60

38. For a patient in status epilepticus, the workup includes the following: G7 p.404:70mm
Hint: abcell
a. a_____   airway
b. b_____   blood pressure
c. c_____   CPR
d. e_____   EKG, EEG, electrolytes
e. I_____   IV
f. l_____   lumbar puncture

39. Complete the following regarding lumbar puncture (LP) after a seizure: G7 p.404:105mm
a. LP after a seizure may show _____.   elevated white count
b. This may be b_____ p_____ p_____.   benign postictal pleocytosis
c. Treat as _____.   infection with antibiotics until cultures return

40. Medications for patients in status epilepticus and their amount are   G7 p.404:115mm
Hint: bAnd DIpt
a. b_____   bicarbonate—2 ampules IV
b. A_____   Ativan—4 mg slowly IV
c. n_____   naloxone—0.4 mg IV
d. d_____   dextrose—25 to 50 mL of a 50% solution
e. D_____   Dilantin—20 mg/kg slowly IV normal saline (NS)
f. I_____   IV NS
g. p_____   phenobarbital—20 mg/kg IV
h. t_____   thiamine—50 to 100 mg IV

41. True or False. The following medications are used in treating status epilepticus: G7 p.405:35mm
a. lorazepam   true
b. phenytoin   true
c. phenobarbital   true
d. general anesthesia   true
e. all of the above   true

42. What is the safe rate?   G7 p.405:35mm
  a. For Dilantin _____ mg/minute   50 mg/minute
  b. For phenobarbital _____ mg/minute   100 mg/minute

43. What IV fluid must be used for giving   normal saline to avoid   G7 p.406:18mm
    Dilantin and why?   precipitation

44. Complete the following about   G7 p.406:135mm
    diazepam:
  a. name (proprietary)   Valium
  b. stops seizures in _____   80% in 5 minutes
  c. preferred drug   no (stored in fat)
  d. seizures recur in _____   in 20 minutes
  e. aborts seizures %   68%
  f. depresses respiration   more
  g. dose   10 mg

45. Complete the following about   G7 p.406:145mm
    lorazepam:
  a. name (proprietary)   Ativan
  b. preferred drug   yes
  c. aborts seizures %   97%
  d. depresses respiration   less
  e. dose   4 mg

46. True or False. The drug of choice for   G7 p.407:40mm
    myoclonic status epilepticus is
  a. lorazepam   true
  b. benzodiazepine   false
  c. Dilantin   false
  d. phenobarbital   false
  e. diazepam   false

47. True or False. The drug of choice for   G7 p.407:55mm
    absence status epilepticus is
  a. valproic acid   true
  b. benzodiazepine   false
  c. dilantin   false
  d. phenobarbital   false
  e. diazepam   false

■ Antiepileptic Drugs

48. What % of patients can achieve   75 to 80%   G7 p.407:80mm
    control of seizures with medical
    therapy?

49. Indicate the drug of choice for each   G7 p.407:145mm
    type of seizure.
  a. generalized tonic-clonic
    i. _____   valproic acid
    ii. _____   Dilantin
  b. absence _____   valproic acid
  c. myloclonic _____   lorazepam

17

d. tonic or atonic _____	lorazepam
e. partial	
i. _____	Tegretol
ii. _____	Dilantin

50. **True or False. Increase a given medication until seizures are controlled or side effects become intolerable, but do not rely solely on therapeutic levels, which are only a range in which most patients have seizure control without side effects.**   true   G7 p.409:35mm

51. **True or False. 75 to 80% of epileptics can be controlled on monotherapy.**   true   G7 p.409:35mm

52. **True or False. Only 10% of epileptics benefit significantly from the addition of a second drug.**   true   G7 p.409:52 mm

53. **True or False. If more than two AEDs are required, consider whether the patient might have nonepileptic seizures.**   true   G7 p.409:52mm

54. **Give the characteristics of Dilantin.**   G7 p.409:155mm

a. half-life _____	24 hours, range 9 to 140 hours
b. oral loading dose _____	300 PO every 4 hours until 17 mg/kg given
c. Can we use IM route?	no
d. rate by IV _____	not more than 50 mg/min
e. permitted solution _____ _____	normal saline
f. How many half-lives until you reach a steady state?	5; therefore, 7 to 21 days

55. **Complete the following about Dilantin:**   G7 p.409:155mm

a. How long does it take for Dilantin to reach a steady state?	7 to 21 days
b. Dilantin can be safely withdrawn over a _____ period gradually.	4-week
c. What is the safe rate at which Dilantin may be given IV?	50 mg/minute

56. **True or False. Fosphenytoin Na (Fos) injection has the following advantages over conventional IV phenytoin:**   G7 p.411:40mm

a. The maximum administration rate is three times as fast (i.e., 150 mg/minute).	true
b. Fos is water soluble and therefore may be infused with saline or dextrose.	true
c. There is less venous irritation due to lower pH of 8.6 to 9 compared with 12 for Dilantin.	true

57. Study Chart.   G7 p.411:85mm
Side effects of Dilantin

i.	a_____	ataxia
ii.	b_____	birth control pills less effective
iii.	c_____	cognitive dysfunction, cerebellar degeneration
iv.	d_____	drug interactions, Prozac
v.	e_____	epidermal necrolysis
vi.	g_____	gingival hyperplasia
vii.	h_____	hirsutism
viii.	l_____	liver granulomas, Lupus
ix.	m_____	megaloblastic anemia
x.	n_____	newborn hemorrhage
xi.	o_____	osteomalacia
xii.	p_____	papular rash
xiii.	r_____	rickets
xiv.	s_____	Stevens-Johnson syndrome/systemic lupus erythematosus (SLE)-like syndrome
xv.	t_____	teratogenic
xvi.	v_____	vitamin D antagonism

58. Describe Tegretol.   G7 p.411:135mm
a. indication

i.	p_____ s_____	partial seizures
ii.	t_____ n_____	trigeminal neuralgia

b. therapeutic level _____ mcg/ml   6 to 12 mcg/ml

c. side effects

i.	a_____	ataxia
ii.	a_____	aplastic anemia
iii.	a_____	agranulocytosis
iv.	b_____	blood dyscrasia
v.	c_____	cymetidine
vi.	d_____	drowsiness
vii.	d_____	diplopia
viii.	D_____	Darvon
ix.	e_____	erythromycin
x.	f_____	fatal hepatitis
xi.	g_____	gastrointestinal upset
xii.	i_____	isoniazid
xiii.	S_____	Stevens-Johnson syndrome
xiv.	S_____	SIADH

17

17

59. Describe carbamazepine.   G7 p.411:136 mm
  a. also known as _____   Tegretol
  b. test for C_____, p_____,   CBC, platelets, iron
     i_____
  c. test according to what schedule
     i.   _____ time(s) per week for   1; 3 months
          _____ _____
     ii. _____ time(s) per month for   1; 3 years
          _____ _____
  d. discontinue drug if levels fall below
     i.   WBC _____   4,000
     ii. RBC _____   3,000,000
     iii. HCT _____   32
     iv. platelets _____   100,000
     v.   reticulocytes _____   0.3%
     vi. iron rises to _____   higher than 150 microgram%
  e. increase dose as follows: _____ pill   1 pill per day per week
     per _____ per _____

60. True or False. When used for   G7 p.412:17mm
     treatment of trigeminal neuralgia or
     partial seizures with or without
     generalization, carbamazepine
     (Tegretol) has both
  a. erratic oral absorption although oral   true   G7 p.412:75mm
     suspension is absorbed more readily
  b. dramatic elevation of CBZ levels with   true
     cimetidine, isoniazid, erythromycin, and
     propoxyphene (Darvon) drug-drug
     interaction

61. Describe valproate.   G7 p.412:155mm
  a. also known as _____   Depakote
  b. indication _____   generalized tonic clonic
  c. therapeutic level _____ to _____   50 to 100 mcg/ml
     mcg/ml
  d. side effects (list at least five)   confusion
                                                drowsy
                                                hyperammonemia
                                                hair loss
                                                liver failure
                                                neural tube defects
                                                platelet dysfunction
                                                teratogenic, tremor
                                                weight gain

62. True or False. Acetylsalicylic acid   true   G7 p.413:44mm
     displaces valproic acid from serum
     protein.

63. True or False. Valproic acid causes   true   G7 p.413:72mm
     neural tube defects in 1 to 2% of
     patients.

64. Describe phenobarbital.
G7 p.413:95mm

a. indication _____ _____ _____   generalized tonic clonic
b. therapeutic level _____ mcg/ml   15 to 30 mcg/ml
c. half-life _____, steady state _____   5 days; 30 days

d. side effects
  i.   c_____   cognitive
  ii. d_____   drowsiness
  iii. p_____ h_____   paradoxical hyperactivity
  iv. h_____ in n_____   hemorrhage in newborns if mother is on phenobarbital

65. True or False. Indicate whether the following statements about antiepileptic drugs are true or false:
G7 p.413:145mm

a. Phenobarbital is a potent inducer of hepatic enzymes that metabolize other AEDs.   true
b. Cognitive impairment may be subtle and may outlast administration of the drug by at least several months.   true
c. They may cause hemorrhage in newborn if mother is on phenobarbital.   true

66. True or False. The following are characteristics of Diamox (acetazolamide):
G7 p.416:70mm

a. It reduces cerebrospinal fluid (CSF) production.   true
b. It may have antiepileptic effect either due to slight central nervous system (CNS) acidosis or due to its direct inhibition of CNS carbonic anhydrase.   true

67. Describe withdrawal of AEDs.
G7 p.418:160mm

a. taper by _____   1 unit every 2 weeks
b. role of EEG _____   if EEG shows epileptiform discharge, discourage AED withdrawal

c. relapse rate_____%   35%
d. over how long? _____ _____   8 months

68. Complete the following about antiepileptic drugs:
G7 p.419:104mm

a. What effect do antiepileptic medications have on birth control pills? They increase the _____ _____ _____.   failure rate fourfold

b. Why?
  i.   AEDs induce liver _____ _____ _____ _____,   microsomal cytochrome P450 enzymes
  ii. which degrades the _____ _____ _____.   birth control medication

17

17

c. What is the effect of an isolated seizure on pregnancy? — little—usually cause no problem

d. The effect of status epilepticus on pregnancy is serious to _____ and _____. — mother and child

69. **Considering seizures, AEDs, and birth defects, describe the following:**　　　　G7 p.419:165mm

a. effect of seizure history on incidence of fetal malformations — double 4 to 5%

b. phenobarbital and malformations — the worst 9.1%—highest rate of malformations

c. teratogenic properties in
   i.   Dilantin — fetal hydantoin syndrome lower IQ
   ii. Tegretol — neural tube defects—rare
   iii. valproate — neural tube defects 1 to 2%

d. therefore, during pregnancy
   i.   first choice is _____ — carbamazepine—lowest dose possible (Tegretol)
   ii. second choice is _____ — valproic acid
   iii. add _____ — folate
   iv. use _____ — monotherapy

■ Seizure Surgery

70. **What percent of patients are not controlled with medication?** — 20%　　　　G7 p.420:85mm

71. **Surgery is for refractory seizures.**　　　　G7 p.420:102mm
a. nature of seizures — severe disabling
b. length of treatment — at least 1 year
c. How many trials? — three (two mono- and one polytherapy)

72. **Name the seizure types for which surgery is appropriate.**　　　　G7 p.420:115mm
Hint: teLi
a. t_____ — temporal
b. e_____ — extratemporal
c. L_____-G_____ — Lennox-Gastaut
d. i_____ h_____ s_____ — infantile hemiplegia syndrome

73. **Complete the following about seizure surgery:**

G7 p.420:175mm

a. Can you see a seizure on diagnostic images?

yes

b. Give examples.

   i. CT with IV contrast _____ _____ _____

focus may enhance

   ii. positron emission tomography (PET) _____ in _____%

hypometabolism; 70%

   iii. single-photon emission computed tomography (SPECT) _____ _____ _____

increased blood flow during a seizure

c. Best test for hippocampal asymmetry for MTS, which produces CPS is m_____ t_____ s_____ c_____ p_____ s_____ in _____.

mesial temporal sclerosis complex partial seizures in MRI

74. **Complete the following about the Wada test:**

G7 p.421:70mm

a. The purpose is to localize _____ _____.

dominant hemisphere (side of language)

b. You can be misled by

   i. a _____ m_____

arteriovenous malformation (AVM)

   ii. p_____ t_____ a_____

persistent trigeminal artery

   iii. h_____ s_____ by p_____ c_____

hippocampus supplied by posterior circulation

75. **Surgical disconnection operations available are**

G7 p.422:60mm

a. c_____

callosotomy

b. h_____

hemispherectomy

c. m_____ s_____ t_____

multiple subpial transections

76. **Complete the following regarding temporal lobectomy limits:**

G7 p.423:100mm

a. on dominant side permitted

   i. _____

4 to 5 cm

   ii. too much _____

injures speech

b. on nondominant side permitted

   i. _____

6 to 7 cm

   ii. too much _____

contralateral partial upper quadrant homonymous hemianopsia (Hint: clpuqhh)

c. greater resection of

   i. _____ will cause

8 to 9 cm

   ii. _____ _____

contralateral complete upper quadrant homonymous hemianopsia (Hint: clcuqhh)

17

77. Complete the following about corpus callosotomy (CC):   G7 p.422:180mm

a. Indication for corpus callosotomy

    i.   d_____ a_____—a_____ s_____   drop attacks—atonic seizures

    ii. i_____ h_____ s_____   infantile hemiplegia syndrome

b. How much of the CC is resected?   anterior two thirds

c. Complication is _____.   akinetic mutism or reduced verbalization temporary

d. Must the anterior commissure also be sectioned?   no—less likely to get disconnection syndrome if spared

e. Contraindication   crossed dominance

f. Exclude by _____ _____ on all _____ _____.   Wada test on all left-handed persons

78. Answer the following about corpus callosotomy: G7 p.423:58mm

a. What test should be done preoperatively?   Wada

b. In which group of patients?   left-handed

c. Why? To identify those with _____ _____.   crossed dominance

79. Answer the following about disconnection syndrome in a left-dominant person (i.e., right-handed):   G7 p.423:70mm

a. usually lasts _____   2 to 3 months

b. effect on

    i.   left hand _____   tactile anomia

    ii.   vision _____   pseudohemianopsia

    iii. smell _____   anomia for smell

    iv. copying figures (i.e., spatial synthesis) _____ _____ _____ _____   poor with right hand

    v.   speech _____   reduced spontaneity

    vi. urinary _____   incontinence

    vii. left-sided _____ (resembles _____)   dyspraxia (resembles hemiparesis)

c. occurs with _____   large lesions of corpus-callosum

d. less likely to occur if _____   anterior commissure is spared

80. Describe seizure surgery outcome expectations.   G7 p.424:125mm

a. incidence of being seizure free _____%   50%

b. seizures reduced by at least 50% in _____%   80%

18

Spine and Spinal Cord

■ Low Back Pain and Radiculopathy

1. **Complete the following about low back pain and radiculopathy:**
   G7 p.428:70mm
   a. True or False. Bed rest beyond 4 days may be more harmful than helpful for patients with low back pain.
      true
   b. True or False. 60% of patients with low back pain will improve clinically within 1 month even without treatment.
      false (89 to 90% will improve in 1 month even without treatment)
   c. Pure radicular symptoms will include upper motor neuron (UMN) signs or lower motor neuron (LMN) signs?
      LMN signs (Radiculopathy will/may show associated decreased reflexes, weakness, and atrophy.)

2. **True or False. The percentage of low-risk back pain patients who will improve without treatment in 1 month's time is**
   G7 p.428:78mm
   a. 10%
      false
   b. 20%
      false
   c. 90%
      true (Most low back patients will resolve and no specific diagnosis can be made in 85% despite aggressive workup.)
   d. none
      false

3. **The nucleus pulposus is a remnant of the embryonic _____.**
   notocord
   G7 p.428:160mm

4. **True or False. The following may be considered a nonpathological condition:**
   G7 p.429:37mm
   a. degenerated disc
      false
   b. protruded disc
      false
   c. bulging disc generalized > 50%
      true (Bulging disc is circumferential symmetrical extension of the disc beyond the end plates. Incidence increases with age.)
   d. herniated disc
      false
   e. focal bulging disc
      false

5. **True of False. Gas in the disc usually is a sign of**   G7 p.429:37mm
   a. disc infection   false
   b. disc generation   true
   c. aka v_____ d_____   vacuum disc

6. **An extruded disc where the free fragment is contained by the posterior longitudinal ligament is called a _____ disc.**   sequestered   G7 p.429:95mm

7. **Give the definition of a sequestered disc.**   G7 p.429:95mm
   a. _____ disc   extruded
   b. that has lost _____   continuity
   c. with its disc of _____   origin
   d. also known as a _____ _____ free fragment

8. **Provide the Modic classification.**   G7 p.430:20mm
   a. Type 1 T1W1_____
       T2W1_____   ↓ ↑
   b. Type 2 T1W1_____
       T2W1_____   ↑ ↓
   c. Type 3 T1W1_____
       T2W1_____   ↓ ↓

9. **Kyphosis**   G7 p.430:35mm
   a. is measured by the _____ angle.   Cobb
   b. Drawn with a line parallel to the
       i.   superior end plate of the body   above
            _____ and the
       ii. inferior end plate of the body   below
            _____.

10. **Scoliosis**   G7 p.430:60mm
   a. is a measure of _____ of the   convexity
       curvature.
   b. Drawn with a line parallel to the superior   uppermost
       end plate of the _____ body and the
   c. inferior end plate of the _____ body   lowermost
       involved.
   d. Draw _____ to these lines   perpendicular
   e. and measure the _____.   angle

11. **Oswestry disability index**   G7 p.430:105mm
   a. is a scale used for _____ _____.   back pain
   b. A score of _____% is essentially   45%
       totally disabled.
   c. A functional score is in the _____.   teens

12. **Signs of cauda equina syndrome include**   G7 p.431:110mm
   a. a_____   anesthesia (saddle)
   b. b_____   bladder incontinence
   c. c_____   continence of stool impaired

d. d_____   dolor leg pain (unilateral/bilateral)

e. l_____   leg weakness (unilateral/bilateral)

13. **True or False. Cauda equina syndrome may include the following:**   G7 p.431:110mm
    a. bladder dysfunction (incontinence or retention)   true
    b. Faber sign or Patrick-Faber sign (flexion abduction external rotation)   false (Positive in hip joint disease and does not exacerbate true nerve root compression.)
    c. saddle anesthesia   true
    d. unilateral/bilateral leg weakness/pain   true
    e. fecal incontinence   true

14. **Name the associated nerve root for each of the following:**   G7 p.432:28mm
    a. great toe strength   L5 and some L4
    b. dorsal foot sensation   L5
    c. lateral foot sensation   S1
    d. medial foot sensation   L4
    e. plantar foot sensation   S1
    f. Achilles reflex   S1

15. **For patients with low back pain, red flags for a serious underlying pathology would include signs consistent with what conditions?**   G7 p.432:65mm
    Hint: cisc
    a. c_____   cauda equina syndrome
    b. i_____   infection
    c. s_____   spinal fracture
    d. c_____   cancer

16. **Electromyography (EMG) is *not* helpful to evaluate for myelopathy, myopathy, or nerve root dysfunction unless the symptoms have been present for at least _____ weeks.**   3 to 4 (Results are variable before this time.)   G7 p.432:65mm

17. **True or False. Regarding plain lumbosacral spine x-rays:**   G7 p.434:70mm
    a. Are recommended for routine evaluation of back pain   false
    b. When indicated AP and lateral views are usually adequate   true
    c. Unexpected findings occur frequently   false
    d. Gonadal radiation is insignificant   false
    e. Appropriate in patients who have "red flags"   true

18. True or False. Red flags include   G7 p.434:105mm
a. patients under age 20   true
b. patients over age 50   false (> 70)
c. drug users   true
d. diabetics   true
e. postop urinary tract patients   true
f. persistent pain for more than 1 week   false (> 4 weeks)

19. Complete the following about low   G7 p.435:60mm
back pain and radiculopathy:
a. Signs on MRI that indicate disc
    degeneration include
    i.   increase or decrease of signal   decrease
         intensity on T2-weighted imaging
         (T2WI)?
    ii. increase or decrease of disc height? decrease
b. Signs on computed tomography (CT)
    that indicate disc herniation include
    i.   increase or decrease of the normal   decrease
         epidural fat?
    ii. _____ of the thecal sac   indentation
c. Will CT show loss of concavity, or   convexity   G7 p.435:96mm
    convexity, of the thecal sac?

20. Other useful tests include the   G7 p.435:155mm
following:
a. myelogram-CT. Identifies contribution to bone
    cause of pressure by _____.
b. discography
    i.   reliability _____   controversial
    ii. interpretation _____   equivocal
    iii. false positives _____   high
    iv. may help in cases of _____   multiple discs
         _____ if one
    v.   produces _____   pain

21. List five signs of psychosocial distress   G7 p.436:138mm
in back pain, remembering that
inappropriate response to any three
suggests distress is present.
Hint: ppaim
a. p_____   physical exam over reaction
b. p_____   pain on superficial palpation
c. a_____   axial loading produces pain
d. i_____   inconsistent SLR
e. m_____   motor or sensory exam
                                             inconsistent

22. Clear indications for urgent lumbar   G7 p.436:175mm
surgery include
a. c_____ e_____ s_____   cauda equina syndrome
b. p_____ n_____ d_____   progressive neurological
                                             deficit
c. p_____ w_____   profound weakness (motor)

23. **True or False. The following conservative therapy treatments have shown proven benefit for patients with back pain:**   G7 p.437:40mm
   a. epidural steroids   false
   b. transcutaneous electrical nerve stimulation (TENS)   false
   c. traction   false
   d. oral steroids   false
   e. spinal manipulation   false
   f. muscle relaxants   false   G7 p.438:50mm

24. **Is there a risk to the use of Parafon Forte? If so what is the risk?**   yes; fatal hepatotoxicity   G7 p.438:62mm

25. **True or False. Standard discectomy and microdiscectomy are of similar efficacy.**   true   G7 p.440:25mm

26. **Injection of chymopapain into herniated discs for treatment carries a significant risk of _____.**   anaphylaxis   G7 p.440:40mm

27. **The patient's chances of returning to work if off for**   G7 p.440:145mm
   a. 6 months is _____%   50%
   b. 1 year is _____%   20%
   c. 2 years is _____%   < 5%

■ Intervertebral Disc Herniation

28. **Enumerate the changes that occur in the intervertebral disc with increasing age.**   G6 p.323:80mm
   Hint: ddddisc   G5 p.295:120mm
   a. d_____   decrease disc height
   b. d_____   decrease in proteoglycan content
   c. d_____   desiccation (loss of hydration)
   d. d_____   degeneration of mucoid
   e. i_____   ingrowth of fibrous tissue
   f. s_____   susceptibility to injury
   g. c_____   circumferential tears of the annulus

29. **Complete the following concerning the aging of a disc:**   G5 p.295:121mm
   a. What decreases?
      i. _____   proteoglycan content
      ii. _____   water
   b. What increases?
      i. _____   mucoid degeneration
      ii. _____   fibrous tissue ingrowth
   c. This results in
      i. _____   annular tears
      ii. _____   nucleus herniation

18

30. Complete the following about sagittal balance: — G7 p.441:130mm

a. Assessment requires a
  i.   s_____ — standing
  ii. l_____ and — lateral
  iii. f_____ spine x-ray. — full

b. A plumb line is drawn
  i.   from the center of _____ — C7
  ii. to the disc space of _____. — L5S1
  iii. Within _____ — 3.2 cm ±
  iv. behind the s_____ p_____ is normal. — sacral promontory

31. Typical disc herniation compresses the nerve exiting _____. — below — G7 p.442:100mm

32. True or False. Surgical indications include — G7 p.442:115mm

a. cauda equina syndrome — true
b. numbness of foot — false
c. progressive symptoms — true
d. abnormal MRI — false
e. neurologic deficits — true
f. abnormal discogram — false
g. failed conservative treatment — true
h. pain when coughing — false
i. severe radicular pain for 2 weeks — false (6 weeks)
j. severe back pain — false

33. The posterior longitudinal ligament — G7 p.442:160mm

a. is strongest in the _____. — midline
b. Therefore, most disc herniations occur off to _____ _____. — one side

34. Complete the following regarding lumbar disc herniation: — G7 p.443:35mm

a. The occurrence of voiding dysfunction in lumbar disc herniation varies from _____ to _____%. — 1 to 18%

b. Concerning bladder symptoms, what is the sequence from the earliest findings?
  i.   d_____ b_____ s_____ — decreased bladder sensation
  ii. u_____ u_____ — urinary urgency
  iii. i_____ f_____ — increased frequency due to increased postvoiding residual
  iv. e_____ and i_____ — enuresis (bed wetting) and incontinence are rare

c. Urinary retention with overflow incontinence is suggestive of what diagnosis? — cauda equina compression

35. What is the most sensitive sign of herniated lumbar disc? — the Lasègue sign — G7 p.443:132mm

36. **The significance of a positive crossed straight-leg raising sign is**

G7 p.443:132mm

a. specificity for nerve root compression of _____%   90%

b. It suggests a more _____ HNP.   central

c. It may correlate with a disc _____ _____ _____ _____ of the contralateral root.   fragment within the axilla

d. Lasègue specificity for root compression is _____%.   83%

e. For crossed Lasègue it is _____%.   90%

37. **Describe a positive Lasègue sign.**

G7 p.443:155mm

a. Patient's position is _____.   supine

b. Raise leg by the ankle until _____.   pain elicited

c. Pain occurs below _____ degrees.   60

d. It is positive in _____% herniated nucleus pulposus (HNP).   83%

38. **Describe the following techniques to elicit indications of nerve root tension:**

G7 p.443:155mm

a. Lasègue sign _____ _____ _____   straight leg raising (SLR)

b. Cram test _____ _____ with _____ _____   extend knee with leg raised

c. Fajersztajn sign _____ _____   crossed SLR (central disc)= 97% HNP (crossed Lasègue test)

d. femoral stretch test _____   prone, knee maximally flexed = L2, L3, L4 root lesions

e. bowstring sign _____ _____ _____ _____   flex knee after SLR, hip pain persists but sciatic pain ceases

f. sitting knee extension _____ _____   sitting SLR

39. **Describe the Faber test.**

G7 p.444:90mm

a. another name?   Patrick sign

b. perform by?   flexion abduction external rotation

c. positive in?   hip pathology

40. **Complete the following regarding the Trendelenburg sign:**

G7 p.444:110mm

a. The affected hip _____ when the patient is walking,   dips

b. which indicates the contralateral thigh adductors are _____.   weak

c. This causes the contralateral pelvis to _____.   tilt

d. which is caused by a lesion of the _____ root.   L5 (Affected hip dips when walking to indicate weakness of contralateral thigh adductors, or while standing on leg with weak adductors causes pelvis to tilt contralateral to weakness [L5 lesion].)

41. **Complete the following about crossed adductors sign:**   G7 p.444:120mm
   a. Crossed adductors sign is positive when knee jerk is elicited and the contralateral thigh _____ _____.   adductors contract
   b. If knee jerk is
      i. hyperactive it suggests _____.   UMN lesion
      ii. hypoactive it suggests _____.   pathological spread due to nerve root irritation

42. **Complete the following about Hoover's sign:**   G7 p.444:133mm
   a. It is a test to learn if patient's leg weakness is _____.   functional
   b. Examiner places hands under patients _____.   heels
   c. Patient is asked to lift each leg from the _____.   bed
   d. If when lifting the normal leg the weak heel pushes _____,   down
   e. we know the leg has _____   strength
   f. and the alleged weakness is _____.   functional

43. **For the listed lumbar disc level, what is the frequency of herniated disc syndrome?**   G7 p.444:133mm
   a. L5-S1 _____%   45 to 50%
   b. L4-5 _____%   40 to 45%
   c. L3-4 _____%   3 to 10%

44. **Name physical findings associated with an L5-S1 disc herniation and where pain radiates.**   G7 p.445:50mm
   a. reflex, a_____ A_____   absent Achilles tendon reflexes
   b. motor, g_____ w_____   gastrocnemius weakness (plantar flexion)
   c. sensory, decreased at l_____ m_____ and l_____ f_____   lateral malleolus and lateral foot
   d. pain, p_____ c_____   posterior aspect of calf to the ankle

45. **How many vertebrae (presacral) are there in the typical human?**   24   G7 p.173:175mm

46. **Name three indicators for emergency lumbar surgery.**
    Hint: ces, pmd, ip

    a. ces _____

    cauda equina syndrome—urinary retention or overflow incontinence, saddle anesthesia

    b. pmd _____

    progressive motor deficit—"foot drop"

    c. ip _____

    intolerable pain (urgent)

G7 p.445:160mm

47. **List potential findings for cauda equina syndrome.**
    Hint: cauda s

    a. c_____

    can't function sexually—sexual dysfunction

    b. a_____

    ankle jerks absent

    c. u_____

    urinary retention/incontinence

    d. d_____

    diminished sphincter tone

    e. a_____

    anesthesia of saddle area

    f. s_____

    strength is decreased

G7 p.446:30mm

48. **True or False. The following is classically recognized as a cause of the cauda equina syndrome:**

    a. tumor   true
    b. epidural spinal hematoma   true
    c. free fat graft following discectomy true
    d. trauma/fracture   true
    e. lumbar stenosis   false (Lumbar stenosis is a more chronic process and therefore would not classically give an acute/subacute presentation of cauda equina syndrome.)

G7 p.446:90mm

49. **True or False. In cauda equina syndrome, surgery should be performed**

    a. stat   false
    b. within 24 hours   false
    c. within 48 hours   true
    d. within 72 hours   false
    e. within a week   false

G7 p.447:35mm

18

50. **True or False. Comparing microdiscectomy to standard discectomy for lumbar disc herniation, which of the following are true?**   G7 p.447:114mm

a. shorter incision   true
b. shorter hospital stay   true
c. less blood loss   true
d. better efficacy   false (Efficacy has been shown to be equivalent between the two techniques.)
e. may be more difficult to retrieve large fragments   true

51. **Success rate at 1 year for surgical discectomy is _____%.**   85%   G7 p.447:143mm

52. **Success rate at 1 year for chemonucleolysis (CNL) is _____%.**   44 to 63%   G7 p.447:146mm

53. **The percentage of patients of chemonucleolysis who eventually undergo surgery for unresolved symptoms is _____%.**   approximately 56% at 6 months   G7 p.447:152mm

54. **Complete the following about intradiscal procedures:**   G7 p.448:23mm

a. What percent of lumbar disc patients considered for surgery could be candidates for intradiscal procedures?   10 to 15%
b. What is the success rate of intradiscal procedures?   37 to 75%   G7 p.448:60mm

55. **True or False. Following discectomy:**   G7 p.448:140mm

a. epidural steroids prior to closure have no benefit.   true
b. systemic steroids and bupivacaine may reduce hospital stay and postop narcotic requirements.   true

56. **True or False. Regarding epidural free fat graft:**   G7 p.448:168mm

a. It can cause nerve root compression.   true
b. It is believed to reduce epidural scar formation.   Opinions on whether it reduces scar formation are mixed.
c. Some believe it may increase epidural scar.   true
d. It increases the incidence of postoperative infection.   false
e. It may cause cauda equina syndrome.   true, rarely

18

57. **Characterize complications of lumbar disc surgery.**   G7 p.449:25mm

a. mortality _____%   0.06% (1/1800 pts)
b. superficial infection _____% usual   1 to 5%; *Staphylococcus aureus*
   organism _____%
c. deep infection _____%   < 1%
d. discitis _____%   0.5%
e. motor deficit _____%   1 to 8%
f. durotomy _____%   0.3 to 13%
g. after redo _____%   18%
h. surgical repair _____   1/1000 pts
i. pseudomeningocele _____%   0.7 to 2%
j. recurrent disc _____%   4% (1.5% first year) 10-year
                                             follow-up

58. **Complete the following about durotomy:**   G7 p.449:60mm

a. What is the incidence of incidental   incidence is 0.3 to 13%
   durotomy in lumbar laminectomy?   (increases up to 18% in
                                          reoperations)

b. Give four possible complications related
   to incidental durotomies
   i.   C_____   CSF fistula-requiring repair in
                                          ⁓10 per 10,000
   ii. p_____   pseudomeningocele
                                          0.7 to 2%
   iii. h_____   herniation of nerve roots
   iv. i_____   increased epidural bleeding

59. **What is the incidence of recurrent herniated lumbar disc?**   G7 p.449:80mm

a. same level either side in first 10 years   ⁓ 4%
   _____%
b. any level over 10 years _____%   3 to 19%
c. first year same level either side   1.5%
   _____%
d. any different incidence depending on   two times more common at
   level   L4-5
e. same level recurrence _____%   74%
f. different level recurrence _____%   26% had herniated disc at
                                               another level

60. **Complete the following regarding the anterior longitudinal ligament:**   G7 p.449:103mm

a. Asymptomatic perforations occur in   12%
   _____% of discectomies.
b. Depth of disc space is _____.   3.3 cm
c. Vascular injury produces bleeding into 50%
   operative field only _____% of the
   time.
d. Great vessel injury mortality is   37 to 67%
   _____%.

61. **Enumerate five complications related to positioning for lumbar discectomies.**

G7 p.450:90mm

Hint: tecup

a. t_____   tibialis anterior compartment syndrome
b. e_____   eyes pressure
c. c_____   cervical spine injury
d. u_____   ulnar nerve compression
e. p_____   peroneal nerve compression

62. **True or False. Regarding unintended durotomy:**

a. Normal ambulation is not considered a cause for failure of dural repair.   true   G7 p.451:135mm
b. Risk of a cerebrospinal fluid (CSF) leak is increased in
   i.   revision surgery   true
   ii. removal of ossification of the posterior longitudinal ligament (OPLL)   true
   iii. high-speed drills   true
c. It is not considered an act of malpractice.   true
d. The use of fibrin glue to close is advantageous.   true
e. It can be due to thinned dura by long-standing stenosis.   true

63. **Enumerate four signs of postoperative cauda equina syndrome (i.e., from epidural hematoma).**

G7 p.452:78mm

Hint: pain

a. p_____   pain out of the ordinary
b. a_____   anesthesia of saddle area
c. i_____   inability to void
d. n_____   numerous muscle groups weak

64. **True or False. Regarding the outcome of surgical treatment of lumbar herniated disc:**

G7 p.452:127mm

a. 5% will be classified as having failed back syndrome.   true
b. At 1 year the surgical group had a better outcome than with conservative treatment.   true

18

c.	The benefit persisted at 10 years.	false (Surgery group had better outcome at 1 year but benefit was no longer statistically significant at 4-year follow-up. At 10 years neither surgical nor conservative treatment group complained of sciatica or back pain.)
d.	63% had complete relief of back pain at 1 year postop.	true
e.	At 5- to 10-year follow-up 86% felt improved.	true

65. **True or False. The percentage of patients with L3-4 disc herniation having a past history of L4-5 or L5-S1 disc herniation is**   G7 p.453:28mm

a. < 10%   false
b. approximately 25%   true
c. approximately 50%   false
d. 60 to 80%   false
e. almost 90%   false

66. **Characterize a herniated upper lumbar disc.**   G7 p.453:33mm

a. What is the incidence?
     i.   L1-2 _____%   0.28%
     ii. L2-3 _____%   1.3%
     iii. L3-4 _____%   3.6%
b. Most common muscle involved?   quadriceps femoris
c. Femoral stretch test _____   may be positive
d. Knee jerk _____   reduced in 50%

67. **Characterize extreme lateral lumbar disc herniations.**   G7 p.453:105mm

a. What is the incidence?   3 to 10%
b. What level is most commonly involved?
     i.   L4-5 _____%   60%
     ii. L3-4 _____%   24%
     iii. L5-S1 _____%   7%
c. Enumerate four differences compared with other common disc herniations
     i.   Straight leg raising (SLR) is negative in _____%.   85 to 90%
     ii. Pain is increased by lateral bending in _____%.   75%
     iii. Pain is more _____.   severe
     iv. Extruded fragments are _____.   more frequent

18

68. Distinguishing features concerning far lateral disc herniation include the following:

a. The root involved is the root _____ _____ _____ _____.
exiting at that level
G7 p.453:118mm

b. SLR is _____.
negative

c. Lateral bending is _____.
likely to produce pain

d. Severity of pain is _____ because _____ _____ _____ is compressed.
greater; dorsal root ganglion

e. Most common levels are _____ and _____.
L4-5 and L3-4

f. Best surgical approach is _____ _____.
standard hemilaminectomy (and follow nerve laterally; perform medial facetectomy)

69. Zones in which disc herniation can occur are
G7 p.453:128mm

a. c_____
central

b. s_____
subarticular

c. f_____
foraminal

d. e_____
extraforaminal

70. True or False. One third of extreme lateral lumbar disc herniations are missed on initial radiologic exams.
true
G7 p.454:70mm

71. To test for far lateral disc what is the value of postdiscography CT scan?
may be a most sensitive test—94%
G7 p.454:94mm

72. Give the incidence of surgery for herniated discs in pediatric patients.
G7 p.455:65mm

a. under 20 years of age _____%
less than 1%

b. under 17 years of age _____%
less than ½ of 1%

73. Characterize intradural disc herniation.
G7 p.455:100mm

a. What is the incidence?
0.04 to 1.1%

b. Can it be diagnosed preoperatively?
rarely

c. It is suspected at surgery because of a _____ _____.
negative exploration

d. Does it require a surgical dural opening?
rarely

74. Characterize juxta facet cysts (JFCs).
G7 p.456:50mm

a. What are the types?

    i. s_____
    synovial

    ii. g_____
    ganglion

b. What is the incidence?
rare (1/500 spinal CTs)

c. Key to diagnosis on myelography or post-myelogram cat scan PMCT is a p_____ f_____ d_____.
posterolateral filling defect

d. Is it uni- or bilateral?
may be bilateral

e. Does juxta facet cysts suggest stability or instability to the spine?
check for stability—may serve as a marker of instability
G7 p.457:5mm

18

75. **Regarding failed back syndrome, the failure rate for lumbar discectomy is _____%.**

8 to 25%

G7 p.457:120mm

76. **True or False. Regarding failed back syndrome, the following is the best test for detecting residual or recurrent disc herniation:**

G7 p.459:45mm

   a. myelography with postmyelogram CT scan

false

   b. CT scan with infusion

false

   c. MRI without and with IV gadolinium

true

   d. unenhanced MRI

false

77. **Answer the following about arachnoiditis:**

G7 p.459:55mm

   a. What test is used to differentiate residual or recurrent disc herniation from scar tissue and adhesive arachnoiditis?

MRI without and with IV gadolinium

   b. Why is it so important to differentiate? Because surgical treatment for scar has _____.

poor results for scar tissue or adhesive arachnoiditis

78. **Characterize recurrent herniated disc.**

G7 p.460:90mm

   a. second herniation _____%

3 to 19%

   b. 10 years same level _____%

4%

   c. 1 year same level _____%

1.5%

   d. second recurrence _____%

1%

79. **Does it take a larger or smaller disc herniation to cause symptoms in recurrent disc? Why? Because _____ _____ prevents the nerve from moving away.**

smaller; scar tissue

G7 p.460:110mm

80. **Where does the cervical root exit in relation to the pedicle?**

in close relation to the undersurface of the pedicle

G7 p.461:42mm

81. **Complete the following table concerning cervical disc syndromes:**

G7 p.461:60mm

	C4-5	C5-6	C6-7	C7-T1
% of cervical discs				
Compressed root				
Reflex diminished				
Motor weakness				
Paresthesias + Hypesthesias				

Table 18.1

	C4-5	C5-6	C6-7	C7-T1
% of cervical discs	2 %	19 %	69 %	10 %
Compressed root	C 5	C 6	C 7	C 8
Reflex diminished	Deltoid and Pectoralis	Biceps and Brachio-radialis	Triceps	Finger jerk
Motor weakness	Deltoid	Forearm Flexion	Forearm Extension Wrist drop	Hand Intrinsics
Paresthesias + Hypesthesias	Shoulder	Upper arm Thumb Radial Forearm	Fingers 2 and 3	Fingers 4 and 5

18

82. **Complete the following about intervertebral disc herniation:**
    a. C6-7 disc causes a C_____ radiculopathy. C7   G7 p.461:70mm
    b. C5-6 disc causes a C_____ radiculopathy. C6
    c. It may simulate a _____. myocardial infarction   G7 p.461:110mm

83. **A left C6 radiculopathy can simulate an _____ _____ _____.** acute myocardial infarction   G7 p.461:110mm

84. **C8 or T1 nerve root involvement (i.e., a C7-T1 or T1-T2 disc) may produce _____.** a partial Horner syndrome   G7 p.461:115mm

85. **The most common scenario for patients with herniated cervical discs is that the symptoms were first noticed upon _____.** awakening in the morning (without identifiable trauma and stress)   G7 p.461:120mm

86. **Complete the following about intervertebral disc herniation:**   G7 p.461:60
    Table 18.18
    a. C 4-5 disc compresses C _____ root _____. C5 root exiting
    b. L 4-5 disc compresses L _____ root _____. L5 root passing

87. **Narrowing the cervical foramen mechanically is called _____ _____.** Spurling sign   G7 p.461:180mm

88. **Complete the following about the Spurling sign:**   G7 p.461:181mm
    a. performed by
       i.   examiner exerting pressure on the _____ vertex
       ii. while patient tilts head toward the _____ _____ symptomatic side
       iii. with neck _____ extended
    b. reproduces _____ _____ radicular pain
    c. analogous to _____ SLR for lumbar disc— a mechanical sign

89. **Give the accuracy of radiological workups.**   G7 p.462:58mm
    a. MRI is _____%. 85 to 90%
    b. CT myelogram is _____%. 98%   G7 p.462:83mm

90. **True or False. To fuse or not to fuse. Fusion is beneficial to**   G7 p.464:15mm
    a. a plate reduces pseudoarthrosis true
    b. a plate reduces graft problems true
    c. a plate maintains lordosis true
    d. improve clinical outcome false
    e. improve arm pain true
    f. provide more rapid relief of arm pain true

g.	maintain foraminal height	false
h.	maintain disc space height	false
i.	reduce post op kyphosis	true
j.	improve fusion rate	true

91. What is the incidence of vocal cord paresis due to injury of the recurrent laryngeal nerve (RLN)? G7 p.465:45mm

a. Temporary _____ %   11%
b. Permanent _____ %   4%

92. True or False. A good way to treat vertebral artery injury is by G7 p.465:70mm

a. packing   false
b. direct suture   true
c. endovascular trapping   true

93. The rare complication of sleep-induced apnea can occur with anterior cervical discectomy and fusion (ACDF) at the level of _____.   C3-4 G7 p.465:140mm

94. Characterize dysphagia following ACDF. G7 p.466:80mm

a. Incidence early is _____ %   60%
b. At 6 months only _____%   5%
c. Most serious cause is _____   hematoma
d. Permanent recurrent laryngeal nerve injury _____%   1.3%

95. Characterize pseudoarthrosis following ACDF. On flexion extension cervical spine x-rays G7 p.467:60mm

a. movement of more than _____ mm   2
b. between the _____ _____   spinous processes
c. lack of _____ across the fusion   trabeculation
d. l_____ around the screws   lucency
e. t_____ of the screws on flexion extension films   toggling
f. n_____ uniformly associated with symptoms   not

96. For patients in certain professions we prefer to do posterior cervical surgery instead of anterior. G7 p.468:125mm

a. Which two professions?   speaker and singer
b. The reason is there is a _____%   5%
c. incidence of _____ _____ after anterior cervical surgery.   voice change

97. Indications for posterior keyhole laminotomy are G7 p.469:95mm

a. s_____ l_____ d_____   soft lateral disc
b. occupation of s_____ or s_____   singer or speaker
c. l_____- or u_____-l_____ d_____   lower- or upper-level disc

18

98. Matching. Match the recommended sequence of bone removal with the recommended sequence for posterior keyhole laminotomy.
Sequence of bone removal recommended:
① superior facet of the vertebra below, ② inferior facet of the vertebra above, ③ lateral aspect of lamina above
Recommended sequence:

a.   1st area of bone removal   ③
b.   2nd area of bone removal   ②
c.   3rd area of bone removal   ①

G7 p.470:20mm

99. The success rate of posterior keyhole laminectomy is in the range of _____ to _____ %.   90 to 96

G7 p.470:150mm

100. Characterize thoracic disc herniation.
a.   It usually occurs below the level of _____.   T8

b.   Because many are calcified it is wise to get a _____ _____.   CT scan

G7 p.470:173mm

101. Characterize thoracic disc herniation.
a.   The incidence is _____% of all disc herniations.   0.25 to 0.75%
b.   _____% occur between ages 30 and 50.   80%
c.   History of trauma is _____%.   25%

G7 p.471:12mm

102. Characterize access to the thoracic spine.
a.   upper _____   sternal splitting
b.   mid _____   right thoracotomy (heart not in way)
c.   lower _____   left–easier to mobilize aorta than vena cava
d.   thoracolumbar _____   right to avoid liver unless pathology is far on left side
e.   lumbar _____   transabdominal

G7 p.471:130mm

103. Complete the following concerning the thoracic spine and spinal cord anterior access to:
a.   lower thoracic spine
    i.   use _____ side thoracotomy   left
    ii.   avoid _____ _____ easier to mobilize   vena cava
    iii.   _____   aorta
b.   thoracolumbar spine
    i.   use _____ side retroperitoneal approach   right
    ii.   thereby avoiding _____   liver

G7 p.471:130mm

■ Degenerative Disc/Spine Disease

104. **For each of the letters listed give the indicated number of terms that collectively describe the pathology of degenerative disc/spine disease.**

G7 p.474:175mm

18

a.	D-3	D dessication
		disruption
		disc herniation
b.	E-0	E
c.	G-1	G growth of fibrous tissue/joint laxity
d.	E-0	E
e.	N-1	N narrowing disc space
f.	E-0	E
g.	R-1	R resorption of disc
h.	A-1	A annular tears
i.	T-1	T torn annulus
j.	I-1	I isthmic spondylolisthesis
k.	V-1	V vertebral body osteophytes
l.	E-0	E
m.	S-1	S spondylosis
n.	P-1	P proteoglycan
o.	I-1	I interarticular (PARS) defects
p.	N-1	N mucoid degeneration
q.	E-0	E

105. **Complete the following about degenerative disc/spine disease:**

G7 p.475:130mm

a. Spondylolisthesis or anterior subluxation of one vertebral body on another is graded according to the percent of _____; therefore, it has   subluxation

b. grades
  i.   I _____%   < 25%
  ii. II _____%   25 to 50%
  iii. III _____%   50 to 75%
  iv. IV _____%   75% to complete

106. **Complete the following about degenerative disc/spine disease:**

G7 p.475:145mm

a. True or False. It is common for listhesis to cause root compression.   false

b. If it does do so it compresses the nerve root that _____ at that level   exits

c. below the _____ above   pedicle

d. compressed by the _____ _____   superior articular facet

e. being displaced _____.   upward

18

107. **What is a pseudo disc?**   G7 p.475:150mm
   a. It is the appearance on _____   MRI
   b. in a patient with _____.   listhesis
   c. More correctly considered a _____   "roll out"
      _____ of the disc
   d. termed _____ by the radiologist.   "uncovered"

108. **What congenital condition is**   achondroplastic dwarfism   G7 p.477:50mm
   associated with spinal stenosis?

109. **True or False. Cervical and lumbar**   G7 p.477:60mm
   stenosis occurs simultaneously in
   what % of patients?
   a. 5%   true
   b. 10%   false
   c. 15%   false
   d. 20%   false

110. **What level is most commonly the site** L4-5 and then L3-4   G7 p.477:110mm
   of lumbar stenosis?

111. **Matching. Match the condition with**   G7 p.477:165mm
   the appropriate clinical feature(s).
   Clinical feature:
   ① pain is dermatomal; ② sensory loss
   stocking; ③ sensory loss is dermatomal;
   ④ pain with exercise; ⑤ pain with
   standing; ⑥ rest relieves pain promptly;
   ⑦ rest relieves pain slowly; ⑧ relief with
   standing; ⑨ relief only with stooping or
   sitting; ⑩ achiness over thigh; ⑪ pain on
   pressure over hip; ⑫ Faber sign positive
   Condition:
   a. neurogenic claudication   ①, ③, ④, ⑤, ⑦, ⑨
   b. vascular claudication   ②, ④, ⑥, ⑧
   c. trochanteric bursitis   ⑩, ⑪, ⑫

112. **What posture may elicit pain in**   hyperextension   G7 p.478:100mm
   lumbar stenosis?

113. **Give the normal lumbar spine CT**   G7 p.479:160mm
   measurements for each of the
   following:
   a. anteroposterior (AP) diameter _____   > 11.5 mm
   b. ligamentum flavum thickness _____   < 4 to 5 mm
   c. height of lateral recess _____   > 3 mm

114. **State the AP diameter of the spine on**   G7 p.479:160mm
   plain films.
   a. normal lumbar spine, lower limits of   15 mm
      normal _____
   b. cervical spine, lower limits of normal   12 mm or less   G7 p.136:133mm
      _____
   c. lumbar severe stenosis _____   less than 11 mm
   d. cervical severe stenosis _____   less than 10 mm   G7 p.489:148mm

115. **Is treatment for asymptomatic moderate stenosis at adjacent levels appropriate?**

yes (They have a likelihood of progressing to become symptomatic.)

G7 p.481:153mm

116. **What percent of patients who undergo decompressive lumbar laminectomies develop instability?**

1%

G7 p.483:40mm

18

117. **Spinal stability is influenced by**
Hint: fads

G7 p.483:52mm

   a. amount of remaining _____

facet: unstable if more than one third or one half facet is removed

   b. patient's _____

age: more unstable in younger patient after decompression

   c. violation of _____ space

disc: intact disc space more stable

   d. decompression _____

surgery: produces instability in 1% of patients

118. **Matching. Following decompression in a patient, which procedures are appropriate?**
① no fusion
② posterolateral fusion
③ adding pedicle screw instrumentation

G7 p.483:103mm

   a. no instability preop   ①
   b. instability preop   ②
   c. spondylolisthesis preop   ②, ③

119. **Give the lumbar spinal stenosis outcomes.**

G7 p.484:48mm

   a. mortality _____%   0.32%
   b. superficial infection _____%   2.3%
   c. deep infection _____%   5.9%
   d. deep vein thrombosis (DVT) _____%   2.8%
   e. postural pain relief _____%   96%
   f. recurrence after 5 years _____%   27%
   g. long-term success at 1 year and 5 years _____%   70%

120. **Non-union risk factors include**

G7 p.484:60mm

   a. s_____   smoking
   b. number of _____ fused   levels
   c. use of _____ type medications   NSAIDs

121. **Characterize lateral recess stenosis.**

G7 p.485:17mm

   a. Is the pain unilateral or bilateral?   can be either
   b. It is due to _____ of the   hypertrophy
   c. _____ _____ facet.   superior articular
   d. The most common level is at _____.   L4-5

18

122. **Give the dimensions of lateral recess on CT.**   G7 p.485:92 mm
   a. lateral recess height _____ mm   3 to 4 mm
   b. suggestive of lateral recess narrowing   < 3 mm
      _____ mm
   c. diagnostic of lateral recess syndrome   < 2 mm
      _____ mm

123. **Complete the following about degenerative disc/spine disease:**   G7 p.488:100mm
   a. What reflex test is said to be pathognomonic of cervical spinal myelopathy?   inverted radial reflex
   b. Elicited by performing the _____
      _____   brachioradialis reflex
   c. and obtaining a response of _____   flexion of the fingers
      _____ _____ _____.

124. **Complete the following regarding hyperactive jaw jerk:**   G7 p.488:118mm
   a. significance is that it indicates an
      i. u_____ m_____ n_____   upper motor neuron lesion
          l_____
      ii. located a_____ t_____   above the pons (It
          p_____   distinguishes this from UMN
                                                 lesions due to lower-level
                                                 causes, i.e., cervical
                                                 myelopathy.)

   b. helps differentiate what diseases?
      i. _____ from   ALS from
      ii. _____ _____   cervical myelopathy

125. **Complete the following table to differentiate amyotrophic lateral sclerosis (ALS) from cervical myelopathy:**   G7 p.489:75 mm

	ALS	CM
Sensory loss		
Sphincter loss		
Jaw jerk		
Dysarthria		
Tongue fasciculations		

	ALS	CM
Sensory loss	No	Yes
Sphincter loss	No	Yes
Jaw jerk	Yes	No
Dysarthria	Yes	No
Tongue fasciculations	Yes	No

126. **True or False. Concerning ALS:**   G7 p.489:75mm
   a. Jaw jerk is present.   true (may be first clue)
   b. Tongue fasciculations are present.   true (as seen on EMG or
                                                visible fasciculations)

127. Complete the following about degenerative disc/spine disease: — G7 p.489:145mm

a. cervical spine myelopathy spinal canal diameter
   i. myelopathic at _____ mm — 10 mm or less
   ii. symptomatic at _____ mm — 11.8 mm
   iii. increased risk at _____ mm — 14.0 mm
b. not symptomatic at _____ mm or more — 14 mm

128. True or False. Regarding MRI abnormalities that correlate with poor prognosis in cervical spondylitic myelopathy: — G7 p.490:15mm

a. T2W1 hyperintensity within the cord — true
b. Spinal cord transverse area less than 60mm^2 — false
c. Spinal cord transverse area less than 45 mm^2 — true
d. "Snake eyes" on axial T2W1 — true

129. True or False. Preop SSEP testing can aid in decision making. — true — G7 p.490:120mm

130. Contraindications to posterior decompression are — G7 p.492:23mm

a. kyphotic angulation, also known as _____ _____. — swan neck
b. subluxation of greater than _____ mm — 3.5 mm
c. or rotation in the sagittal plane of more than _____ degrees. — 20 degrees — G7 p.492:65mm

131. Characterize cervical sprodylitic myelopathy. — G7 p.493 :100mm

a. Postop palsy after anterior or posterior decompression occurs in _____%. — 3 to 5%
b. It involves the d_____ or b_____ muscles — deltoid, biceps
c. and C5 region; that is _____ area sensory symptoms. — shoulder
d. It usually occurs within _____ _____ of surgery. — 1 week
e. Prognosis for recovery is _____. — good

■ Craniovertebral Junction and Upper Cervical Spine Abnormalities

132. Name 13 causes of craniovertebral abnormalities.

G7 p.494:40mm

Hint: attaCK roMinDs

a. a_____   ankylosing spondylitis
b. t_____   trauma
c. t_____   tumor
d. a_____   atlantoaxial dislocation
e. C_____   Chiari malformation
f. K_____   Klippel-Feil
g. r_____   rheumatoid arthritis
h. o_____   occipitalization of the atlas
i. M_____   Morquio syndrome (a mucopolysaccharidosis)
j. i_____   infection
k. n_____   neoplasm
l. D_____   Down syndrome
m. s_____   surgery (transoral odontoidectomy)

133. What are some of the abnormalities at the craniocervical junction?

G7 p.494:90mm

Hint: baaoa

a. b_____ i_____   basilar impression
b. a_____-o _____ d_____   atlanto-occipital dislocation
c. a_____ d_____   atlantoaxial dislocation
d. o_____ of the a_____   occipitalization of the atlas
e. a_____ p_____ a_____ of C1   absent posterior arch

■ Rheumatoid Arthritis

134. Name four upper cervical spine abnormalities associated with rheumatoid arthritis.

G7 p.494:170mm

a. b_____ i_____   basilar impression
b. a_____ s_____   atlantoaxial subluxation
c. s_____ s_____   subaxial subluxation (less common)
d. v_____ a_____ i_____ vertebral artery insufficiency— due to changes at the craniocervical junction (less common)

135. **What are the three stages in pathophysiology that lead to atlantoaxial subluxation in rheumatoid arthritis?**
Hint: iel

G5 p.495:50mm

a. infl_____ at a_____ s_____ j_____ — inflammation at atlantoaxial synovial joints
b. ero_____ c_____ in o_____ — erosive changes in odontoid
c. loo_____ of the t_____ l_____ — loosening of the transverse ligament

136. **What percentage of rheumatoid arthritis patients develop subluxation?**   Atlantoaxial subluxation occurs in 25% of patients with rheumatoid arthritis.

G5 p.495:60mm

137. **Complete the following regarding atlantoaxial subluxation in rheumatoid arthritis:**

G7 p.495:125mm

a. The odontoid C1 interval is normal when less than _____ mm.   4 mm
b. The asymptomatic patient needs surgery if distance is greater than _____ mm.   8 mm
c. To do transoral odontoidectomy the mouth needs to open at least _____ mm.   25 mm
d. Mortality of C1-C2 wiring is _____%.   5 to 15%

138. **Characterize posterior atlantodental interval (PADI).**

G7 p.495:135mm

a. Correlates with the presence of _____   paralysis
b. Predicts neurologic recovery following _____   surgery
c. No recovery occurs if the PADI is less than _____ mm   10
d. An indication for surgery is a PADI less than _____ mm   14

139. **What degree of atlantodental interval is a generally accepted surgical indication in asymptomatic patients?**   8 mm (6 to 10 mm is the range)

G7 p.496:60mm

140. **What is the percentage of nonfusion for C1-C2 fusions in rheumatoid arthritis?**   18 to 50%

G7 p.496:160mm

141. **Characterize basilar impression in rheumatoid arthritis.**

G7 p.497:30mm

a. Changes in lateral masses are called e_____.   erosive
b. Permitting relationship of C1-C2 to change is called t_____.   telescoping
c. Position of dens moves u_____   upward
    i. causes compression of p_____ and m_____   pons and medulla
    ii. compression contributed to by p_____   pannus
    iii. located _____ to dens   posterior

18

18

142. **Matching. List the most common symptoms and signs of basilar impression of patients with rheumatoid arthritis and match with their order of frequency.**   G7 p.497:65mm
① _____, 100%; ② _____, 80%;
③ _____, 80%; ④ _____, 71%;
⑤ _____, 30%; ⑥ _____, 22%
   a. limb paresthesias _____%   ④ 71%
   b. Babinski, hyperreflexia _____%   ② 80%
   c. bladder incontinence/retention   ⑤ 30%
      _____%
   d. cranial nerve dysfunction _____%   ⑥ 22%
   e. headache _____%   ① 100%
   f. ambulatory problems _____%   ③ 80%

143. **Characterize basilar impression in rheumatoid arthritis.**   G7 p.797:65mm
   a. Pain may be a result of _____ of C1   compression
      and C2 nerves.
   b. Cranial nerve dysfunction results from   medulla
      compression of the _____.

144. **What is the treatment for basilar impression?**   G7 p.497:175mm
   a. if reducible with _____   traction
      i.   C1 d_____ l_____ followed   decompressive laminectomy
           by
      ii. o_____-c_____ f_____   occipital-cervical fusion
   b. in nonreducible patients
      i.   t_____ o_____ r_____   transoral odontoid resection
           followed by   followed by
      ii. o_____-c_____ f_____   occipital-cervical fusion

■ Paget Disease

145. **Characterize Paget disease.**   G7 p.498:130mm
   a. Also known as o_____ d_____   osteitis deformans
   b. Disorder of o_____   osteoclasts
   c. Results in r_____ of bone   resorption
   d. Reactive osteoblasts o_____ produce   over
   e. Sclerotic, radiodense, brittle bone called   ivory bone
      i_____ b_____

146. **Recommended laboratory tests include**   G7 p.499:100mm
   a. a_____ ph_____   alkaline phosphatase
   b. ur_____ hy_____   urinary hydroxyproline
   c. bone scan _____ _____ areas of   lights up
      abnormality
   d. and treatment with c_____   calcitonin

147. **What are the neurosurgical indications in Paget disease of the spine?** G7 p.501:95mm
   a. spinal _____   instability
   b. uncertain _____   diagnosis
   c. failure of _____ _____   medical management

18

■ Ankylosing Spondylosis

148. **Characterize ankylosing spondylosis.** G7 p.502:45mm
   a. It is also known as M_____   Marie Strümpell disease
      S_____ d_____.
   b. Locus of involvement is the _____   entheses
   c. replacement of _____ with   ligaments with bone
      _____.
   d. Bone is very _____.   osteoporotic
   e. On x-ray it is called _____ _____.   bamboo spine
   f. To differentiate from rheumatoid   negative for rheumatoid
      arthritis (RA) serum is _____ for   factor
      _____ _____.
   g. Fracture may occur with _____   minimal trauma
      _____.
   h. Screws for fusion may _____   not hold
      _____.
   i. Enthesis   G7 p.502:60mm
      i.   is the _____ _____   attachment point
      ii. of ligaments, tendons or capsules on bones
           _____.

149. **What are radiologic considerations in ankylosing spondylosis?** G7 p.503:15mm
   a. Rotary _____ may occur in high   subluxation
      cervical area.
   b. Last area to stay mobile is the   occipito-atlanto
      o_____-a_____
   c. and a_____ joints.   atlantoaxial
   d. Minor trauma may result in spine   fracture
      _____.
   e. Vertebral fractures occur through the   ossified disc
      _____ _____.
   f. An early site of involvement is the   SI joint
      _____ _____.
   g. If suspicious, x-ray the _____   entire spine
      _____.

■ Ossification of the Posterior Longitudinal Ligament

150.   Insert a term starting with the indicated letter to characterize the pathologic process of ossification of the posterior longitudinal ligament (OPLL).   G7 p.504:77mm

    a.   c_____   calcification
    b.   d_____   dura
    c.   e_____   evolves from C34
    d.   f_____   fibrosis
    e.   g_____   grows 0.6 mm and 4.1 mm/year
    f.   h_____   hypervascular
    g.   p_____   periosteal
    h.   o_____   ossification

151.   True or False. OPLL progresses in the following order: G7 p.504:78mm
        1. ossification
        2. fibrosis
        3. calcification
    a.   1,3,2   false
    b.   2,1,3   false
    c.   3,1,2   false
    d.   2,3,1   true

152.   OPLL grows at a rate of   G7 p.504:90mm
    a.   _____ mm in the anterior posterior (AP) direction and   0.6 mm
    b.   _____ mm longitudinally per year   4.1 mm

153.   Provide the pathologic classification.   G7 p.504:125mm
    a.   Confined to space behind vertebral body.   segmental
    b.   Extends from body to body spanning disc is called _____.   continuous
    c.   Combines both of the above and has skip areas is called _____.   mixed

154.   Describe the evaluation of OPLL.   G7 p.504:175mm
    a.   Plain x-rays _____ _____ to demonstrate OPLL.   often fail
    b.
        i.   MRI: OPLL is difficult to appreciate until it is _____ mm thick.   5mm
        ii.   T2W1 may be very _____.   helpful
    c.   CT, especially with 3D reconstruction, is the _____ method.   best

155. List the clinical grading of OPLL.   G7 p.505:30mm
  a. class 1   x-ray only—radiographically evident; no symptoms or signs
  b. class 2   minimal—myelopathy A/O radiculopathy minimal or stable deficit
  c. class 3A   myelopathy—moderate to severe myelopathy
  d. class 3B   quadriplegia—moderate to severe quadriplegia

156. Complete the following regarding Nurick grades of cervical spondylosis: G7 p.505:82mm
  a. Assess the extent of _____.   disability
  b. Surgery showed no benefit for Nurick grades _____ and _____.   1 and 2
  c. Surgery was valuable for Nurick grades _____ and _____.   3 and 4
  d. Surgery was ineffective for Nurick grade _____.   5

■ Diffuse Idiopathic Skeletal Hyperostosis

157. Characterize diffuse idiopathic skeletal hyperostosis (DISH).   G7 p.506:83mm
  a. Areas of spine affected by %
    i.   thoracic _____%   97%
    ii. lumbar _____%   90%
    iii. cervical _____%   78%
    iv. all three segments _____%   70%
  b. Area spared   sacroiliac joints
  c. Is the area spared in ankylosing spondylitis?   no

■ Scheuermann's Kyphosis

158. Complete the following regarding Scheuermann's Kyphosis: G7 p.506:158mm
  a. Which age group does it affect?   adolescents
  b. It is defined as
    i.   _____ wedging   anterior
    ii. of at least _____ degrees   5
    iii. of _____ or more _____   3; adjacent
    iv. _____ vertebral bodies.   thoracic

■ Spinal Arteriovenous Malformation

159. Characterize spinal AVM classification.   G7 p.507:65mm
- a. Type I
    - i. known as _____ _____   dural AVM
    - ii. IA: has _____ _____ arterial   a single
      feeder
    - iii. IB: has _____ or _____   2 or more
      arterial feeders
    - iv. Formed at the _____ _____   dural root
      sleeve
- b. Intradural AVMs
    - i. Flow is _____   high
    - ii. _____% with acute symptoms   75%
- c. Type II
    - i. aka spinal _____ AVM   glomus
    - ii. located _____   intramedullary
    - iii. true _____ of the cord   AVM
    - iv. has a _____ _____   compact nidus
    - v. prognosis is _____ than dural   worse
      AVM
- d. Type III
    - i. aka _____ spinal AVM   juvenile
    - ii. essentially on enlarged _____   glomus
    - iii. occupies _____ _____ cross   the entire
      section
- e. Type IV
    - i. aka _____ spinal AVM   perimedullary
    - ii. aka _____ fistula   arteriovenous
    - iii. presents with _____ hemorrhage   catastrophic

160. What is the most common type of   G7 p.507:70mm
spinal AVM?
- a. type _____   type 1
- b. dural _____   AVM
- c. fed by a _____   dural artery
- d. and draining into a _____   spinal vein
- e. on the _____ aspect of the cord   posterior
- f. _____ % are males   90

161. What is the most common   G7 p.508:80mm
presentation of a spinal AVM?
- a. onset of _____   back pain
- b. progressive lower extremity _____   weakness and sensory loss—
  and _____   acute onset of back pain
  associated with progressive
  LE weakness and sensory loss
  (may be over months to
  years)

18

162. **Spinal AVM with pain may have this syndrome.** G7 p.508:90mm
    a. Patient with onset of subarachnoid hemorrhage (SAH), and sudden excruciating back pain is also called c_____ d_____ p_____ of Michon. coup de poignard
    b. This is considered clinical evidence of _____ _____. spinal AVM

163. **What is Foix-Alajouanine syndrome?** G7 p.508:95mm
    a. acute or subacute _____ _____ neurologic deterioration
    b. in a patient with a _____ _____ spinal AVM
    c. without evidence of _____ hemorrhage
    d. caused by _____ _____ venous hypertension
    e. with secondary _____ ischemia

■ Spinal Meningeal Cyst

164. **What is a Tarlov cyst?** spinal meningeal cyst G7 p.509:97mm

165. **What are the different types of spinal meningeal cyst, and which compartment are they located in?** G7 p.509:110mm
    a. type I superficial compartment extradural without root fibers
    b. type II middle compartment extradural with spinal root fibers—diverticulum
    c. type III central compartment intradural arachnoid cyst

166. **Complete the following statements about spinal meningeal cyst:** G7 p.509:120 mm
    a. Type II spinal meningeal cyst is also known as _____ _____. Tarlov cyst
    b. It occurs on the _____ roots. dorsal

167. **What are the treatment options for spinal meningeal cyst?** G7 p.510:40mm
    a. e_____ excise the cyst
    b. o_____ obliterate the ostium between cyst and subarachnoid space
    c. m_____ marsupialize if excision is not possible

■ Syringomyelia

168. Complete the following about syringomyelia: G7 p.510:75mm

a. _____ cavitation of the spinal cord   cystic
b. associated with Chiari I in _____%   70%
c. affects upper or lower extremities first?   upper
d. More rapid neurologic progression is   5 mm; edema
   predicted by a cavity more than
   _____mm in diameter and with
   associated cord _____.

169. Rostral extension into brainstem is called _____.   syringobulbia   G7 p.510:105mm

170. Distinguish from similar entities.   G7 p.510:115mm

a. Tumor cyst
   i.   Most _____   enhance
   ii. Fluid is _____   proteinaceous
   iii. Syrinx fluid has MRI characteristics of   CSF
        _____

b. Residual spinal canal
   i.   Central canal usually _____   involutes
   ii. No more than _____ to   2; 4
        _____ mm wide
   iii. Perfectly _____ on cross section   round
   iv. Perfectly in the _____ on axial   center
        MRI

171. Dilatation of central canal with ependymal lining is called _____.   hydromyelia   G7 p.510:160mm

172. Communicating syringomyelia is commonly associated with what congenital conditions?   G7 p.511:75mm
Hint: bCDe

a. b_____   basilar impression
b. C_____   Chiari malformation
c. D_____   Dandy-Walker syndrome
d. e_____   ectopia of cerebellum

173. What are the main presenting symptoms and signs of a syrinx?   G7 p.511:175mm
Hint: accC

a. a_____ w_____   arm/hand weakness
b. c_____ s_____ l_____   sensory loss with suspended
                                                    "cape" dissociated sensory
                                                    loss (loss of pain and
                                                    temperature with preserved
                                                    joint position sense)
c. c_____ o_____ p_____   cervical/occipital pain
d. C_____ j_____ p_____   Charcot joints—painless
   a_____   arthropathies

174. **True or False. The level of spinal injury that has the highest incidence of posttraumatic syringomyelia is**
    G7 p.513:125mm
    a. cervical — false — G7 p.513:155mm
    b. thoracic — true — G7 p.513:163mm
    c. lumbar — false

175. **Characterize posttraumatic syringomyelia.**
    G7 p.514:28mm
    a. Most common symptom is _____. — pain, not relieved by analgesics
    b. Most common sign is _____ _____ _____. — ascending sensory level — G7 p.514:55mm

176. **What may be the only feature of descending syringomyelia in patients with complete cord lesions?** — hyperhidrosis — G7 p.513:163mm

177. **Complete the following statements about syringomyelia:**
    G7 p.513:155mm
    a. What should raise the index of suspicion for a syrinx in a patient who is paraplegic from trauma?
        i. The _____ development — late
        ii. in a _____ patient — paraplegic
        iii. of _____ _____ weakness. — upper extremity
    b. Incidence is _____. — 0.3 to 3.0%
    c. Latency is _____. — 3 months to 30 years

178. **Complete the following statements about syringobulbia:**
    G7 p.510:106mm
    a. What is a common symptom in syringobulbia?
        i. p_____ p_____ — perioral paresthesias bilaterally (bilateral perioral tingling and numbness)
        ii. located _____
    b. due to compression of _____ _____ _____. — spinal trigeminal tracts

■ Spinal Epidural Hematoma

179. **What is the most common cause of spinal epidural hematoma?**
    G7 p.515:38mm
    a. _____ plus — trauma (almost exclusively in patients with)
    b. _____ — higher bleeding tendency (anticoagulated, bleeding diathesis, etc.)

18

180. **Complete the following about spinal epidural hematoma:**   G7 p.515:15mm
  a. The most common area of occurrence is   thoracic
      _____.
  b. Is it anterior or posterior?   often posterior (which facilitates removal)
  c. The most common category of patient is   anticoagulated
      _____.

181. **What is the usual presentation of spinal epidural hematoma?**   severe back pain (with radicular component)   G7 p.515:83mm

---

■ Spinal Subdural Hematoma

182. **Complete the following regarding spinal subdural hematoma:**   G7 p.515:150mm
  a. They occur _____.   rarely
  b. They are often related to _____.   trauma
  c. Patients are usually on _____ medication.   anticoagulant
  d. It may sometimes be treatable _____.   conservatively

■ Spinal Epidural Lipomatosis (SEL)

183. **Characterize spinal epidural lipomatosis (SEL).**   G7 p.516:30mm
  a. Due to _____ of epidural fat   hypertrophy
  b. Due to
      i. _____ and/or   obesity
      ii. exogenous _____   steroids
  c. Symptoms
      i. first is _____ _____   back pain
      ii. progressive _____ _____   lower extremity
      iii. and _____ weakness.   sensory
  d. Most occur in the _____ spine.   thoracic
  e. Diagnose by use of _____ or _____.   CT or MRI
  f. Should be at least _____ mm thick to be SEL.   7
  g. Treat by
      i. Reduce the use of _____ or _____.   steroids
      ii. Lose _____.   weight
      iii. Remove _____.   surgically
  h. Complication rate is _____.   high

◼ Coccydynia

184. **Answer the following about coccydynia:**   G7 p.516:130mm

  a. True or False. It is more common in males.

  false (It is more common in females.)

  b. Due to _____.

  a more prominent coccyx (In fact, if found in males in absence of trauma, search for underlying cause should be performed.)

185. **What are some causes of coccydynia?**   G7 p.516:140 mm

  a. t_____

  trauma

  b. n_____

  neoplasm

  c. r_____ p_____

  referred pain

186. **What is the primary treatment for typical coccydynia?**   G7 p.517:87mm

  conservative comfort measures: nonsteroidal antiinflammatory drugs, analgesics, sitting cushion, and lumbar support for 3 months

187. **What percentage of conservatively treated coccydynia will recur?**   G7 p.517:100mm

  20%; usually within first year

188. **What ganglion will be targeted for blockade or neurolysis in treatment of refractory coccydynia?**   G7 p.517:132mm

  Hint: Wilps

  a. Ganglion of _____,

  Walther

  b. also known as the ganglion _____,

  impar

  c. is the _____ ganglion of the

  lowest

  d. _____ _____,

  parasympathetic chain

  e. just anterior to the _____ _____.

  sacrococcygeal joint

18

19

Functional Neurosurgery

■ Deep Brain Stimulation

1. Characterize Parkinson disease.   G7 p.532:72mm
a. Best target is the _____ _____   subthalamic nucleus
b. It has similar efficacy to _____   levodopa
c. with fewer _____ _____.   side effects
d. ablative surgery is giving way to   deep brain stimulators   G7 p.534:50mm
    _____.

■ Surgical Treatment of Parkinson Disease

2. Matching. Regarding surgical ablative   G7 p.532:150mm
treatment of Parkinson disease and its
historical background, match the
listed procedures with the appropriate
phrase(s) and benefits.
Abandoned because:
① unpredictable results; ② tremor did
not improve; ③ bradykinesia did not
improve; ④ rigidity did not improve;
⑤ ipsilateral tremor persists; ⑥ side
effects/resistance; ⑦ only modest
benefits
Procedure:
a. anterior choroidal artery ligation   ①
b. anterodorsal pallidotomy   ②, ③
c. ventrolateral thalamotomy   ③, ④, ⑤
d. L-dopa   ⑥
e. transplantation   ⑦

3. How beneficial is pallidotomy of   G7 p.534:65mm
globus pallidus interna for the
following (percentage)?
a. Dyskinesia is _____%.   90%
b. Bradykinesia is _____%.   85%
c. Rigidity is _____%.   75%
d. Tremor is _____%.   57%

4. **True or False. The following symptoms improve after anterodorsal pallidotomy:**
   a. tremor ipsilateral   false
   b. rigidity   true
   c. bradykinesia   false
   d. ataxia   false
   e. tremor contralateral   false

   G7 p.532:157mm

5. **Ventrolateral thalamotomy can improve tremor; it can*not* be performed bilaterally because bilateral thalamotomy causes**
   a. d_____ and   dysarthria
   b. g_____ d_____. gait disturbance (Incidence of postoperative dysarthria and gait disturbance is high.)

   G7 p.532:162 mm

6. **Complete the following about surgical treatment of Parkinson disease:**
   a. The target today is the _____ _____   posteroventral pallidum
   b. specifically the
      i. _____   GPi—internal segment of the globus pallidus
      ii. which blocks the input from the _____   STN—subthalamic nucleus

   G7 p.533:165mm

7. **How might pallidotomy work?**
   a. direct destruction of the _____   GPi
   b. interrupt _____ fibers   pallidofugal
   c. diminish input from the _____   subthalamic nucleus

   G7 p.534:66mm

8. **Answer the following about surgical treatment of Parkinson disease:**
   a. What was an early procedure for the treatment of Parkinson disease?   ligation of the anterior choroidal artery
   b. What are the mechanisms by which pallidotomy may work?
      i.   destroy _____   GPi or
      ii. interrupt p_____ p_____   pallidofugal pathways
      iii. reduce input into m_____ p_____   medial pallidum

   c. What is the target for the tremor treatment?   ventralis intermedius nucleus (VIM) of the thalamus
   d. True or False. Pallidotomy is primarily focused on the treatment of motor symptoms.   true
   e. What are the most common complications of pallidotomy? Hint: vhid
      i.   v_____   visual field deficit
      ii. h_____   hemiparesis
      iii. i_____ h_____   intracerebral hemorrhage
      iv. d_____   dysarthria

   G7 p.532:150mm
   G7 p.534:65mm
   G7 p.534:120mm
   G7 p.536:62mm

19

9. **Characterize thalamic lesions.**   G7 p.536:80mm
   a. Lesioning in the thalamic _____   intermedius
      nucleus
   b. reduces parkinsonian _____,   tremor
   c. however it does not improve _____   bradykinesia
   d. and may worsen
      i. g_____ s_____ and   gait symptoms
      ii. s_____ p_____.   speech problems

10. **Characterize subthalamatomy.**   G7 p.536:105mm
   a. Lesions in the STN classically produced   hemiballism
      _____.
   b. Selective lesions may give relief on a par   pallidotomy
      with _____.

11. **Characterize dystonia.**   G7 p.536:135mm
   a. Stimulation of the _____ is the   pallidum
      primary surgical treatment for the
      dystonia.
   b. Results are better for _____   tardive
      dyskinesia.
   c. The most common target is _____.   GPi

12. **True or False. Stimulation has**   G7 p.534:83mm
    attracted increasing interest in
    patients with Parkinson disease who
    are refractory to medical drug
    treatment. The deep brain stimulator
    (the electrode) is placed in which of
    the following locations? (There are
    three true answers.)
    a. zona incerta   false
    b. posterior ventral pallidum (PV)   false
    c. substantia nigra (SN)   false
    d. Forel field (H)   false
    e. subthalamic nucleus (STN)   true
    f. globus pallidus internus (GPi)   true
    g. pedunculopontine nucleus   true   G7 p.534:92mm

13. **True or False. Indications for**   G7 p.534:100mm
    pallidotomy in parkinsonism include
    a. refractory to drug therapy   true
    b. drug-induced dyskinesia   true
    c. rigidity   true
    d. tremor   false
    e. dementia   false

14. **Ipsilateral hemianopsia is a**   optic tract injury; blind (Visual   G7 p.534:150mm
    contraindication to ventral   field defects could occur in
    pallidotomy because one of the side   2.5% of patients; blindness
    effects of the procedure could be   could result.)
    o_____ t_____ i_____
    and would cause the patient to be
    _____.

15. **Bilateral pallidotomies carry an increased risk of**   G7 p.535:168mm
    a. s_____ d_____ and   speech difficulties
    b. c_____ d_____.   cognitive decline

16. **True or False. What are the benefits for the patient from posteroventral pallidotomy as done currently?**   G7 p.536:18mm
    a. motor symptoms   true
    b. dyskinesia   true
    c. rigidity   true
    d. bradykinesia   true
    e. tremor   true

17. **True or False. Common complications of pallidotomy (unilateral) include**   G7 p.536:62mm
    a. visual field deficit   true
    b. dysarthria   true
    c. hemisensory deficit   false (Hemisensory deficit is not a common complication.)
    d. hemiparesis   true

■ Spasticity

18. **True or False. A spastic bladder will**   G7 p.537:40mm
    a. have high capacity and empty spontaneously   false
    b. have high capacity and empty with difficulty   false
    c. have low capacity and empty spontaneously   true (Low capacity and spontaneous emptying are the hallmarks of the spastic bladder.)
    d. have low capacity and empty with difficulty   false

19. **True or False. The onset of a spastic bladder after spinal cord injury is**   G7 p.537:48mm
    a. immediate   false
    b. delayed   true (Delayed onset is typical because the acute phase of spinal shock is hyporeflexic and hypotonic.)
    c. can occur at any time   false

20. **True or False. The Ashworth score can grade severity of spasticity. The highest score in this system is given when there is**   G7 p.537:80mm
    a. no increase in tone (full movement)   false
    b. rigidity in all flexors   false
    c. rigidity in all extensors   false
    d. rigidity in flexion and extension   true

19

21. The Ashworth score is the clinical grading of the _____ _____ _____.

severity of spasticity

G7 p.537:90mm

22. What are the medications used in the treatment of spasticity?
    a. b_____
    b. d_____
    c. d_____
    d. p_____

baclofen
diazepam
dantrolene
progabide

G7 p.537:140mm

23. What are the nonablative procedures used for the treatment of spasticity?
    a. i_____ b_____
    b. i_____ m_____
    c. e_____ e_____ s_____

intrathecal baclofen
intrathecal morphine
epidural electrical stimulation

G7 p.538:72mm

24. What are the ablative procedures with preservation of ambulation used for the treatment of spasticity? Name one.

motor point block, phenol nerve block, selective neurectomy, percutaneous radiofrequency foraminal rhizotomy, Bischof myelotomy, selective dorsal rhizotomy, stereotactic thalamotomy, or dentatotomy

G7 p.538:83mm

25. True or False. Fibers that are more sensitive to radiofrequency rhizotomy are
    a. small unmyelinated sensory fibers
    b. large myelinated alpha motor fibers

true
false

G7 p.538:120mm

26. What are the ablative procedures with sacrifice of ambulation used for the treatment of spasticity? Name one.

intrathecal injection of phenol, selective anterior rhizotomy, neurectomy, intramuscular neurolysis, cordectomy, cordotomy

G7 p.539:32mm

27. True or False. Spasticity can be treated with intrathecal baclofen pumps. Complications are mainly
    a. pump underinfusion
    b. wound complications
    c. catheter complications

    d. drug resistance

false
false
true (Catheter complications may have a frequency of up to 30% in baclofen pumps.)
false

G7 p.540:45mm

19

■ Torticollis

28.	What is another name for torticollis?	wry neck	G7 p.541:50 mm
29.	What muscle is usually affected in spasmodic torticollis?	sternocleidomastoid	G7 p.541:69mm

30. **What are the surgical procedures used for the treatment of spasmodic torticollis?**   G7 p.541:130mm

19

  a. stimulate _____ _____   dorsal cord
  b. inject _____ _____   botulinum toxin
  c. cut _____   rhizotomy
  d. coagulate _____ _____   Forel's H1

31. **What artery is most commonly implicated in the torticollis of the eleventh nerve origin?**   vertebral   G7 p.541:185mm

■ Neurovascular Compression Syndromes

32. **Characterize root entry zone.**   G7 p.542:35mm
  a. Syndromes due to compression of
    i. _____ _____   cranial nerves
    ii. at the _____ _____   root entry zone
    _____
  b. This site, also known as the _____-_____ zone,   Obersteiner-Redlich
  c. is the point where the central myelin from the _____ cells.   oligodendroglial
  d. Changes to the peripheral myelin of the _____ cells   Schwann

33. **True or False. Hemifacial spasm (HFS) starts from the lower half of the face and spreads to the upper half of the face.**   false (starts with the orbicularis oculi)   G7 p.542:98mm

34. **Complete the following about neurovascular compression syndromes:**   G7 p.542:110mm
  a. On what side is HFS more common?   left
  b. What is the age and gender predilection?   women, after the teen ages
  c. What is the most commonly involved artery?   AICA
  d. True or False. Carbamazepine and phenytoin are generally effective treatment.   false
  e. What is the material used as a cushion in the microvascular decompression (MVD)?   Ivalon, polyvinyl formyl alcohol foam

35. What is the only other involuntary movement disorder besides HFS that persists during sleep?

palatal myoclonus

G7 p.542:125mm

36. What distinguishes HFS from blepharospasm?

G7 p.542:155mm

a. HFS is _____.

unilateral

b. Blepharospasm is _____.

bilateral

37. What distinguishes HFS from facial myokymia (FM)?

G7 p.542:172mm

a. Hemifacial spasm (HFS) is _____.

intermittent

b. Facial myokymia (FM) is _____.

continuous

38. True or False. The vessel most commonly associated with hemifacial spasm is

G7 p.543:15mm

a. posterior inferior cerebellar artery (PICA)   false

b. superior cerebellar artery (SCA)   false

c. anterior inferior cerebellar artery (AICA)   true

d. posterior cerebral artery (PCA)   false

e. vertebral artery   false

f. basilar artery   false

39. Hemifacial spasm

G7 p.543:48mm

a. is caused by compression at the _____ _____ _____

root entry zone

b. of the _____ _____

facial nerve

c. by the _____.

AICA

d. This does not cause _____ conduction but

ephaptic

e. produces _____

kindling

f. and _____.

synkinesis

40. Synkinesis is a phenomenon where

G7 p.543:57mm

a. stimulation of _____ _____ of the facial nerve

one branch

b. results in _____ _____

delayed discharges

c. through _____ _____.

another branch

41. True or False. Postoperatively after microvascular decompression for hemifacial spasm the patient can expect

G7 p.543:145mm

a. immediate cessation of facial spasms   false

b. reduction starting 2 to 3 days later   true

c. better results the longer the patient has had HFS   false

d. better results the older the patient is   false

e. complete resolution of spasms eventually   true (in 81 to 93% of patients)

f. possible relapse even if free of spasms for a full 2 years   false (relapse after 2 years only 1%)

42. **Complications of hemifacial spasm (HFS) surgery include the following:**
G7 p.544:70mm
Hint: hemifacial s

i.	h_____	hoarseness
ii.	e_____	elderly do less well
iii.	m_____	meningitis (aseptic)
iv.	i_____	ipsilateral hearing loss
v.	f_____	facial weakness
vi.	a_____	ataxia
vii.	c_____	CSF rhinorrhea
viii.	i_____	incomplete relief—
ix.	a_____	aseptic meningitis
x.	l_____	lip (perioral) herpes
xi.	s_____	swallowing (dysphagia)

■ Hyperhidrosis

43. **Complete the following statements about hyperhidrosis:**
G7 p.544:132mm
a. It is due to overactivity of the _____ _____ glands.   eccrine sweat
b. These glands are under control of the _____ _____ _____.   sympathetic nervous system
c. The neurotransmitter is _____.   acetylcholine   G7 p.544:140mm
d. Most _____ end organs are _____.   sympathetic; adrenergic
e. Some cases warrant _____ _____.   surgical sympathectomy

■ Sympathectomy

44. **Name five indications for upper extremity (UE) sympathectomy.**
G7 p.545:75mm
Hint: "crash" the sympathetic ganglia
a. c_____   causalgia major primary
b. R_____   Raynaud disease
c. a_____   intractable angina
d. s_____   shoulder-hand syndrome
e. h_____   hyperhidrosis

45. **Complete the following statements about sympathectomy:**
G7 p.545:60mm
a. What is the level for cardiac sympathectomy?   from stellate ganglion
b. What is the level for UE sympathectomy?   second thoracic ganglia T2   G7 p.545:82mm
c. What is the level for lumbar sympathectomy?   L2 and L3 sympathetic ganglia   G7 p.545:147mm
d. What is the most commonly used approach for lumbar sympathectomy?   retroperitoneal

19

46.   What are the complications of UE   G7 p.545:100mm
sympathectomy?
   a.   p_____   pneumothorax
   b.   i_____ n_____   intercostal neuralgia
   c.   s_____ c_____ i_____ spinal cord injury
   d.   H_____ s_____   Horner syndrome

19

20

Pain

■ Neuropathic Pain Syndromes

1. **Complete the following statements about pain:**

   G7 p.548:40mm

   a. Three types of pain are
      i. n_____   nociceptive
      ii. d_____   deafferentation
      iii. s_____ m_____   sympathetically maintained
   b. Two types of nociceptive pain are
      i. s_____   somatic
      ii. v_____   visceral
   c. Two sites of electrical stimulation for pain in deep brain are
      i. peria_____ _____   periaqueductal gray   G7 p.567:135mm
      ii. periv_____ _____   periventricular gray

■ Craniofacial Pain Syndromes

2. **Complete the following statements about craniofacial pain syndromes:**

   G7 p.549:83mm

   a. Tic convulsif is g_____ neuralgia plus h_____ spasm.   geniculate; hemifacial
   b. Ramsay Hunt syndrome is p_____ g_____ n_____.   postherpetic geniculate neuralgia
   c. Tolosa-Hunt syndrome is s_____ o_____ f_____ i_____.   superior orbital fissure inflammation
   d. Raeder neuralgia is p_____ n_____.   paratrigeminal neuralgia

3. **Characterize craniofacial pain syndromes.**

   G7 p.549:120mm

   Hint: sunct

   a. s_____ _____   short lasting
   b. u_____   unilateral
   c. n_____ _____ with   neuralgiform headache
   d. c_____ _____ and   conjunctival injection
   e. t_____   tearing
   f. brief—about _____   2 minutes

g. near the _____   eye
h. occurs _____ _____ per day   multiple times
i. affects _____   males

4. **Complete the following regarding**   G7 p.550: 40mm
   primary otalgia:
a. It may have its origin from which nerves?   fifth, seventh, ninth, tenth,
                                               and occipital nerves
b. Cocainization of the pharynx producing   glossopharyngeal neuralgia
   pain relief suggests _____ _____
   instead of primary otalgia.
c. Treatment includes
   i. medicines: T_____, D_____,   Tegretol, Dilantin, and
       and b_____   baclofen
   ii. surgical procedures of   microvascular decompression
       decompression by m_____   (MVD), nerve fibers, nervus
       d_____ or sectioning n_____ intermedius, ninth and tenth
       f_____ of the n_____   CN
       i_____ and n_____ and
       t_____ CN

5. **Characterize trigeminal neuralgia**   G7 p.551:120mm
   (TGN).
a. The incidence is _____.   4/100,000
b. The percentage of multiple sclerosis (MS)   2%
   patients who have TGN is _____%.
c. The percentage of bilateral TGN patients   18%
   who also have MS is _____%.
d. It is pathophysiologically caused by   ephaptic transmission from
   _____.   large myelinated A fibers to
                                               poorly myelinated A delta and
                                               C fibers
e. It is caused
   i.   most commonly by _____   superior cerebellar artery
        _____ _____   (SCA)
   ii. or _____ _____ _____   persistent primitive
        _____   trigeminal artery
   iii. or _____ _____.   basilar artery

6. **Complete the following statements**   G7 p.552:80mm
   about craniofacial pain syndromes:
a. What should the neurologic exam be in a   entirely normal
   patient with trigeminal neuralgia?
b. How effective is Tegretol?   pain relief in 69%
c. What if Tegretol has no effect?   The diagnosis of trigeminal
                                             neuralgia is suspect.
d. What is the second drug of choice for   baclofen (Lioresal)
   trigeminal neuralgia?
e. The two special precautions needed with
   the use of this medication are as follows:
   i. It may be _____.   teratogenic
   ii. Don't _____ _____.   stop abruptly

7. **Medicines for trigeminal neuralgia include the following:** G7 p.552:155mm
   a. a_____ — amitriptyline (old)
   b. b_____ — baclofen
   c. c_____ — carbamazepine, clonazepam, capsaicin
   d. D_____ — Dilantin
   e. E_____ — Elavil
   f. g_____ — gabapentin
   g. L_____ — Lamictal
   h. o_____ — oxcarbazepine

8. **Oxcarbazepine** G7 p.553:20mm
   a. aka _____ — trileptal
   b. is metabolized into_____. — carbazepine
   c. It is useful because patients can tolerate _____ _____. — higher doses

20

9. **What is the basis upon which percutaneous procedures treat trigeminal neuralgia?** G7 p.553:167mm
   a. They destroy _____ _____, — nociceptive fibers
   b. which are _____ _____ — A Δ and C
   c. and preserve _____, — touch fibers
   d. which are _____ _____. — A α and β

10. **Which treatment procedure is most helpful in trigeminal neuralgia in multiple sclerosis patients?** — percutaneous techniques (Microvascular decompression [MVD] does not work well for multiple sclerosis [MS] patients with trigeminal neuralgia [TGN].) G7 p.553:167mm

11. **State the benefits of percutaneous microcompression (PMC).** G7 p.554:175mm
   a. Patient can choose to avoid _____ _____. — major surgery
   b. With multiple sclerosis and trigeminal neuralgia treatment
      i. Which procedure is best? — balloon PMC
      ii. Does it respond to microvascular decompression? — not well
   c. Occurrences of intraoperative hypertension are _____. — less with PMC than with radiofrequency
   d. Reports of intracranial hemorrhage? — none reported with PMC

12. **Answer the following concerning trigeminal neuralgia (TGN) and microvascular decompression (MVD):** G7 p.554:175 mm
   a. True or False. It is appropriate for an older age group. — false (not to be used on persons over 65)
   b. True or False. It may produce anesthesia dolorosa. — false (It does not occur with MVD.)
   c. It has a mortality rate of _____%. — 1%
   d. It has a major neurologic morbidity of _____%. — 1 to 10%

20

e. It has a failure rate of _____%.   20 to 25%

f. True or False. It is the procedure of   false (MS patients do not
    choice in MS patients.   respond to MVD.)

g. What is the procedure of choice in MS   percutaneous
    patients?   microcompression (PMC)
                                                           (i.e., balloon)

h. What is the recurrence rate in MS   50% in 3 years with
    patients?   percutaneous techniques

13. Complete the following about TGN   *G7 p.555:78mm*
    and the benefits of stereotactic
    radiosurgery:

a. Complete pain relief is achieved in   65%
    _____%.

b. There is significant pain reduction in an   15 to 30%
    additional _____%.

14. Complete the following about TGN   *G7 p.556:140mm*
    and electrode positioning:

a. Positioning for percutaneous approach
    i.   lip: _____   lateral to lip 2 to 3 cm
    ii. eye: _____   medial aspect of pupil
    iii. ear: _____   3 cm anterior to external
                                                           auditory meatus

b. X-ray landmarks
    i.   anteroposterior (AP)—submental   foramen ovale
         vertex, aim for _____
    ii. lateral x-ray, aim for _____   10 mm below floor of sella
                                                           along clivus

15. Characterize complications of   *G7 p.558:55mm*
    radiofrequency trigeminal rhizotomy.

a. masseter weakness _____%   24%
b. anesthesia dolorosa _____%   4%
c. neuroparalytic keratitis _____%   4%
d. oculomotor paresis _____%   2%
e. How would you identify pterygoid
    muscle weakness?
    i.   ask patient to _____   open mouth
    ii. chin deviates to side of _____   weak pterygoid

16. Describe microvascular   *G7 p.561:150mm*
    decompression (MVD) complications.

a. mortality _____%   0.22 to 2%
b. morbidity _____%   1 to 10%
c. hearing loss _____%   3%
d. infarction _____%   0.6%
e. success rate _____%   75 to 80%, approximately
                                                           60% of original group

17. Complete the following about   *G7 p.562:115mm*
    supraorbital and supratrochlear
    nerves:

a. They arise from the _____ nerve.   frontal
b. The larger of the two is the _____.   supraorbital
c. It exits the orbit via the _____ notch.   supraorbital

d. It is located within the _____ third of   medial
    the orbital roof.
e. Which nerve is most medial?   supratrochlear

18. Complete the following about   G7 p.563:36mm
supraorbital neuralgia (SON):
a. True or False. SON can be differentiated   true
    from trigeminal neuralgia.
b. SON lacks _____ zones.   trigger
c. SON lacks _____ _____–like pain.   electric shock

19. Characterize glossopharyngeal   G7 p.563:100mm
neuralgia.

a. Pain is located in
    i.   base of t_____ = g_____ and   tongue = glosso
    ii. t_____ = p_____   throat = pharyngeal
b. Other symptoms
    i.   h_____   hypotension—vagus
    ii. s_____   syncope
    iii. c_____ a_____   cardiac arrest

20. Describe glossopharyngeal neuralgia.   G7 p.563:110mm
a. The incidence is _____ in _____   1 in 1,775,000 (1/70 as
    persons.   frequent as trigeminal
                                                      neuralgia; trigeminal
                                                      neuralgia occurs 4/100,000
                                                      [i.e., 1/25,000])
b. Pain occurs in t_____, b_____ of   throat, base of tongue, ear,
    t_____, e_____, n_____   neck
c. Treatment includes
    i.   medicine: c_____   cocainization
    ii. surgery: m_____ d_____   microvascular decompression
    iii. section of n_____ and   ninth and upper third of tenth
         u_____ t_____ of t_____   nerve
         n_____

21. Complete the following concerning   G7 p.563:180mm
geniculate neuralgia:
a. Pain is located _____.   deep in the ear, eye, cheek
b. It is called _____.   prosopalgia
c. If there are herpetic lesions this is called   Ramsey Hunt syndrome
    R_____ H_____ s_____.
d. If combined with hemifacial spasm it is   tic convulsif
    called t_____ c_____.
e. Treatment
    i.   medicine _____   same as trigeminal neuralgia
    ii. surgery _____ _____   microvascular decompression
                                                      of seventh nerve
    iii. What vessel is involved?   AICA—compressing sensory
                                                      and motor roots of seventh
                                                      nerve

■ Postherpetic Neuralgia

22. **Complete the following about herpes zoster:**   G7 p.564:120mm
    a. The etiologic agent is h_____ v_____ z_____ v_____.   herpes varicella zoster virus
    b. It involves the eye in _____%.   10%
    c. Pain lasts _____.   2 to 4 weeks
    d. Long-term pain persists in _____%,   10%
    e. called p_____ n_____.   postherpetic neuralgia
    f. Vesicles and pain run in the
       i. distribution of the d_____   dermatome
       ii. not the p_____ n_____.   peripheral nerve
    g. Treatment is with
       i. c_____ and   capsaicin
       ii. a_____.   amitriptyline

23. **Complete the following about postherpetic neuralgia:**   G7 p.465:105mm
    a. With an acute attack of herpes zoster, you may treat with e_____ or i_____ i_____.   epidural or intercostal injection
    b. For acute treatment use
       i. a_____ or   acyclovir
       ii. v_____   valacyclovir
    c. For postherpetic neuralgia use
       i. Z_____ (c_____)   Zostrix (capsaicin)
       ii. N_____ (g_____)   Neurontin (gabapentin)
       iii. E_____ (a_____)   Elavil (amitriptyline)
    d. Start treatment with
       i. l_____ p_____, which is   lidocaine patches   G7 p.465:170mm
       ii. better tolerated in the _____.   elderly   G7 p.465:155mm

■ Pain Procedures

24. **Usual maximum oral narcotic dose tolerated is _____.**   MS contin (up to 300 to 400 mg/day)   G7 p.567:95mm

25. **Name intracranial ablative procedures to treat the following pains:**   G7 p.567:157mm
    a. cancer pain: m_____ t_____   medial thalamotomy (stereotactic procedure used for nociceptive cancer pain)
    b. head, neck, face pain: s_____ m_____   stereotactic mesencephalon lesion 5 mm lateral to aqueduct at level of inferior colliculus; diplopia may occur
    c. suffering from pain: c_____   cingulotomy—bilaterally (modifies affect use MRI— recurs in approximately 3 months)

20

26. **Matching. Match the procedure and its application (some have more than one).**

    Applications for pain from:
    ① spinal cord injuries; ② post-laminectomy pain; ③ pelvic pain with incontinence; ④ at or below C5; ⑤ head, face, neck, upper extremity; ⑥ bilateral below diaphragm; ⑦ causalgia; ⑧ bilateral below thoracic dermatomes; ⑨ avulsion injuries; ⑩ not for cancer pain

    Procedure:
    a. stereotactic mesencephalotomy ⑤
    b. cordotomy ④
    c. spinal intrathecal ⑥
    d. sacral cordotomy ③
    e. sympathectomy ⑦
    f. commissural myelotomy ⑧
    g. dorsal root entry zone (DREZ) ①, ⑨, ⑩
    h. spinal cord stimulator ②, ⑩

    G7 p.567:170mm

27. **Complete the following concerning cordotomy:**
    G7 p.568:80mm
    a. Your objective is to interrupt the fibers of the _____ _____ _____ _____ on the side _____ to the pain.

    lateral spinal thalamic tract; contralateral

    b. Cordotomy is the procedure of choice for _____ pain below the _____ dermatome.

    unilateral; C5

    c. Two ways to perform cordotomy are
    i. _____
    ii. _____

    open
    percutaneous

    d. Loss of automatic breathing can occur after _____ _____ and is called _____ _____.

    bilateral cordotomy; Ondine curse

    e. What is the cutoff percentage on pulmonary function test before patients can undergo cordotomy?

    50%

28. **Answer the following about pain procedures:**
    G7 p.568:165mm
    a. What kind of patients are candidates for cordotomy?

    terminally ill patients

    b. On which side should the cordotomy be performed?

    contralateral to the pain

    c. What happens to impedance as the needle penetrates the cord?

    jumps from 300 to 500 ohms to 1200 to 1500 ohms.

    d. What response should stop cordotomy from being performed?

    muscle tetany upon stimulation

    e. If you look at the eye what will you learn?

    if there is a Horner syndrome ipsilaterally the procedure is satisfactory

    f. What percent will have pain relief?

    94%

29. Answer the following concerning commissural myelotomy:

a. What is the indication for commissural myelotomy?

bilateral or midline pain

G7 p.570:75mm

b. What is the rate of complete pain relief after commissural myelotomy?

60%

c. What is the special requirement for intrathecal morphine?

preservative-free 0.9% saline

30. Answer the following regarding central nervous system (CNS) narcotic administration:

G7 p.571:88mm

a. Requirement for implantation of a morphine pump is _____ _____ _____.

preoperative testing dose

b. _____ _____ can shorten the delay time for a morphine pump to function; otherwise the relief may not occur for _____.

Bolus infusion; days

c. Is meningitis common after pump placement?

no

d. Is respiratory failure common after pump placement?

no

31. Complete the following concerning spinal cord stimulation:

G7 p.572:175mm

a. Site of spinal cord stimulation is the _____ _____.

dorsal column

   i. The most common indication is _____ _____ _____.

postlaminectomy pain syndrome

G7 p.573:28mm

   ii. It is not usually indicated for _____ _____.

cancer pain

b. Two kinds of electrodes are

   i. p_____-like

plate

G7 p.573:60mm

   ii. w_____-like

wire

32. Complete the following regarding deep brain stimulation:

G7 p.575:15mm

a. Periventricular stimulation will be beneficial for _____ pain.

nociceptive

b. A lesion at the _____ _____ _____ _____ can help phantom limb pain.

dorsal root entry zone

c. Rate of recurrence after thalamotomy for pain is _____% in _____.

60% in 6 months

Dorsal Root Entry Zone Lesions

33. **Complete the following about dorsal root entry zone (DREZ) lesions:**   G7 p575 :45mm
a. They are useful for _____ pain.   deafferentation
b. They result from nerve root _____.   avulsion
c. They most commonly occur from _____ accidents.   motorcycle
d. For such an injury, pain relief can be expected in _____%.   80 to 90 %   G7 p575 :115mm

Thalamotomy

34. **Complete the following about thalamotomy:**   G7 p.575:143mm
a. It is used _____.   rarely
b. Target is the _____ thalamus.   medial
c. Cancer pain control occurs in _____%   50%   G7 p.575:143mm
d. but by 6 months only in _____%.   20%
e. Neuropathologic pain control is successful in only _____%.   20%

Complex Regional Pain Syndrome

35. **Complete the following statements about causalgia:**   G7 p.576:54mm
a. Triad to diagnose causalgia
   i.   a_____ d_____   autonomic dysfunction
   ii. b_____ p_____   burning pain
   iii. t_____ c_____   trophic changes
b. What is the cause of major causalgia?   high-velocity missile injury
c. Allodynia is pain induced by _____ _____.   non-noxious stimulus
d. Signs of causalgia are
   i.   tapered _____   fingers
   ii. hands are _____ and _____   cold and moist
   iii. touching causes _____   pain
   iv. also known as _____   allodynia   G7 p.576:170mm
e. Current name for causalgia is _____ _____ _____ _____.   complex regional pain syndrome (CRPS)

36. **Complete the following statements about causalgia:**   G7 p.577:84mm
a. Medical treatment for causalgia uses _____ _____.   tricyclic antidepressants
b. A common agent used for intravenous injection for causalgia is _____.   guanethedine
c. Surgical sympathectomy may relieve the pain of causalgia in _____%.   90%   G7 p.577:103mm

20

21

Tumor

■ General Information

1. **True or False. The following tumor is considered to be a World Health Organization (WHO) grade IV:**   G7 p.582:97mm
   a. anaplastic astrocytoma — false (Anaplastic astrocytoma is a grade III.)   G7 p.582:117mm
   b. gliosarcoma — true   G7 p.582:12mm
   c. fibrillary astrocytoma — false (Fibrillary astrocytoma is a grade II.)
   d. subependymal giant cell astrocytoma — false (Subependymal giant cell astrocytoma is a grade II.)   G7 p.582:148mm

2. **True or False. Tumors of mixed neuronal-glial origin include the following:**   G7 p.583:45mm
   a. ganglioglioma — true
   b. central neurocytoma — true
   c. primitive neuroectodermal tumor (PNET) — false (Primitive neuroectodermal tumor [PNET] is listed under embryonal tumors. Old nomenclature is medulloblastoma—small round blue cell tumor.)
   d. desmoplastic infantile ganglioglioma (DIG) — true

3. **Complete the following about general tumor information:**   G7 p.583:95mm
   a. Medulloblastoma is considered to be what type of tumor? — embryonal
   b. It is also known as _____. — PNET

4. **What are the two types of craniopharyngioma?**   G7 p.584:180mm
   a. a_____ — adamantinomatous ("Adam Antinomatous")
   b. p_____ — papillary

5. **List the four most common presentations of brain tumor and their frequency.**   G7 p.585:160mm
    a. p_____ n_____ d_____—_____%   progressive neurologic deficit—68%
    b. h_____—_____%   headache—54%
    c. m_____ w_____—_____%   motor weakness—45%
    d. s_____—_____%   seizure—26%

6. **When encountering a first-time seizure in a patient older than 20 years of age, think _____ until proven otherwise.**   tumor   G7 p.586:38mm

■ Infratentorial Tumors

21

7. **What is the name of the so-called vomiting center?**   area postrema   G7 p.586:145mm

8. **What nerve has the longest intracranial course?**   sixth nerve (abducens)   G7 p.586:160mm

9. **Matching. Match the area of cerebellum with symptoms.**   G7 p.586:165mm
    Area of cerebellum:
    ① hemisphere, ② vermis, ③ brain stem
    Symptoms:
    a. Ataxia of extremities   ①
    b. Broad-based gait   ②
    c. Truncal ataxia   ②
    d. Dysmetria   ①
    e. Intention tremor   ①
    f. Nystagmus   ③
    g. Cranial nerve dysfunction   ③

10. **Complete the following concerning a > 20-year-old patient presenting with a headache:**   G7 p.587:120mm
    a. The classical headache of brain tumor includes
        i.   a.m. _____   worse
        ii. strain cough _____   increases
        iii. bending forward _____   increases
        iv. associated with n_____ and/or   nausea and/or vomiting
             v_____
    b. Is this constellation truly suggestive of brain tumor?   no
    c. What percentage have these "classic" headaches?   8% (77% had headache similar to tension headache, 9% were similar to migraine, only 8% showed classic brain tumor headache; two thirds of these had high intracranial pressure [ICP])

11. Familial syndromes
G7 p.588:40mm

a. are associated with _____ _____ CNS tumors
b. which are (Hint: vntLT):
   i. v_____ _____-_____ von Hippel-Lindau
   ii. n_____ neurofibromatosis
   iii. t_____ _____ tuberous sclerosis
   iv. L_____-_____ Li-Fraumeni
   v. T_____ Turcot

12. Matching. Match the familial syndromes with the associated CNS tumors.
G7 p.588:40mm

Syndromes:
① von Hippel-Lindau, ② neurofibromatosis, ③ tuberous sclerosis, ④ Li-Fraumeni, ⑤ Turcot
CNS tumors:
a. PNET ④
b. glioblastoma multiforme (gbm) ⑤
c. hemangioblastoma ①
d. subependymal grant cell astrocytoma ③
e. vestibular schwannoma ②

13. True or False. The following central nervous system (CNS) tumors occur in neurofibromatosis (NF):
G7 p.588:108mm

a. acoustic (vestibular schwannoma) true (bilateral)
b. meningioma true
c. ependymoma true
d. astrocytoma true (otherwise known as multiple inherited schwannomas, meningiomas, and ependymomas)
e. ganglioglioma false

14. True or False. The beneficial effect of steroids is greater for
G7 p.588:115mm

a. metastatic tumor true
b. primary tumor false

15. What brain tumor has a generally favorable response to chemotherapy? oligodendroglioma
G7 p.589:90 mm

16. What tactics can be used to circumvent the blood-brain barrier (BBB)?
G7 p.589:115mm

Hint: lhdb
a. l_____ lipophilic agent nitrosoureas
b. h_____ higher doses of medications
c. d_____ disrupt BBB with mannitol
d. b_____ bypass BBB with intrathecal methotrexate for primary lymphoma

17. What common medication can be used to disrupt the BBB for chemotherapy delivery? mannitol
G7 p.589:135mm

21

18. **Complete the following about general tumors:**   G7 p.589:160mm
   a. What is the proper time to obtain postop computed tomographic (CT) scan after brain tumor surgery?
      i. to check for bleeding use contrast immediately. True or false?   false
      ii. to check for residual tumor use contrast _____?   in the first 2 days postop
   b. What period of time would be inappropriate to obtain a postop head CT scan with contrast to assess for residual tumor?   during the period 2 days to 8 weeks after surgery is not a reliable testing time for CT or MRI
   c. Any exception to this timing rule of thumb?   yes
      i. In what case?   pituitary tumors
      ii. How long to wait?   4 months' delay is recommended

19. **Complete the following about general tumors:**   G7 p.590:45mm
   a. In a pediatric patient with a posterior fossa tumor, what additional test should be done preoperatively?   MRI of lumbosacral spine with contrast
   b. Why?   to rule out drop metastases
   c. Why not do it postoperatively when you are sure the test is needed?   because postoperative blood may cause an artifact
   d. Artifact will last for _____.   3 weeks

20. **Should we place a shunt or external ventricular drain (EVD) into a pediatric patient with a posterior fossa tumor and hydrocephalus?**   G7 p.590: 60mm
   a. pros
      i. possible lower o_____ m_____   operative mortality
   b. cons
      i. l_____ shunt   lifelong
      ii. s_____ of peritoneum   seeding
      iii. u_____ _____ herniation   upward transtentorial
      iv. i_____ in shunt   infection
      v. d_____ in definitive treatment   delay

■ Primary Brain Tumors

21. **Characterize low-grade gliomas.**   G7 p.591:58mm
   a. On T1-weighted image (T1WI), they are _____.   hypointense
   b. On T2WI, they are _____.   hyperintense
   c. What percentage enhance?   30% only
   d. A positron emission tomographic (PET) scan may demonstrate _____.   hypometabolism
   e. Can they be diagnosed radiologically?   no (Biopsy is needed for definitive diagnosis.)

21

22. Under the WHO classification an astrocytoma with necrosis is called a _____.

GBM

G7 p.594:168 mm

23. Complete the following about astrocytoma:

G7 p.595:50mm

a. grade I
   i. frequency _____%   0.7%
   ii. frequency rule of thumb _____%   1%
   iii. median survival _____ years   10
   iv. peak age incidence _____ years   20
b. grade II
   i. frequency _____%   16%
   ii. frequency rule of thumb _____%   15%
   iii. median survival _____ years   4
   iv. peak age incidence _____ years   30
c. grade III
   i. frequency _____%   17%
   ii. frequency rule of thumb _____%   15%
   iii. median survival _____ years   1.6
   iv. peak age incidence _____ years   40
d. grade IV
   i. frequency _____%   65%
   ii. frequency rule of thumb _____%   65%
   iii. median survival _____ years   0.7 (8.5 months)
   iv. peak age incidence _____ years   50

24. Complete the following regarding astrocytoma:

G7 p.595:122mm

a. longevity with low-grade astrocytoma
   i. aged 45 or younger _____   ~5 years
   ii. aged 45 or older _____   ~1½ years
b. why?
   i. Because low-grade astrocytomas undergo _____ _____   malignant transformation
   ii. _____-fold more rapidly after   six
   iii. age _____   45

25. List astrocytoma GBM microscopic characteristics.
Hint: cgppmnn

G7 p.596:73mm

a. c_____   cellular
b. g_____ a_____   gemistocytic astrocytes
c. p_____   pleomorphism
d. p_____   pseudopallisading
e. m_____   mitosis
f. n_____   necrosis
g. n_____   neovascularization

26. True or False. The following fluid clots:

G7 p.596:120mm

a. cerebrospinal fluid (CSF)   false
b. cyst fluid   true
c. subdural fluid   false
d. blood   true

27. **Describe astrocytoma CT and MRI characteristics.**   G7 p.596:165mm
   a. grade I
      i. CT   low
      ii. MRI   abnormal
      iii. mass?   no
      iv. enhancement?   no
   b. grade II
      i. CT   low
      ii. MRI   abnormal
      iii. mass?   yes
      iv. enhancement?   no
   c. grade III
      i. CT   low
      ii. MRI   abnormal
      iii. mass?   yes
      iv. enhancement?   yes
   d. grade IV
      i. CT   low
      ii. MRI   abnormal
      iii. mass?   yes
      iv. enhancement?   ring
   e. In ring enhancement the center represents
      i. n_____ and the rim is   necrosis   G7 p.597:88mm
      ii. c_____ t_____.   cellular tumor

28. **Meningeal gliomatosis occurs in _____% of high-grade gliomas at autopsy.**   20%   G7 p.598:52mm

29. **True or False. Treatments for low-grade gliomas should generally include**   G7 p.598:145mm
   a. biopsy or surgery for tissue diagnosis   true
   b. excisional biopsy   false
   c. radiation   false
   d. chemotherapy   false
   e. excision of pilocytic astrocytomas   true
   f. removal because the more tumor removed improves longevity   false (not clearly proven)   G7:p.599:15mm

30. **Complete the following regarding stereotactic biopsy:**   G7 p.600:20mm
   a. It underestimates the occurrence of GBM by _____%.   25%
   b. Some CNS _____ mimic GBM radiographically.   lymphomas
   c. Yield of biopsy is highest when
      i. low density _____ and   center
      ii. enhancing _____ are both sampled.   rim
   d. If Karnosky rating is higher than _____   70
   e. it portends a _____ prognosis.   better

31. Answer the following concerning malignant astrocytoma grade III or IV: G7 p.600:120mm

a. True or False. Treatment is surgical excision when possible.   true

b. Prognosis from surgical excision and radiotherapy is _____ weeks in the elderly.   30

c. Prognosis from biopsy and radiotherapy is _____ weeks in the elderly.   17

d. Type of radiotherapy advised is _____.   focal

e. Amount is _____ Gy.   50 to 60

32. Characterize wounded glioma syndrome.   G7 p.600:175mm

a. Partial resection of a GBM carries significant risk of _____   hemorrhage

b. or _____   edema

c. with resultant _____.   herniation

d. The benefit of subtotal resection is _____.   dubious

e. Surgical excision should be considered if total removal is _____.   feasible

33. Characteristic radiation therapy for   G7 p.601:35mm

a. malignant gliomas is _____Gy.   50 to 60

b. Is whole brain x-ray treatment (XRT) valuable?   no (It does not increase survival.)

34. Considering malignant gliomas, what is the only protocol fully validated by a phase 3 study for treatment of malignant glioma?   G7 p.601:125mm

a. s_____   surgery—maximal resection

b. r_____, _____ Gy   radiation, 60 Gy

c. c_____ (B_____)   chemotherapy (BCNU at 6-week intervals)

35. Matching. Match level of risk with patient characteristics.   G7 p.603:45mm

Risk:
① low risk, ② low moderate risk, ③ moderate high risk, ④ high risk
Patient characteristics:

a. Age under 40   ①
b. Age between 40 and 65   ③
c. Frontal tumor   ①
d. Tumor outside frontal lobe   ②
e. Karnofsky scale < 80   ④
f. Age above 65   ④
g. Subtotal resection (STR)   ③
h. Gross total resection (GTR)   ③

36. **What are the common locations of pilocytic astrocytoma?**
    Hint: hoc

    a. h_____   hypothalamus
    b. o_____ _____   optic chiasm
    c. c_____   cerebellum

37. **Characterize pilocytic astrocytoma.**
    a. Appearance on CT and MRI
       i. True or False. It enhances.   true (enhancing lesion)
       ii. True or False. It is solid.   false (often cystic)
       iii. It may have a _____ nodule.   mural
       iv. True or False. It is diffuse.   false (well circumscribed)
    b. You should resect the wall of the cyst if   enhances
       the wall _____.

38. **Characterize the radiologic appearance of pilocytic astrocytoma.**
    a. What is their shape?   well circumscribed
    b. Do they enhance?   yes—on MRI and CT
    c. Are they cystic?   yes
    d. Is there anything in the cyst?   mural nodule
    e. Are they surrounded by edema?   no
    f. Where are they located?   periventricular

39. **Complete the following about primary brain tumor:**
    a. cystic cerebellar astrocytoma
       i. incidence in adults _____%   10% of CNS tumors
       ii. percentage of childhood tumors   27 to 40% of posterior fossa
          _____%
    b. optic glioma
       i. incidence in adults _____%   2% of gliomas
       ii. percentage of childhood tumors   7% of gliomas
          _____%
    c. brain stem gliomas
       i. incidence in adults _____%   1% of CNS tumors
       ii. percentage of childhood tumors   10 to 20% of CNS tumors
          _____%
    d. oligodendroglioma
       i. incidence in adults _____%   2 to 4% of CNS tumors and
                                                 35% of all gliomas
       ii. percentage of childhood tumors   small%
          _____%
    e. meningioma
       i. incidence in adults _____%   15 to 20%
       ii. percentage of childhood tumors   1.5% of CNS tumors
          _____%
    f. vestibular schwannoma
       i. incidence in adults _____%   8 to 10%
       ii. percentage of childhood tumors   0%
          _____%

21

40. **According to Collins' law, a patient's tumor is considered cured if**   G7 p.605:160mm
a. it does _____ recur   not
b. after a postop period equal to the   age
    patient's _____
c. plus _____.   9 months

41. **Consider treatments for optic glioma.**   G7 p.606:85mm
a. One optic nerve involved sparing chiasm,   craniotomy and orbital
    painless proptosis, gliosis of optic nerve exploration
    head on funduscopy perform _____
    and _____ _____.
    i.   Treatment should be to e_____   excise optic nerve
         o_____ n_____
    ii. from g_____ b_____   globe back
    iii. to c_____.   chiasm
b. More posterior lesions with nonspecific   chiasmal lesion
    visual defects, no proptosis,
    hypothalamic dysfunction, pituitary
    dysfunction, hydrocephalus, it is likely a
    _____ _____.
    i.   Treatment should be b_____   biopsy
         and
    ii. X_____.   XRT

42. **Diencephalic syndrome consists of**   G7 p.606:135mm
Hint: diencephalic
    i.   d_____ s_____   diencephalic syndrome
    ii.   i_____ a_____ r_____   intraventricular appearance
                                              radiographically
    iii. e_____ e_____   excessively energetic
    iv.   n_____   macrocephaly
    v.   c_____   cachexia
    vi.   e_____   euphoria
    vii. p_____   failure to thrive
    viii. h_____   hypoglycemia
    ix.   a_____ h_____   anterior hypothalamus
    x.   l_____ of s_____ f_____ loss of subcutaneous fat
    xi.   i_____   infiltrating
    xii. c_____ u_____   children usually

43. **Characterize brain stem glioma.**   G7 p.607:28mm
a. Lower-grade tumors tend to occur in the   higher
    _____ brain stem.
b. Higher-grade tumors tend to occur in the   lower
    _____ brain stem.
c. They present with _____ _____   multiple cranial nerve palsies
    _____ _____.
d. True or False. Most are surgical   false
    candidates.

44. **How do upper brain stem gliomas present?**   G7 p.607:65mm
a. c_____ f_____   cerebellar findings
b. h_____   hydrocephalus

45. **How do lower brain stem gliomas present?**
    G7 p.607:65mm
    a. l_____ c_____ n_____   lower cranial nerves
    b. l_____ t_____ f_____   long tract findings

46. **Characterize four categories of brain stem gliomas.**
    G7 p.607:120mm
    a. diffuse
       i.   location _____, _____, _____   pons, medulla, cord
       ii. glioma grade _____   malignant
       iii. percent _____%   100%
       iv. treatment _____ _____   no surgery
    b. cervicomedullary
       i.   location _____   cervicomedullary
       ii. glioma grade _____   low
       iii. percent _____%   72%
       iv. treatment _____ _____   surgery if exophitic
            _____
    c. focal
       i.   location _____   medulla
       ii. glioma grade _____   low
       iii. percent _____%   66%
       iv. treatment _____ _____   surgery if exophitic
            _____
    d. exophytic
       i.   location _____, _____ _____   medulla, spinal cord
       ii. glioma grade _____   low
       iii. percent _____%   60%
       iv. treatment _____ _____   surgery is okay
            _____

47. **How do brain stem gliomas appear on MRI?**
    G7 p.607:175mm
    a. T1 _____   hypointense
    b. T2 _____   increased signal
    c. gad _____   gadolinium highly variable

48. **Complete the following about brain stem gliomas:**
    G7 p.608:140mm
    a. Prognosis of most patients is _____ months.   6 to 12
    b. Subgroup of dorsally exophytic pilocytic astrocytomas have a longer survival of up to _____ years.   5
    G7 p.608:150mm

49. **Characterize tectal gliomas.**
    G7 p.608:165mm
    a. Pathology is usually _____-_____ _____ that   low-grade astrocytoma
    b. presents with _____.   hydrocephalus
    c. Diagnostic study of choice is _____.   MRI
    d. Symptoms resolve with treatment of the _____.   hydrocephalus

21

e. MRI appearance
   i. mass arising from the q_____   quadrigeminal plate
      p_____
   ii. on T1 _____   isointense
   iii. on T2 _____   iso- or hyperintense
   iv. gadolinium _____% _____   18% enhance
f. Treatment
   i. s_____ or   shunt
   ii. t_____ v_____   third ventriculostomy

50. Characterize oligodendroglioma.   G7 p.609:120mm
   a. Presenting symptom is _____ in   seizure in 50 to 80%
      _____%.
   b. Calcified on
      i. _____% of skull x-rays   30 to 60%
      ii. _____% of CT scan   90%
   c. Oligodendroglioma cells in a tumor   a better prognosis
      suggests what for the patient?

51. Characterize oligodendrogliomas.   G7 p.609:155mm
   a. They have a predilection for the   frontal lobes
      f_____ l_____.
   b. A classic description of cytoplasm is   fried egg
      f_____ e_____.
   c. The role of chemotherapy is the   primary treatment
      p_____ t_____
   d. after s_____ r_____.   surgical resection

52. What are the chemotherapy agents   G7 p.611:30mm
   used for oligodendrogliomas?
   Hint: Cvpt
   a. C_____   CCNU
   b. v_____   vincristine
   c. p_____   procarbazine
   d. t_____   temozolomide

53. Prognosis: best, middle, worst. Relate.   G7 p.611:130mm
   a. Pure oligodendroglioma   best
   b. Mixed oligodendroglioma   middle
   c. Pure astrocytoma   worst

54. Complete the following regarding   G7 p.611:130mm
   prognosis:
   a. An oligodendroglial component conveys   better
      a _____ prognosis.
   b. Pure oligo 10-year survival is _____%.   10 to 30%
   c. Postop survival is _____ to _____   35 to 52
      months.
   d. Calcification in an oligodendroglioma   better
      (ODG) conveys a _____ prognosis.
   e. Loss of chromosome 1p conveys a   better
      _____ prognosis.
   f. Loss of chromosome 1p and 19q conveys   better
      a _____ prognosis.

21

55. Describe central neurocytoma.
   a. It is located in the l_____ v_____   lateral ventricles
   b. or in the s_____ p_____.   septum pellucidum
   c. It tends to affect y_____ a_____   young adults
   d. and is curable by t_____ r_____.   total resection

G7 p.612:105mm

56. Characterize meningiomas.
   a. They arise from what cell of origin?   arachnoid cap cell
   b. What percentage of meningiomas occur at the falx? (includes parasagittal)   60 to 70%
   c. With foot drop plus hyperreflexia, think _____ _____.   parasagittal meningioma
   d. Olfactory groove meningiomas
      i. can produce what syndrome?   Foster Kennedy
      ii. consisting of a_____, i_____ o_____ a_____, and c_____ p_____   anosmia, ipsilateral optic atrophy, and contralateral papilledema
      iii. What other syndrome?   frontal lobe
      iv. consisting of a_____, i_____   apathy, incontinence

G7 p.613:90mm
G7 p.613:155mm
G7 p.614:50mm
G7 p.614:68mm

57. Abulia is
   a. l_____ o_____ w_____.   lack of willpower
   b. characteristic of damage to f_____ l_____.   frontal lobes
   c. can occur with a meningioma of the o_____ g_____.   olfactory groove

G7 p.614:85mm

58. Give a description of asymptomatic meningiomas.
   a. The most common primary intracranial tumor is _____.   meningioma
   b. Percent of primary brain tumors that are meningiomas _____%   32%
   c. Percent that are stable in size over 2½ years _____%   66%
   d. Percent that increase in size when observed for 2½ years _____%   33%
   e. What does calcification tell us about rate of growth?   slower
   f. Operative morbidity in patients under 70 _____%   3.5%
   g. Above 70 _____%   23%
   h. Classic histological finding is the p_____ b_____.   psammoma body

G7 p.615:30mm

59. Complete the following about MRI and meningioma:
   a. Meningioma on T1W1 and T2W1 may be _____.   isodense
   b. With contrast most will _____.   enhance
   c. Accurately predicts sinus involvement in _____%.   90%
   d. A common finding is a d_____ t_____.   dural tail

G7 p.616:175mm

21

60. What metastatic cancer can mimic meningioma in the bone on MRI?

prostate

G7 p.617:40mm

61. Olfactory groove meningiomas tend to be fed by the

a. _____ arteries

ethmoidal

b. which are branches of the _____ artery.

ophthalmic

G7 p.617:52mm

62. The artery of B_____ and C_____ is enlarged in lesions involving the tentorium (i.e., tentorial meningiomas).

Bernasconi and Cassinari (a branch of the meningohypophyseal trunk)

G7 p.617:65mm

63. True or False. The artery most likely to be enlarged on an angiogram depicting a tentorial meningioma is the

a. superficial temporal artery

false

b. artery of Bernasconi and Cassinari

true

c. occipital artery

false

d. posterior inferior cerebellar artery

false

e. anterior choroidal artery

false

G7 p.617:65mm

64. Regarding meningiomas and plain x-rays, the plain x-rays may show

a. b_____ _____ _____

blistering of bone

b. c_____ _____ _____

calcification in tumor 10%

c. d_____ _____ — _____

density changes—hyperostosis

d. e_____ _____ _____

enlarged vascular grooves

e. f_____ _____ _____

frontal fossa hyperostosis

G7 p.617:110mm

65. Complete the following regarding sinus involvement:

a. Occlusion of middle third of the SSS is _____.

treacherous

b. Morbidity/mortality is _____ / _____%,

8/3%

c. due to v_____ i_____.

venous infarction

G7 p.618:20mm

66. Complete the following regarding sinus involvement:

a. The sinus may be divided safely anterior to the _____ _____.

coronal suture

b. Posterior to this site the sinus _____ _____ be divided.

must not

c. If tumor is attached, it is best to leave _____ _____.

residual tumor

G7 p.618:82mm

d. True or False. It is safe to occlude the dominant transverse sinus.

false

G7 p.618:92mm

G7 p.618:60mm

21

67. Complete the following about the removal of meningiomas: G7 p.619:140mm

a. The Simpson grading system grades the degree of removal of _____. meningiomas

b. It is important because it correlates with _____ _____. recurrence rate

c. Components of the system are In order of complexity, from minimal surgery to complete removal:

   i. s_____ r_____, b_____ small removal, biopsy
   ii. p_____ r_____ partial removal
   iii. c_____ r_____ complete removal
   iv. c_____ d_____ coagulate dura
   v. r_____ d_____ and b_____ and s_____ remove dura and bone and sinus

d. Correlates with grade
   i. _____ V
   ii. _____ IV
   iii. _____ III
   iv. _____ II
   v. _____ I

e. What is the most important factor regarding recurrence? extent of tumor removal

68. Five year survival for patients with menigioma is _____%. 91.3% G7 p.619:150mm

■ Vestibular Schwannoma

69. True or False. Vestibular schwannomas (VS) usually arise from which nerve? G7 p.620:145mm

a. facial nerve false
b. cochlear nerve false
c. nervus intermedius false
d. vestibular nerve, inferior division false
e. vestibular nerve, superior division true

70. Vestibular schwannomas arise from the junction of the _____ and _____ myelin called the _____-_____ zone. central and peripheral; Obersteiner-Redlich G6 p.429:170mm

71. Complete the following about primary brain tumors: G6 p.429:175mm

a. What is the Obersteiner-Redlich zone? site of junction of central and peripheral myelin

b. Where is it located? 8 to 12 mm from brain stem
c. From what cells do acoustic tumors arise? from the neurilemmal sheath

d. On what structure do they arise? the superior division of the vestibular nerve

e. Therefore, are they schwannomas or neuromas? schwannomas

f. They are the result of a chromosomal
defect that leads to

   i.   loss of a t_____ s_____ gene   tumor suppressor   G7 p.620:148mm
on the

   ii.   l_____ arm of c_____   long arm of chromosome 22
#_____.

72. True or False. What is the most G7 p.620:150mm
common chromosomal defect in
vestibular schwannomas?

  a.   P53 mutation   false
  b.   gain of function mutation on Ch 3   false
  c.   loss of tumor suppressor gene on Ch 22   true
  d.   loss of tumor suppressor gene on Ch 17   false
  e.   loss of heterozygosity on Ch 10   false

73. List the common triad of symptoms G7 p.621:40mm
seen with vestibular schwannomas.

  a.   h_____—_____%   hearing loss—98%
  b.   t_____—_____%   tinnitus—70%
  c.   d_____—_____%   dysequilibrium—67%
                                        (insidious, progressive, 70%
                                        have high-frequency loss,
                                        word discrimination
                                        difficulties)

74. A patient with good hearing has an G7 p.621:65mm
MRI study that shows a
cerebellopontine angle mass.

  a.   Is this compatible with a vestibular   no (At the time of diagnosis
schwannoma?   virtually all VS have otologic
                                          symptoms.)

  b.   When hearing is involved in VS, what is
lost?

     i.   low frequencies?   no
     ii.   high frequencies?   yes (70% have a high-
                                          frequency loss pattern.)

     iii. word discrimination?   yes (Most have impaired word
                                          discrimination, e.g.,
                                          telephone conversation.)

75. What cranial nerve deficits, other than G7 p.621:125mm
CN VIII, occur with vestibular
schwannomas?

  a.   CN _____; o_____, f_____   CN V; otalgia, facial
n_____, and t_____ c_____   numbness, and taste changes
  b.   CN _____; f_____ w_____   CN VII; facial weakness
  c.   CN _____; h_____ and   CN IX, X, XII; hoarseness and
d_____   dysphagia

21

76. Answer the following about vestibular schwannoma:

G7 p.621:135mm

a. As tumor increases in size the following occur in what sequence?
   A. facial weakness
   B. facial numbness
   C. impaired hearing

C, B, A (Facial numbness occurs earlier than facial weakness even though CN V is only slightly compressed, whereas CN VII is severely distorted early—a paradox. Why? Differential resilience of motor nerves relative to sensory nerves.)

b. What size tumor causes fifth and seventh nerve compression?

larger than 2 cm

77. Complete the following about vestibular schwannomas:

G7 p.621:170mm

21

a. What percentage of patients have no abnormal physical findings except for hearing loss?

66%

b. The Weber test lateralizes to the _____ side.

uninvolved (Hearing loss is sensorineural.)

c. Is the Rinne test positive or negative if hearing is preserved?

positive

d. What is normal for the Rinne test?

air conduction > bone conduction = positive means normal. (Note: An A is better than a B.)

78. Complete the following about primary brain tumors:

G7 p.622:75mm

a. In VS what causes nystagmus?

vestibular involvement

b. What fibers constitute VS?
   i. A_____ _____ n_____
       e_____ b_____ f_____
   ii. A_____ _____ l_____
       r_____ f_____

Antoni A narrow elongated bipolar fibers
Antoni B loose reticulated fibers

c. What is the growth rate for VS?

1 to 10 mm/year

d. What is the proper follow-up protocol, if no surgery is done?

repeat scan at 6-month intervals for 2 years then once each year

e. Recommend surgery if what occurs?
   i. size changes by _____
   ii. or symptoms _____

> 2 mm/year
progress

79. Answer the following about the House and Brackmann scale: G7 p.622:15mm

a. What does the House-Brackmann scale measure?

clinical measurement of facial nerve function

b. What are the categories?

normal
mild
moderate
moderate-severe
severe
no movement

c. Synkinesis is defined as i_____ m_____ accompanying a v_____ m_____.

involuntary movement accompanying a voluntary movement

80. Answer the following about vestibular schwannomas: G7 p.625:30mm and G6 p.431:110mm

a. What is the growth rate of vestibular schwannomas?

slow (1 to 10 mm/year)

b. Do some shrink?

yes (6%)

c. Can they remain stable?

yes

d. Can they grow faster?

yes (2 to 3 cm/year)

e. If followed most will show _____ in 3 years.

enlargement

81. Describe the audiometric findings for "useful" hearing in vestibular schwannomas.

50/50 rule G7 p.623:90mm

a. pure-tone audiogram threshold of _____

≤ 50%

b. speech discrimination of _____

≥ 50%

82. Complete the following regarding the Gardener-Robertson system: G7 p.623:108mm

a. The Gardener-Robertson system is used to grade h_____ p_____.

hearing preservation

b. It consists of

i. testing patient with _____ _____ of increasing loudness.

pure tones (decibels [db]) (If patient hears dB 0 to 30—excellent hearing; 30 to 50 dB—serviceable; 50 to 90 dB—nonserviceable; 90 dB max—poor; not testable—none)

ii. Evaluating patient ability to understand spoken words is called _____ _____.

speech discrimination (understands words spoken to him or her correct 100 to 70%—excellent; 70 to 50%—serviceable; 50 to 5%—nonserviceable)

c. Useful hearing is judged to be present up to a cutoff point of _____.

50/50 patient can hear at 50 dB or less and understands at least 50% of words spoken to him or her

83. **Name the findings for the following tests in vestibular schwannomas:**
G7 p.622:175mm

   a. pure-tone audiogram — hearing difference between each ear > 10 to 15 dB

   b. speech discrimination — 4 to 8% score (normal is 92 to 100%)
G7 p.623:45mm

   c. brain stem auditory evoked response (BSAER) — prolonged I-III and I-V interpeak latencies
G7 p.624:45mm

   d. electronystagmography (ENG) — abnormal if one ear has ≤ 35% of total (Normally, 50% of response is from each ear.)
G7 p.624:20mm

84. **Complete the following concerning vestibular schwannoma:**
G7 p.623:20mm

   a. It causes what kind of hearing loss? — sensorineural loss of high tones

   b. This is the same as the loss from
      i. _____ — old age
      ii. _____ — loud noise exposure

   c. Think tumor if the difference between the ears on audiogram is more than _____ dB. — 10 to 15

85. **True or False. A 55-year-old male is referred for evaluation of a 4.0 cm right cerebellopontine angle (CPA) mass. You conclude it is a vestibular schwannoma. The following is *least* likely to be a factor in your treatment. Give rationale for each.**
G7 p.624:65mm

   a. pure-tone audiogram score of 95 dB — false (Audiogram with hearing threshold < 50 dB may allow consideration of hearing—sparing procedure, but with a score of 95 dB hearing—saving procedure is not an option.)
G7 p.622:175mm

   b. effacement of the fourth ventricle with modest ventriculomegaly — false (Evidence of hydrocephalus warrants CSF diversion—needs a shunt.)
G7 p.621:170mm

   c. stereotactic surgery 2 years previously — true (Stereotactic radiosurgery 2 years previously is long enough for SRS effect to be over. Surgery should be avoided during the interval 6 to 18 months after SRS because this is the time of maximum damage from the radiation.)

21

21

| d. | contralateral (left) vestibular schwannoma, 1.0 cm in diameter | false (Bilateral VS unable to preserve right hearing [95 dB], will need to plan for second procedure to address the left-sided lesion. Chance of preserving left hearing—35 to 71% for a 1 cm tumor.) |
| e. | angiogram showing absence of right transverse sinus | false (Atretic/obstructed right transverse sinus allows consideration of translabyrinthine and suboccipital approach as a combined procedure.) |

86. True or False. Possible treatments for vestibular schwannomas include   G7 p.624:120mm

a. expectant observation, following symptoms, hearing testing, serial CT, or MRI — true
b. radiation therapy, external beam radiation therapy (EBRT) — true
c. radiation therapy, stereotactic radiosurgery (SRS) — true
d. retrosigmoid (suboccipital) resection — true
e. translabyrinthine resection — true
f. extradural subtemporal (middle fossa approach) resection — true

87. Complete the following about vestibular schwannoma treatment: G7 p.625:115mm

a. Under 20 mm can be _____, — observed
b. Protocol is to retest at 6, 12, 18, 24, 36, 48, 60, 84, 108, and 168 _____. — months
c. Growth of more than _____ mm between studies deserves treatment. — 2
d. Tumors larger than 15 to 20 mm should be _____. — treated
e. Tumors with cysts can ____ ____. — grow dramatically   G7 p.625:103mm

88. Matching. Match outcome with technique with microsurgery and SRS.   G7 p.625:170mm
Outcome:
① hearing, ② facial nerve function, ③ trigeminal neuropathy, ④ tumor control
Technique:
a. microsurgery — ③, ④
b. stereotactic radiosurgery — ①
c. equal — ②

89. Classically, vestibular schwannomas push the facial nerve in which direction? Pushed _____ and _____ in _____% of cases. — forward and superiorly in 75%   G7 p.627:92mm

90. **Complete the following about** G7 p.627:145mm
   vestibular schwannomas:
   a. Small, laterally located intracanalicular   subtemporal extradural (also
   vestibular schwannomas can be removed   known as middle fossa
   by what surgical approach?   approach)
   b. A disadvantage is that the seventh nerve   injured at the geniculate
   may be _____ at the _____
   ganglion.
   c. An advantage is that hearing function   preserved
   may be _____.

91. **What is the size vestibular**   < 2 to 2.5 cm   G7 p.627:80mm
   schwannomas should be considered
   for hearing and CN VII preservation
   procedures?

92. **What are the advantages of**   G7 p.628:65mm
   translabyrinthine approach for
   resecting vestibular schwannomas?
   a. early identification of the _____   facial nerve
   b. less risk to _____ and _____   cerebellum and lower cranial
   _____ _____   nerves
   c. best for VS that are located _____   intracanalicular

93. **What are the disadvantages of a**   G7 p.628:65mm
   translabyrinthine approach for
   resecting vestibular schwannomas?
   a. Hearing is _____.   sacrificed
   b. Exposure is _____.   limited
   c. CSF leak is _____.   more common

94. **Complete the following about**   G7 p.628:135mm
and also
G6 p.434:122mm
   vestibular schwannomas:

   a. What are the disadvantages of
   suboccipital approach (also known as
   retrosigmoid) for vestibular
   schwannomas?
      i.   higher _____ when compared   morbidity
          with the translabyrinthine approach
      ii. small tumors _____   difficult to remove in lateral
          recess of internal auditory
          canal (IAC)
      iii. facial nerve is located _____   on blind side deep to the
          tumor
   b. The advantage is the possibility of   hearing preservation
   h_____ p_____.

21

95. Complete the following about localizing the VII nerve origin: G7 p.629:145mm

a. The seventh nerve originates in the _____ sulcus,   pontomedullary

b. anterior to the eighth nerve by _____ mm.   2

c. It lies just anterior to the foramen of _____   Lushka

d. and anterior to a tuft of _____.   choroid

e. It originates _____ mm cephalad to the ninth nerve.   4

96. How do you treat postoperative facial nerve weakness after vestibular schwannoma resection?   G7 p.630:130mm

a. N_____ T_____   Natural Tears (2 drops to eye every 2 hours as needed)

b. L_____   Lacrilube (to eye and tape eye at bedtime)

c. t_____   tarsorrhaphy within a few days if there is a complete CN VII palsy

d. Anastomose by attaching a portion of the _____ nerve to the _____ nerve   hypoglossal
facial

e. When there is no CN VII function and
   i. nerve is known to be divided you may anastomose in _____   2 months
   ii. nerve is known to be intact you may anastomose in _____   1 year

97. True or False. The following symptoms of brain stem compression from a vestibular schwannoma if present postop is not likely to improve: G7 p.630:155mm

a. nausea   false (Nausea resolves with time.)

b. vomiting   false (Vomiting resolves with time.)

c. balance difficulties   false (Balance difficulties clear rapidly.)

d. ataxia   true (Ataxia from brain stem dysfunction may be permanent.)

98. **True or False. The routes of CSF leakage after vestibular schwannoma resection can be via the**

G7 p.631:20mm

a. apical cells — true (to tympanic cavities or eustachian tube—most common)

b. vestibule — true (Posterior SCC is usually entered by drilling—via the oral window.)

c. perilabyrinthine cells — true (and tracks to mastoid antrum)

d. mastoid air cells — true (at craniotomy site)

99. **True or False. The following is the *most likely* source of a postoperative CSF fistula after resection of a vestibular schwannoma:**

G7 p.631:20mm

a. mastoid air cells via craniotomy site — false

b. through the vestibule of the bony labyrinth via the oval window — false

c. perilabyrinthine cells to the mastoid antrum — false

d. apical cells to the tympanic cavity or eustachian tube — true (All are potential routes but this is the most frequent.)

100. **With vestibular schwannoma, postoperative routes for rhinorrhea are**
Hint: avam

G7 p.631:20mm

a. a_____ — apical cells to tympanic cavity and down the eustachian tube

b. v_____ — vestibule after drilling the ICA into the semicircular canal via oval window

c. a_____ — to antrum of mastoid via the perilabyrinthine cells

d. m_____ — mastoid air cells at site of craniotomy

101. **What are treatment strategies for CSF leakage after vestibular schwannoma resection?**

G7 p.631:92mm

a. What percent stop spontaneously? — 25 to 35%

b. Do what with the head of the bed? — elevate

c. Place a drain where? — lumbar

d. If hydrocephalus is present place a _____. — CSF shunt

e. If leak persists _____. — reexplore surgical site to pack with tissue or apply bone wax

21

21

102. What are common complications of vestibular schwannoma surgery?
G7 p.631:175 mm

a. CSF leak in _____%   4 to 27%
b. infection in _____%   5.7% meningitis
c. stroke in _____%   0.7% cerebrovascular accident (CVA)
d. CN VII palsy in _____%   0 to 50%
e. hearing loss in _____%   34 to 43%
f. death in _____%   1%

103. Complete the following concerning hearing loss and CN VII weakness after suboccipital removal of VS:
G7 p.632:25mm

a. Tumor < 1 cm
  i. CN VII preserved, _____%   95 to 100%
  ii. CN VIII preserved, _____%   57%
b. Tumor 1 to 2 cm
  i. CN VII preserved, _____%   80 to 92%
  ii. CN VIII preserved, _____%   33%
c. Tumor > 2 cm
  i. CN VII preserved, _____%   50 to 76%
  ii. CN VIII preserved, _____%   6%

104. Complete the following concerning hearing loss after suboccipital removal of VS:
G7 p.632:25mm

a. Hearing preserved _____% with tumors < 1.5 cm   14 to 48%
b. After SRS hearing preserved _____% with tumors < 3 cm   26%

105. Concerning acoustic neuroma (i.e., vestibular schwannoma), recurrence following microsurgery is
G7 p.633:18mm

a. _____% after   10
b. _____ years follow-up.   15

106. Complete the following concerning SRS for vestibular schwannoma:
G7 p.633:47mm

a. Dose recommended is _____.   14 Gy
b. Local control achieved is _____%.   94%

107. For vestibular schwannoma, what are local control rates for?
G7 p.633:60mm

a. microsurgery   97%
b. SRS   94%

108. When is the time of maximal damage (possible tumor enlargement) from radiation to vestibular schwannomas?
G7 p.633:75mm

a. from _____ to _____ months   6 to 18
b. This is important to know because it can produce a false appearance of tumor _____.   enlargement (Surgery should be avoided during the interval of 6 to 18 months after SRS because of damage from radiation and the appearance of tumor enlargement.)

109. **Most pituitary tumors are benign tumors that arise from the _____.**

adenohypophysis

G7 p.634:25 mm

110. **Answer the following about pituitary tumors:**

G7 p.634:37mm

a. By definition what is the maximal size of a pituitary microadenoma?

1 cm

b. Larger tumors are called _____.

macroadenomas

c. 50% of pituitary tumors are less than _____ mm.

5 mm

111. **Complete the following about pituitary carcinoma:**

G7 p.634:48mm

a. Occurence is _____.

rare

b. They are usually i_____.

invasive

c. They are usually s_____.

secretory

d. The most common hormones are

i. a_____

adrenocorticotropic hormone (ACTH)

ii. P_____

PRL

e. True or false. They can metastasize.

true

f. Prognosis of 1-year mortality is _____%.

66%

112. **True or False. Regarding pituitary tumors:**

G7 p.634:67mm

a. 10% of intracranial tumors

true

b. most common in third to fourth decades

true

c. affect females more often

false (Pituitary tumors affect both sexes equally.)

d. higher incidence in MEN or MEA syndrome

true

e. usually present due to endocrine disturbance or mass effect

true

113. **Complete the following about pituitary tumors:**

G7 p.634:70mm

a. MEN stands for _____ _____ _____.

multiple endocrine neoplasms

b. MEA stands for _____ _____ _____.

multiple endocrine adenomatosis

c. Incidence of pituitary tumors in MEN is _____.

increased

114. **Complete the following about clinical presentation of pituitary tumors:**

G7 p.634:125mm

a. Hormone hypersecretion

i. _____% of adenomas secrete active hormone

65%

ii. prolactin _____%

48%

iii. growth hormone _____%

10%

iv. ACTH _____%

6%

v. thyroid-stimulating hormone (TSH) _____%

1%

21

b. Growth hormone
    i.   If elevated it is due to a _____   pituitary adenoma
         _____
    ii. More than _____% of the time.   95%
c. Corticotropin
    i.   aka _____   ACTH
    ii. Excess causes _____ _____   Cushing disease
    iii. Nelson syndrome can develop only   adrenalectomy
         in patients who have had an
         _____.

115. Complete the following about   G7 p.634:180mm
     hormone hyposecretion:
a. Due to _____ of the normal pituitary   compression
b. In order of sensitivity to compression
    Hint: *go look for the adenoma*
    i.   G_____   GH
    ii. L_____   LH
    iii. F_____   FSH
    iv. T_____   TSH
    v.   A_____   ACTH
c. Most common symptom   G7 p.635:52mm
    i.   o_____ h_____   orthostatic hypotension
    ii. e_____ f_____   easy fatigability
d. selective loss of one hormone consider   hypophysitis
    _____
    i.   A_____   ACTH
    ii. A_____   ADH
e. True or False. Diabetes insipidus is seen   false
    with preop pituitary tumors.

116. Complete the following about mass   G7 p.635:95mm
     effect:
a. The pituitary tumor that gains the
    greatest size is
    i.   non-secreting. (True or False)   true
    ii. of the secreting type is the   prolactinoma
         _____
b. The tumor that is usually the smallest is   ACTH
    the _____ tumor.

117. Patient presents with sudden onset of   G7 p.635:155mm
     headache, visual disturbance,
     ophthalmoplegia, and reduced mental
     status.
a. Consider diagnosis of p_____   pituitary apoplexy (due to
    a_____.   expanding mass in sella
                      turcica resulting from
                      hemorrhage or necrosis)
b. This may occur in macroadenomas in as   3 to 17%   G7 p.636:110mm
    many as _____%.

118. **Complete the following about primary brain tumors:**

G7 p.636:150mm

a. What are the indications for rapid decompression after pituitary apoplexy?
  i. s_____ c_____ — sudden constriction of visual field (VF)
  ii. s_____ — severe deterioration of acuity
  iii. mental status changes due to h_____ — hydrocephalus (complete tumor removal usually not necessary)

b. What else needs to be done? — treat with corticosteroids

119. **Complete the following about the anatomic classification of pituitary adenoma:**

G7 p.637:15mm

21

a. Named the _____ system — Hardy
b. Suprasellar extension
  i. O — none
  ii. A expanding into the _____ cistern — suprasellar
  iii. B anterior recesses of third ventricle _____ — obliterated
  iv. C _____ of third ventricle _____ — floor; displaced
c. Floor of sella
  i. Intact or _____ _____ — focally expanded
  ii. Sella _____ — enlarged
d. Sphenoid extension
  i. Localized _____ of sella floor — perforation
  ii. Diffuse _____ of sella floor — destruction

120. **Complete the following about functional pituitary tumors:**

G7 p.637:135mm

a. What is the most common functional pituitary tumor? — prolactinoma
b. What are its most common symptoms?
  i. In females, _____-_____ — amenorrhea-galactorrhea
  ii. called the syndrome of _____-_____ — Forbes-Albright
  iii. causes _____ in males — impotency
c. It arises from anterior pituitary l_____. — lactotrophs
d. The most common cause of amenorrhea is p_____. — pregnancy

121. **Answer the following about Cushing syndrome:**

G7 p.638:25mm

a. Which hormone? — ACTH
b. It is produced by a _____ tumor. — pituitary
c. It is called Cushing _____. — disease (if tumor is in the pituitary hypercorticalism, it is called Cushing disease)

122. Complete the following about pituitary adenoma: G7 p.638:25mm

a. Adrenocorticotropic hormone (ACTH)—secreting pituitary adenoma is known as _____ _____.   Cushing disease

b. Other causes of hypercortisolism are known as _____ _____.   Cushing syndrome

c. Nelson disease manifests by   G7 p.639:30mm
  i. hyper-_____ due to   hyperpigmentation
  ii. cross reactivity of m_____-s_____ h_____ with _____.   melanocyte-stimulating hormone (MSH) with ACTH

123. Complete the following about Nelson syndrome: G7 p.639:30mm

a. Follows bilateral _____   adrenalectomy
b. In only _____ to _____% of cases   10 to 30%
c. Classic triad of
  i. h_____   hyperpigmentation
  ii. ↑ in _____   ACTH
  iii. Enlargement of the _____   pituitary tumor
  iv. Usually occurs _____ to _____ years after adrenalectomy   1 to 40 years

d.   G7 p.639:90mm
  i. The earliest sign is the _____   linea negra
  ii. Midline pigmentation from the pubis to _____   umbilicus
  iii. And hyperpigmentation of _____ _____ and areolae   scars, gingivae

e. Have an ACTH level greater than _____ Ng/L   200   G7 p.639:130mm
f. The normal being less than _____ Ng/l   54

124. Complete the following about pituitary adenoma (Cushing syndrome):   G7 p.638:25mm

a. caused by _____   hypercortisolism—from any source
b. exogenous source _____   ingestion of steroids
c. endogenous sources
  i. p_____ t_____, _____%   pituitary tumor, 60 to 80%
  ii. a_____ t_____, _____%   adrenal tumor, 10 to 20%, 15 to 25%
  iii. e_____ t_____, _____%   ectopic tumor, 1 to 10%, 5 to 10%

125. Characterize the typical Nelson syndrome scenario.   G7 p.639:53mm

a. patient who had _____ _____   Cushing syndrome
b. had a surgical procedure _____   adrenalectomy
c. develops _____   hyperpigmentation
d. occurs in _____% of such patients   10 to 30%
e. due to _____-_____ of _____ and _____   cross-reactivity of ACTH and MSH

21

126. **To remember Cushing syndrome versus disease:**

G7 p.638:36mm

a. syndrome due to _____   steroids from any source
                                    Hint: syndrome = steroids
b. disease due to _____   pituitary only

127. **List the findings in Cushing syndrome.**
Hint: steroids

G7 p.638:115mm

a. s_____   striae
b. t_____   thin skin
c. e_____   ecchymosis
d. r_____   reduced libido
e. o_____   obesity
f. i_____   impotence, increased blood
                     pressure
g. d_____   diabetes
h. s_____   skin hyperpigmentation

128. **List the findings in Cushing syndrome.**
Hint: Ectopic sources of acth secretions
Hint: (a) c^3 t^2 h

G7 p.639:15mm

a. (a)
b. c_____   carcinoma small cell lung
c. c_____   carcinoid
d. c_____   (pheo) chromocytoma
e. t_____   thymoma
f. t_____   thyroid carcinoma
g. h_____   islet cell pancreas

129. **Characterize pituitary adenoma in Cushing disease.**

G7 p.638:36mm

a. secretion of _____   ACTH
b. most are small < _____ mm   5 mm
c. only _____% are large enough to   10%
   produce mass effect
d. cells produce _____   proopiomelanocortin (POMC)
e. which contains the precursors for:
   i.   A_____   ACTH
   ii. a_____   alpha-MSH
   iii. b_____   beta-lipotropin
   iv. b_____   beta-endorphin
   v.   e_____   met-enkephalin

130. **Criteria for biochemical cure is IGF-1 level less than _____ Ng/mL.**   5

G7 p.639:180mm

21

131. Chart. List the effects of excess growth hormone alphabetically.

G7 p.640:50mm

arthropathy
acromegaly
bone
cartilage
cardiomyopathy
diabetes
entrapment of nerve syndromes
frontal bossing
fatigue
glucose intolerance
gigantism
hyperhydrosis
hypertension
headaches
infection
increased hand and foot size
joint pain
macroglossia
malignancies
neoplasia
neuropathy
oily skin
polyps
paresthesias
prognathism
palmar hyperhydrosis
respiratory obstruction
rings no longer fit
shoe size enlarges
sleep apnea
skeletal changes
soft tissue swelling
thickened heel pad
thyromegaly with normal thyroid studies

132. Describe the hypothalamic pituitary axis dysfunction in acromegaly.

G6 p.441:55mm

a. Hypothalamus produces _____.

GHRH

b. _____ causes the pituitary to make _____.

GHRH; GH

c. _____ affects the liver, which produces _____ also known as _____.

GH, somatomedin-C, IGF–1 (hypothalamic GHRH stimulates pituitary GH secretion. Excess GH induces IGF-1 secretion from liver.)

d. What medication can suppress GH release?

somatostatin (Acromegaly findings are due to IGF-1, also known as somatomedin-C.)

133. **Complete the following about acromegaly growth hormone releasing hormone (GHRH):**

G6 p.441:56mm

  a. produced in the _____   hypothalamus

  b. causes

      i.   sy_____   synthesis of growth hormone

      ii. se_____   secretion

      iii. re_____   release

  c. somatomedin-C

      i.   produced in the _____   liver

      ii. due to stimulus of _____   GH

      iii. produces _____ _____   systemic effects

      iv. also known as _____ _____ _____   insulin-like growth factor (IGF-1, also known as somatomedin-C)

134. **True or False. Regarding acromegaly, somatostatin suppresses growth hormone by interfering with**

G6 p.441:60mm

  a. synthesis   false

  b. secretion   false

  c. release of the hormone   true

135. **Answer the following about acromegaly:**

G7 p.640:18mm

  a. Is there any possible ectopic source of growth hormone?   yes

  b. If so, what?   carcinoid tumor

136. **Answer the following about acromegaly:**

G7 p.640:135mm

  a. What effect on mortality does elevated GH levels have? Mortality rates are _____ to _____ times normal   2 to 3 times

  b. due to

      i.   c_____   cancer

      ii. c_____   cardiomyopathy

      iii. d_____   diabetes

      iv. h_____   hypertension

      v.   i_____   infection

      vi. n_____ _____   neural entrapment

137. **Concerning growth hormone, what effects does GH have on the following?**

G7 p.640:136 mm

  a. mortality rates   ↑

  b. blood pressure   ↑

  c. diabetes   ↑

  d. infections   ↑

  e. cancer   ↑

  f. cardiomyopathy   ↑

  g. closure of epiphyseal plates in children   delays closure

138. **Which pituitary tumor is**

G7 p.638:90mm

  a. least likely to cause mass effect?   ACTH-producing tumor

  b. most likely to cause mass effect?   prolactin-producing tumor

21

21

139. Describe the mass effects of pituitary tumors.   G7 p.637:80 mm
  a. What are the structures compressed?
     Hint: cop
     i.   c_____ s_____   cavernous sinus
     ii. o_____ c_____   optic chiasm
     iii. p_____   pituitary
  b. What are the mass effects usually seen in nonfunctioning pituitary tumors?
     i.   p_____, f_____ p_____,   ptosis, facial pain, diplopia
          d_____
     ii. b_____ h_____   bitemporal hemianopsia
     iii. h_____   hypopituitarism

140. Describe the Hardy system of pituitary adenoma classification.   G7 p.637:14mm
  a. suprasellar extension of tumor
     i.   _____   no suprasellar extension
     ii. _____   fills suprasellar cistern
     iii. _____   anterior recess of III ventricle
     iv. _____   displaces floor of III ventricle
     v.   _____   intracranial (intradural)
     vi. _____   intracavernous sinus
                             (extradural)
  b. invasion
     i.   I s_____ n_____   sella normal
     ii. II s_____ e_____   sella enlarged
     iii. III l_____ p_____ of   localized perforation of sella
          s_____ f_____   floor
     iv. IV d_____ d_____ of   diffuse destruction of sella
          s_____ f_____   floor
     v.   V s_____ via C_____   spread via CSF

141. What percentage of pituitary adenomas become locally invasive?   5%   G7 p.637:15mm

142. Cavernous sinus invasion   G7 p.637:60mm
  a. can be *suspected* if medial wall of sinus is   pushed laterally
     _____ _____.
  b. can be *diagnosed* if carotid artery is   encased
     _____.

143. What is the most definite sign of cavernous sinus invasion?   carotid artery encasement   G7 p.637:70mm

144. Matching. Match the light microscopic appearance of each of the following pituitary tumors with its most common secretory product.   G7 p.641:60mm
     Secretory product:
     ① growth hormone; ② ACTH;
     ③ prolactin; ④ TSH; ⑤ nonsecretory
     Appearance:
  a. chromophobe   ⑤
  b. acidophil   ①
  c. basophil   ②

145. What percentage of pituitary tumors are   G7 p.641:30mm

   a. endocrine-secretorily active?   70%

   b. endocrine-secretorily inactive?   30%

146. Complete the following about tumors of the neurohypophysis and infundibulum: G7 p.641:105mm

   a. Most common tumor in the posterior pituitary is _____.   metastasis

   b. Most common primary tumor is the _____ _____ _____.   granular cell tumor (GCT)

   c. If this tumor is suspected, operative approach is _____.   transcranial

   d. MRI appearance is identical to _____.   adenoma

147. True or False. Baseline endocrinologic evaluation of patients presenting with pituitary tumors includes the following among others: G7 p.642:80mm

   a. 8 a.m. cortisol (24 hours is better)   true

   b. serum prolactin level   true

   c. somatomedin-C   true

   d. serum thyroid-stimulating hormone (TSH)   true

   e. serum T3   false

148. List the baseline pituitary function tests.   G7 p.642:81mm

   Hint: pqrsTT

   a. p_____   prolactin serum level

   b. q_____   Q-cortisol 24 hour

   c. r_____   rest FSH LH FBS (rest means the rest of the endocrine studies) (reproductive)

   d. s_____   somatomedin C

   e. T_____   TSH serum level

   f. T_____   T4 serum level

149. What is the chiasm location in relationship to the sella and the resulting visual field defect?   G7 p.642:80mm

   a. prefixed _____%   5%, homonymous hemianopsia

   b. above _____%   80%, bitemporal hemianopsia

   c. postfixed _____%   5%, ipsilateral loss of vision, junctional scotoma contralaterally, so-called "pie in the sky," due to compression of the anterior knee of Willebrand

21

21

150. Visual fields is tested using a small red stimulus because desaturation of color is an early sign of _____ compression.

chiasmal

G7 p.642:170mm

151. Answer the following about pituitary adenoma:

G7 p.643:24mm

a. What is the classic finding when a tumor compresses the optic chiasm?

bitemporal hemianopsia

b. What occurs in patients with a postfixed chiasm?

   i. s_____ o_____ q_____

superior outer (temporal) quadrantanopsia

   ii. j_____ s_____

junctional scotoma

c. due to compression of the k_____ of v_____ w_____

knee of von Willebrand

d. What occurs in patients with a prefixed chiasm?

homonymous hemianopsia (complete or incomplete)

e. due to compression of _____ or _____ optic tracts

one or both

152. Characterize the pattern of progressive visual field defect caused by pituitary tumor.

G7 p.643:24mm

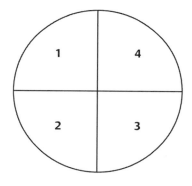

Left Field
Counterclockwise

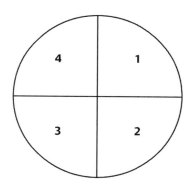

Right Field
Clockwise

Fig. 21.1

a. first

superior temporal field

b. second

inferior temporal field

c. third

inferior nasal field

d. fourth

superior nasal field

e. clockwise in the _____ field

right

f. counterclockwise in the _____ field

left

153. **Describe baseline pituitary evaluation before surgery. (*Note: Results not listed here are also not listed in the Greenberg 6th edition because results vary with age, gender, and menstrual cycle.)**

G7 p643:70mm

a. Hint: $P_8R^3st^2$

   i.   p_____   prolactin
       normal   < 30
       measured in   ng/mL
       maybe abnormal   25 to 150
       abnormal value   > 150

   ii.   (sounds like q) c_____   cortisol 8 a.m.
       normal   6 to 18
       measured in   µg/100 mL
       maybe abnormal   5 to 10
       abnormal value   > 10

   iii.   *(r rest) f_____-s_____ _____   follicle-stimulating hormone (FSH)
       normal
       measured in
       maybe abnormal
       abnormal

   iv.   *(r rest) l_____   luteinizing hormone
       normal
       measured in
       maybe abnormal
       abnormal

   v.   (r rest) f_____ b_____ s_____   fasting blood sugar
       normal   65 to 99
       measured in   mg/dL
       maybe abnormal
       abnormal

   vi.   *s_____   somatomedin-C
       normal   0.31 to 1.4
       measured in   U/mL
       maybe abnormal
       abnormal

   vii.   *T_____   TSH   G7 p.445:15mm
       normal   0.4 to 5.5 mg
       measured in   µg
       maybe abnormal   peak 2x normal
       abnormal   if TSH stimulation test causes peak 2x normal

   viii.   *T_____   TH thyroid hormone
       normal   0.8 to 15
       measured in   free T4 index
       maybe abnormal
       abnormal

21

b. Also include diagnostic studies of
- i. f_____ v_____ f_____ — formal visual fields
- ii. M_____ w_____ and w_____ e_____ — MRI with and without enhancement
- iii. C_____-c_____ v_____ — CT-coronal views (11 tests in all)

154. **Thickening of the pituitary stalk and loss of a single pituitary hormone is strongly suggestive of l_____ h_____.**

lymphocytic hypophysitis

G7 p.643:83mm
also see
G7 p.1217:55mm

155. **True or False. Regarding lymphocytic hypophysitis:**

G7 p.643:83mm
also see
G7 p.1217:55mm

- a. more common in men than women — false (more common in women; only 5 cases reported in men)
- b. associated with postpartum state — true
- c. affects multiple pituitary hormones — false (affects single hormone)
- d. rarely causes diabetes insipidus — false (often causes diabetes insipidus)

156. **Characterize screening for Cushing syndrome.**

G7 p.643:92mm

- a. 8 a.m. cortisol level: normal value is _____ — 6 to 18 µg/100 mL
- b. 24-hour urine-free cortisol _____ — more accurate—almost 100% sensitive and specific

157. **True or False. Findings of primary hypothyroidism with secondary pituitary hyperplasia include the following:**

G7 p.645:45mm

- a. prolonged and elevated TSH response to TRH stimulation — true
- b. low T4 — true
- c. hypoglycemia — false (Hypoglycemia is not part of the syndrome.)
- d. elevated TSH — true
- e. elevated prolactin — true (Enlarged pituitary causes stalk effect and prolactin increases.)
- f. pituitary enlarges because of hypertrophy of the _____ producing cells — thyrotropin releasing hormone (TRH)
- g. pituitary enlargement occurs because of the loss of _____ _____ from _____ _____ — negative feedback from thyroid hormones

21

158. Considering pituitary tumors, prolactin is under:

G7 p.644:35mm

a. inhibitory control of the _____ and the infundibular stalk.

hypothalamus

b. Therefore, injury to the hypothalamus or injury to the pituitary stalk causes loss of the inhibitory chemical _____.

prolactin inhibitory factor (PRIF)

c. Does this lead to an increase or decrease in prolactin in the patient?

increase

159. After surgery for prolactin-secreting tumor, what should you think if prolactin is still elevated

G7 p.644:33mm

a. but less than 90 ng/mL _____?

injury to stalk and/or hypothalamus due to loss of prolactin inhibitory factor (PRIF), which is present in the intact stalk and hypothalamus

b. but more than 150 ng/mL _____?

persistent tumor

160. Answer the following about large adenomas with normal prolactin:

G7 p.644:160 mm

a. What should you instruct the laboratory to do?

perform several dilutions and rerun the PRL (This may be a false negative.)

b. This false negative is called the _____ effect.

hook

161. True or False. Extremely high prolactin levels may produce false negatives due to the tendency for large numbers of PRL molecules to prevent formation of PRL-antibody-signal complexes in assays.

true (hook effect)

G7 p.644:160mm

162. Complete the following about cortisol reserve insulin tolerance test:

G7 p.647:115mm

a. Insulin IV will promptly lower _____.

blood sugar

b. Hypoglycemia is a _____.

stressor

c. In response the body produces _____.

cortisol

d.

  i. An increment in baseline more than _____ mg/dL

6

  ii. to a peak of _____ mg/dL is normal.

20

e.

  i. An increment of less than _____ mg/dL

6

  ii. to a peak less than _____ mg/dL

16

  iii. indicates a need for g_____ r_____.

glucocorticoid replacement

163. The most useful test for acromegaly is an _____ level.

IGF-1

G7 p.647:170mm

164. **Complete the following about acromegaly and somatomedin-C:**   G7 p.647:170mm
   a. also known as _____   IGF-1
   b. normal fasting level _____   0.67 U/mL (range 0.31 to 1.4 U/mL)
   c. in acromegalics level is _____   6.8 U/mL (range 2.6 to 21.7 U/mL)

165. **Some growth hormone-secreting pituitary tumors also secrete _____.**   prolactin   G7 p.653:20mm also G6 p.447:115mm

166. **Complete the following about growth hormone:**   G7 p.648:15mm
   a. Normal basal fasting level is _____.   less than 5 ng/mL
   b. Acromegalic patients have levels _____ than _____.   greater than 10 ng/mL
   c. Due to pulsatile secretion of GH sporadic peaks up to _____ can occur.   50 ng/mL
   d. Is this a reliable test?   no

167. **Complete the following about the size of the pituitary gland:**   G7 p.648:115mm
   a. Size of pituitary gland
      i. in men up to _____ mm   10
      ii. in women up to _____ mm   9, 11
         child-bearing age up to _____ mm
      iii. in adolescent girls up to _____ mm   15
   b. size of stalk is same size as b_____   basilar artery
   c. differential diagnosis of large stalk
      i. l_____   lymphoma
      ii. l_____ h_____   lymphocytic hypophysitis
      iii. g_____ d_____   granulomatous disease
      iv. h_____ g_____   hypothalamic glioma

168. **Findings compatible with pituitary microadenoma on MRI include the following:**   G7 p.648:145mm
   a. True or False. Lack of early (< 5 minute) gadolinium enhancement   true
   b. True or False. Pituitary stalk deviation   true
   c. True or False. Thickened pituitary stalk   false (A thickened pituitary stalk is not compatible with adenoma.)
   d. True or False. Late (after 30 minute) gadolinium enhancement   true
   e. True or False. Timing of scan after gadolinium infusion is important.   true (In early scanning, under 5 minutes, tumor will not enhance but gland will. In late scanning, after 30 minutes, tumor will enhance as well and may not be seen because the gland is also enhanced.)

21

f. The best time to scan for pituitary tumor is _____ minutes after infusion. — 5

g. At that time what enhances? — normal pituitary tissue

h. Microadenoma is seen since it does _____ _____. — not enhance

169. Characterize the neurohypophysis.
    a. normally on T1WI is _____ _____ — high signal
    b. possibly because it contains _____ — phospholipids
    c. absence of this sign suggests _____ _____ — diabetes insipidus

G7 p.648:160 mm

170. For pituitary tumors, what is the benefit of coronal CT slices?
    a. sphenoid series _____ — midline (can be identified by the anatomy of sphenoid sinus septa)
    b. sella floor _____ — erosion (of the sella floor to indicate presence of the tumor on one side)

G7 p.649:42mm

171. What is the medical treatment for the following?
    a. growth hormone-secreting tumors _____ — octreotide
    b. ACTH-secreting tumors _____ — ketoconazole
    c. prolactin-secreting tumors _____ — bromocriptine

G7 p.653:45mm
G7 p.654:148mm
G7 p.651:60mm

172. Complete the following about nonsecreting pituitary adenomas:
    a. Usual treatment is with _____ or _____ — Sx or XRT
    b.
        i. Medication (bromocriptine) may reduce tumor size by _____% — 20%
        ii. Due to the paucity of _____ receptors — dopaminergic
    c. Octreotide reduces the tumor by _____% — 10%
    d. Follow-up by MRI at: _____, _____, _____, and _____ years — 0.5, 1, 2, and 5

G7 p.649:100mm

173. Surgical indications are v_____ f_____ d_____. — visual field defects

G7 p.649:165mm

174. Tumors secreting GH or ACTH
    a. warrant _____ treatment — surgical
    b. because the secretion is _____ — harmful
    c. and there is no effective _____ _____. — medical treatment

G7 p.650:70mm

175. Complete the following about hormone replacement therapy:
    a. corticosteroids
        i. am replacement dose is _____ mg and — 20
        ii. pm replacement dose is _____ mg — 10

G7 p.650:125mm

21

b. thyroid hormone
    i.   Do not replace if patient has   adrenal insufficiency
         _____ _____
    ii. Synthroid _____ µg/d   125

176. **Complete the following about primary brain tumors:**   G7 p.651:24mm
    a. Above what level of prolactin is surgery unlikely to normalize the prolactin?   above 500 ng/mL
    b. In such a case what should your treatment be?   medication—dopamine agonists bromocriptine—not surgery

177. **Complete the following about prolactinoma as treatment with bromocriptine:**   G7 p.651:40mm
    a. Response should be evident in _____ to _____ weeks.   4 to 6
    b. _____% will not respond.   18%
    c. _____% will continue to enlarge on bromocriptine.   1%
    d. Upon discontinuation tumor may _____ _____.   rapidly enlarge

178. **What does bromocriptine do?**   G7 p.651:80 mm
    a. binds to r_____   receptors
    b. inhibits s_____ and s_____ of _____   synthesis and secretion of PRL
    c. lowers prolactin to about _____% of its elevated amount   ~10%
    d. reduces tumor size by _____% in _____   75% in 6 to 8 weeks
    e. restores _____   fertility
    f. harms patient by _____   producing fibrosis
    g. This reduces good surgical results by _____%.   50%
    h. Therefore, decide about surgery within _____ _____ of starting bromocriptine.   6 months
    i. Prolactinomas may _____ _____ upon discontinuation of the drug.   enlarge rapidly

179. **If response to dopamine agonists is satisfactory**   G7 p.652:90mm
    a. continue to treat for _____ to _____ years and   1 to 4
    b. check prolactin every _____.   year
    c. If tumor not visible on MRI may _____.   discontinue
    d. Recurrence rate is highest in the _____ _____.   first year

180. **True or False. Surgery is not indicated in elderly asymptomatic patients with GH-secreting pituitary tumors.**   true   G7 p.652:125mm

181. **Answer the following about pituitary tumors:**   G7 p.652:130mm

a. best treatment for prolactinoma PRL < 500 — transsphenoidal surgery

b. best treatment for prolactinoma PRL > 500 — surgery not recommended if PRL > 500

c. best treatment if prolactin is < 500 try _____ first — medical treatment

d. meds will fail in _____% — 18%

e. treat the failures with _____ — transsphenoidal surgery

f. acromegaly best treatment is _____ — transsphenoidal surgery (Surgery is not recommended for elderly; instead use bromocriptine and/or octreotide.)

g. cure for microadenoma _____% — 85%

h. cure for macroadenoma _____% — 30%

i. Cushing disease best treatment is _____. — transsphenoidal surgery

182. **In acromegaly, IGF-1 stabilizes after surgery in _____.** — months   G7 p.652:185mm

183. **Complete the following about acromegaly and octreotide:**   G7 p.652:98mm

a. suppresses _____ _____ — growth hormone

b. reduces _____, _____% to _____% become _____ — GH in 71%, 50 to 66% become normal

c. reduces _____ in _____%, _____% become _____ — GF-1 in 93%, 66% become normal

d. requires injection _____ — 3 times per day

e. side effects can be _____ — cholelithiasis (10 to 25% of patients)

f. may also be useful in _____ — thyrotropic (TSH)-secreting tumors

184. **True or False. Common side effects of octreotide include the following:**   G7 p.653:120mm

a. decreased GI motility — true

b. sweating — false

c. diarrhea — true

d. steatorrhea — true

e. bradycardia — true

f. cholelithiasis — true

185. **Complete the following about Cushing disease and ketoconazole:**   G7 p.654:148mm

a. blocks _____ _____ synthesis — adrenal steroid

b. normalizes _____% of patients — 75%

c. normalizes _____ _____ cortisol — urinary free

d. normalizes _____ steroids — hydroxycortico

e. may cause

i. adrenal _____ — insufficiency

ii. hepato-_____ — hepatotoxicity

21

186. **True or False. Regarding bilateral total adrenalectomy:**   G7 p.654:90mm

a. It is better tolerated than transsphenoidal pituitary surgery.   false

b. Lifelong glucocorticoid replacement is required.   true

c. Lifelong mineralocorticoid replacement is not required.   false   G7 p.654:94mm

d. Development of Nelson syndrome is rare.   false (Not rare; it occurs in 30%.)

187. **Complete the following about thyrotropin-secreting adenomas:**   G7 p.655:85mm

a. First-line treatment is _____ _____.   transsphenoidal surgery

b. The tumor may be difficult to remove and _____.   fibrous

c.
  i. Medical treatment is with the same agent as for _____   acromegaly
  ii. namely, _____.   octreotide

188. **Complete the following about pituitary tumors and radiation therapy side effects on:**   G7 p.655:147mm

a. cognition
  i. m_____ d_____   memory disturbances
  ii. l_____   lethargy
b. vision
  i. o_____ n_____ and c_____ i_____   optic nerve and chiasm injury
  ii. b_____   blindness
c. endocrine
  i. h_____   hypocorticalism
  ii. h_____   hypothyroidism
d. tumor
  i. n_____   necrosis
  ii. a_____   apoplexy

189. **Radiation therapy should be routinely used:**   G7 p.655:160mm

a. True or False. Following surgical removal of pituitary adenomas   false

b. True or False. If recurrence occurs   false (Repeat surgery is recommended.)

c. Radiation is appropriate in the following circumstances
  i. if recurrence _____ _____ _____   can't be removed

  ii. if recurrence _____ _____ _____ _____   mass continues to grow

21

190. Answer the following about radiation for acromegaly:

G7 p.656:35mm

a. True or False. It is the preferred treatment. — false

b. 90% of patients reach normal growth hormone levels in _____ years. — 20

c. During this time they are exposed to _____ levels of GH — unacceptable

d. and are also exposed to the risks of _____. — radiation

191. True or False. Indications for pituitary surgery include

G7 p.649:164mm
also
G6 p.452:140mm

a. prolactinomas with levels greater than 500 ng/mL not controlled with surgery — true (Medical treatment will not suffice; both are needed in 18%.)

b. Cushing disease — true (Medical therapy is not adequate.)

c. acromegaly — true

d. macroadenoma — true (if not PRL secreting)

e. visual field defect — true

f. sudden visual loss — true

g. to obtain tissue for diagnosis — true

h. hypopituitarism — false

i. Nelson syndrome — true

192. What is the medical preparation for surgery?

G7 p656 :90mm

a. Steroids _____ _____ — stress doses

b. Hypothyroid patients ideally to be treated before surgery for _____ _____ — 4 weeks

193. Regarding pituitary tumors, what artery might you encounter laterally as you open the Hardy speculum and expose the keel of the sphenoid bone? — the sphenopalatine artery—a branch of the maxillary artery, which is the eighth branch of the external carotid artery

G7 p. 656:117mm

194. Concerning the sublabial approach for pituitary adenoma, what structures can be injured?

G7 p.656:118mm

a. artery g_____ p_____ — greater palatine artery branches (AKA) descending palatal arteries (They enter the incisive foramina and incisive canals.)

b. nerve n_____ — nasopalatine nerves (Branch of maxillary nerve [V2] serves roof of mouth, upper lip, and teeth.)

195. True or False. Regarding pituitary tumors:

G7 p.656:150mm

a. Minimal enlargement of the sella and a large suprasellar mass indicate a transcranial approach. — true

21

b. The subtemporal approach provides good visualization of the optic nerves, chiasm, and carotid arteries.

false (The subfrontal approach is better to see this anatomy.)

c. The subfrontal approach may be more difficult with prefixed chiasm.

true

d. The transsphenoidal approach is preferred for microadenomas.

true

196. **Conditions indicating transsphenoidal approach that may not be appropriate for this pituitary tumor include:**   G7 p.656:151mm

a. sella not _____   enlarged
b. large _____ mass   suprasellar
c. e_____ tumor   extrasellar
d. sphenoid _____   sinusitis

197. **Complete the following about transspehenoidal surgery:**   G7 p.657:185mm

a. Open the sella exactly in the _____.   midline
b. Use the _____ _____ as your landmark.   nasal septum
c. Is the sphenoid sinus septum also reliable?   no, it is unreliable

198. **Complete the following about intraoperative disaster:**   G7 p.659:100mm

a. Profuse arterial bleeding suggests _____ _____.   carotid injury

b. It can usually be controlled by _____.   packing

c.
   i. The operation should _____   be stopped
   ii. and _____ be done.   angiography

d.
   i. If _____ is found   pseudoaneurysm
   ii. the patient is at risk for _____ _____.   lethal rupture

e.
   i. It must be eliminated by _____   endovascular techniques
   ii. or surgical _____.   trapping

199. **True or False. Common complications of transsphenoidal pituitary surgery include**   G7 p.659:135mm

a. transient diabetes insipidus   true (common but lasts less than 3 months)

b. basilar artery injury   false (Basilar artery injury is rare.)

c. cerebrospinal fluid leakage   true (Cerebrospinal fluid leakage is common, 3.5%.)

d. carotid artery rupture   false (Carotid artery rupture is rare.)

200. True or False. Treatment for diabetes insipidus includes the following: *G7 p.661:125mm*

a. desmopressin 2 to 4 mg daily (subcutaneous)   true

b. vasopressin 5 U (IV) every 6 hours   true

c. desmopressin 10 to 40 mg twice a day   true

d. clofibrate 500 mg four times a day by mouth   true

201. Complete the following regarding postoperative pituitary surgery: *G7 p.661:26mm*

a. diabetes insipidus

   i. can be diagnosed if urine output is more than _____ cc   250 cc

   ii. for _____   1 to 2 hours

b. ACTH (corticotropin) reserve

   i. take patient off steroids for _____ hours   24 hours

   ii. check _____ a.m. cortisol level   6 a.m.

   iii. normal cortisol level at 6 a.m. is _____   above 9 µg/dL

   iv. suspect low cortisol is _____   3 to 9 µg/dL

   v. definitely low cortisol is _____   below 3 µg/dL

c. To assess for residual tumor don't do CT until _____ _____ postoperative.   4 months   *G7 p.661:40mm*

202. Characterize the good outcomes of transsphenoidal surgery.   *G7 p.662:60mm*

a. vision _____ _____   much improved

b. prolactin secreting tumors in _____%   25%

c. growth hormone secreting tumors in _____%   20%

d. Cushing disease—microadenomas in _____%   85%

e. acromegaly

   i. microadenoma in _____%   85%

   ii. macroadenoma in _____%   30%

   iii. all acromegalics in _____%   50%

f. recurrence _____%   12%

203. Regarding acromegaly, cure requires: *G7 p.662:130mm*

a. basal (morning) serum GH of less than _____   5 ng/mL

b. suppression after ingesting glucose less than _____   2 ng/mL

c. somatomedin-C (I-GF-1) of normal _____ acromegalics _____   normal range—0.31 to 1.4 ng/mL; acromegalics 2.6 to 21.7 ng/mL

204. Characterize biochemical outcome acromegaly.   *G7 p.662:120mm*

a. Recommended is a _____ serum GH level.   morning

b. Cure is considered GH level of less than _____ ng/ml.   5

21

  c. In tumors less than 10 mm this is 85%
    achieved in _____%.

  d. In all acrogmegalics cure is achieved in 50%
    _____%.

  e. Macroadenomas cure is achieved in 30%
    _____%.

  f. These patients should be seen for follow- 6 to 12
    up every _____ to _____ months.

205. **Answer the following about**   G7 p.663:130mm
   craniopharyngiomas:

  a. Craniopharyngiomas are lined with what stratified squamous
    types of cells?   epithelium

  b. They arise from _____ _____ anterior superior margin
    _____ of the pituitary.

  c. Show calcification
    i. on histology in _____% 50%
    ii. on plain x-ray in children in 85%
      _____%
    iii. on plain x-ray in adults in _____% 40%

  d. Do they contain cysts?   yes
  e. Do they contain solid components also? yes
  f. Do they undergo malignant   no
    degeneration?

206. **The pituitary stalk can be recognized**   G7 p.664:95mm
   by its pattern

  a. of l_____ s_____   longitudinal striations
  b. which are the long _____ _____. portal veins

207. **Describe the Rathke cleft cyst (RCC).**   G7 p.665:25mm

  a. Where are they located?   intrasellar—pars intermedia
  b. How common are they?   incidental finding in 20% of
                autopsies

  c. Do you find RCC together with pituitary no
    adenomas?

  d. Why?   They arise from the same
                tissue, which goes one way or
                the other but not both.

  e. appearance on CT
    i. cystic?   yes
    ii. density?   low density
    iii. enhancement?   may have capsular
                enhancement

208. **True or False. Rathke cleft cysts arise**   G7 p.665:35mm
   in/at the:

  a. anterior superior margin of pituitary false
  b. neurohypophysis   false
  c. pars intermedia   true
  d. none of the above   false

209. Answer the following about Rathke cleft cyst:

G7 p.665:35mm

a. Where is a Rathke cleft cyst located? — in the pars intermedia of pituitary

b. From what does Rathke cleft cyst originate? — remnant of Rathke pouch—stomodeum

210. True or False. A 14-year-old patient is found to have a 3 cm low-density lesion in the sella turcica. Surgical excision reveals a single-layer cuboidal epithelium. The most likely diagnosis is

G7 p.665:45mm

a. mucocele — false
b. epidermoid — false
c. craniopharyngioma — false
d. Rathke cleft cyst — true

211. With a colloid cyst, hydrocephalus involves only the _____ _____. — lateral ventricles

G7 p.665:90mm

212. Complete the following about primary brain tumors:

G7 p.665:120mm

a. True or False. A 40-year-old male complains of intermittent headaches and gait difficulty. CT scan of head shows a cystic mass in the third ventricle. The most likely diagnosis is
  i. neurocystercercosis — false
  ii. meningioma — false
  iii. choroid plexus papilloma — false
  iv. colloid cyst — true

b. the site of origin of this cystic mass is the
  i. d_____ e_____ of the recess of the postvelar arch called — diencephalic ependyma
  ii. the p_____ — paraphysis (that is, an evagination of the roof of the third ventricle)

213. True or False. A 27-year-old male with a history of a colloid cyst who underwent a right frontal ventriculoperitoneal shunt 3 days ago returns to the emergency room (ER) with recurrence of severe headaches and gait difficulty. Treatment at this time could be

G7 p.110:110mm

a. removal of ventriculoperitoneal shunt — false
b. externalization of shunt — false
c. placement of left frontal ventricular drainage — true (Colloid cysts can obstruct both foramina of Monro; thus, bilateral ventricular drainage is needed.)
d. medical management and reassurance — false
e. fenestration of the septum pellucidum — true
f. removal of colloid cyst — true

21

21

214. **Complete the following about colloid cyst:** G7 p. X:111mm
a. shunt
    i.   r_____ b_____ s_____ requires bilateral shunts
    ii. or f_____ of s_____ fenestration of septum
         p_____ plus o_____ s_____ pellucidum plus one shunt
b. transcallosal approach complications
    i.   v_____ i_____ venous infarction
    ii. f_____ i_____ fornix injury
c. transcortical approach complications
    i.   s_____ _____% seizures 5%
d. stereotactic aspiration
    i.   f_____—r_____ failure—recurrence
e. ventriculoscopy
    i.   f_____—r_____ failure—recurrence

215. **Answer the following about hemangioblastoma:** G7 p.667:80mm
a. What is the most common primary intraaxial tumor in the adult posterior fossa? hemangioblastoma
b. It can occur sporadically or as part of v_____ _____-_____ disease. von Hippel-Lindau
c. What blood problem is associated?
    i.   P_____ also known as polycythemia
    ii. e_____ due to erythropoietin
    iii. e_____. erythropoitin
d. Incidence of brain tumors _____% 1 to 2%
e. Characteristic appearance c_____ c_____ m_____ w_____ m_____ n_____ cystic cerebellar mass with mural nodule
f. Should you remove the cyst wall? no

216. **True or False. A 42-year-old male presents with headache, nausea, vomiting, and right-sided dysmetria. Laboratory studies revealed a hemoglobin of 17. The likely diagnosis is** G7 p.667:80mm
a. metastatic lesion false
b. renal cell carcinoma false
c. hemangioblastoma true (headache, nausea, vomiting-hydrocephalus-dysmetria-cerebellum high hemoglobin-polycythemia)
d. high-grade astrocytoma false

217. **Complete the following about the posterior fossa hemangioblastoma:** G7 p.667:80mm
a. May be associated with
    i.   p_____, e_____ polycythemia, erythrocytosis
    ii. v_____ H_____-L_____ d_____ von Hippel-Lindau disease

218. **Complete the following about von Hippel-Lindau disease (VHL):**
G7 p.667:130mm

Has hemangioblastomas tumors or cysts in the following sites:

a. c_____   cerebellum
b. r_____   retina
c. b_____   brain stem
d. s_____   spinal cord
e. p_____   pheochromocytomas
f. c_____   cysts in kidneys

219. **Complete the following about von Hippel-Lindau disease (VHL):**
G7 p.667:135mm

a. Most common in the _____   cerebellum
b. Second most common in the _____   retina
c. Always manifests before age _____   60
d. Incidence is 1 in every _____ persons   35,000

220. **True or False. The mode of inheritance of von Hippel-Lindau disease is:**
G7 p.667:175mm

a. autosomal recessive   false
b. autosomal dominant   true
c. sex linked   false
d. multifactorial   false

221. **What is the diagnostic criteria for VHL?**
G7 p.668:60mm

a.
  i. One sign of VHL is needed if there is a _____ _____   family history
  ii. It will be present in _____%   80%
b. Two signs of VHL if it is a _____ _____ mutation   de novo

222. **Complete the following about tumors associated with VHL:**
G7 p.668:105mm

a. Occur in younger persons if patient has _____   VHL

b. True or False. Cysts are associated with HGBs.   true

c. Cerebellar HGBs are located in the
  i. s_____   superficial
  ii. p_____   posterior
  iii. s_____ half of the hemisphere   superior
d. _____% of cerebellar HGBs were found in the _____   7%, vermis

223. **Complete the following about spinal cord hemangioblastoma:**
G7 p.668:145mm

a. _____% are in the cervical and thoracic cord.   90%
b. _____% are located in the posterior cord.   96%
c. _____% of spinal HGBs are associated with VHL.   90%
d. _____% symptoms are associated with syringomyelia.   95%

224. The only disease with bilateral endolymphatic sac tumors is _____.

VHL

G7 p.668:180mm

225. Complete the following about VHL:

G7 p. : mm

a. Retinal hemangioblastomas occur in _____%

50%

b. Typically located in the _____

periphery

c. Frequently _____

multiple

d. Treat with laser _____

photocoagulation

226. Complete the following about renal cell carcinoma (RCC):

G7 p.669:130mm

a. Which is the most common malignant tumor in VHL?

RCC

b. Usually it is a _____ _____ _____.

clear cell carcinoma (CCC)

c. It is the cause of death in _____ to _____% of VHL patients.

15 to 50%

227. Complete the following about surgical treatment of HGB:

G7 p. : mm

a. Reserved until _____

symptomatic

b. Treatment of choice for _____ _____ HGBs

accessible cystic

c. True or False. The wall must be removed.

false

d. The _____ _____ must be removed.

mural nodule

228. Answer the following about hemangioblastoma (HGB):

G7 p.671:17mm

a. True or False. Starts at an earlier age in

　i.   von Hippel-Lindau disease

true

　ii. sporadic cases

false

b. In sporadic cases

　i.   Most originate in the _____

cerebellum

　ii. Next most common is the s_____ c_____

spinal cord

　iii. _____% of patients with cerebellar HGB have VHL

30%

c. Erythropoitin liberated by the tumor may be responsible for the _____

erythrocytosis

G7 p.671:53mm

d. If one HGB is suspected we should do an

G7 p.671:140mm

　i.   MRI scan of the _____ _____.

entire neuraxis

　ii. Vertebral angiography usually demonstrates _____ _____.

intense vascularity

　iii. CBC reveals _____.

polycythemia

229. Complete the following about surgery on a solitary HGB:

G7 p.672:22mm

a. It may be _____ in sporadic HGB

curative

b. but not in _____.

VHL

c. Preoperative _____ may be helpful.

embolization

21

230. **Complete the following about surgery on HGB:**   G7 p.672:40mm
  a. They should be removed using _____ technique.   AVM
  b. Avoid _____ removal.   piecemeal
  c. Work along the _____   margin
  d. and _____ the blood supply.   devascularize

■ CNS Lymphoma

231. **Complete the following about CNS lymphoma:**   G7 p.672:95mm
  a. Associated with an eye condition called _____   uveitis

  b. How frequently does it occur?   1 to 2% of all brain tumors
  c. What relationship does CNS lymphoma have with the ventricles?   up close to ventricles
  d. CT characteristics
    i. plain CT tumor is _____   hyperdense to brain
    ii. contrast CT tumor _____   enhances homogeneously
    iii. reminiscent of _____ _____ _____   "fluffy cotton balls"

  e. reaction to steroids _____   tumor may completely resolve
  f. CSF is positive for lymphoma cells in _____%.   only 10%
  g. What form of radiation therapy is given?   whole brain

232. **True or False. A 70-year-old male with a homogeneously enhancing lesion in the central gray matter and corpus callosum is suspected of having CNS lymphoma. What would make this diagnosis more likely and how is it properly diagnosed?**   G7 p.672:107mm
  a. hydrocephalus   false
  b. café au lait spots   false
  c. uveitis   true (diagnosed with slit lamp)
  d. proximal muscle weakness   false

233. **A 73-year-old male with a history of recently diagnosed CNS lymphoma by biopsy presents to the ER with stupor and progressively deteriorating mental status. CT of the brain reveals the mass but no other abnormalities.**   G7 p.675:55mm
  a. True or False.
    i. emergent surgical excision   false
    ii. radiation therapy   true (CNS lymphomas are very sensitive to radiation.)
    iii. chemotherapy   false
    iv. steroids   false
  b. followed by _____   chemotherapy

21

■ Chordoma

234. Complete the following about chordoma: G7 p.675:165mm

a. It has a characteristic cell type called _____.   physaliphorous

b. It occurs in the clivus in _____%.   35%

c. It occurs in the sacrococcygeal area in _____%.   55%

d. The recurrence rate after surgery is _____%.   85%

e. X-rays show _____ lesions with _____.   lytic lesions with calcifications

f. Is there any gender predominance?   yes, male predominance for sacral chordomas

g. What are the risks to bladder and bowel control

   i. from a sacrectomy between S1 and S2?   most will be impaired

   ii. from a sacrectomy between S2 and S3?   50% will be impaired

■ Ganglioglioma

235. True or False. Physaliphorous cells are distinctive features of   G7 p.675:165mm

a. schwannomas   false

b. pinealoblastomas   false

c. gangliogliomas   false

d. chordomas   true

236. Answer the following about gangliogliomas: G7 p.677:165mm

a. True or False. Peak age of occurrence for gangliogliomas is

   i. children   true (Peak age is 11.)

   ii. elderly   false

   iii. no age predilection   false

   iv. unknown   false

b. presenting symptom is _____   seizure

■ Paraganglioma

237. Complete the following about paraganglioma: G7 p.678:175mm

a. used to be called _____   chemodectomas

b. now also called what if at

   i. carotid bifurcation: c_____ b_____ t_____   carotid body tumor

   ii. jugular foramen: g_____ j_____   glomus jugulare

   iii. adrenal medulla: p_____   pheochromocytoma

21

c. may secrete
  i.   e_____   epinephrine
  ii. n_____   norepinephrine
  iii. c_____   catecholamines
d. Resection of carotid body tumor has a
  i.   morbidity of up to _____%   50%
  ii. mortality of _____%   5 to 13%

238. Complete the following about   G7 p.679:80mm
pheochromocytoma:
a. We used to study _____   catecholamines
b. Better test now is
  i.   f_____   fractioned
  ii. p_____   plasma
  iii. m_____   metanephrines
c. Imaging is _____ with _____   MRI; contrast

239. Carotid body tumor   G7 p.679:140mm
a. and _____ are the most common   pheochromocytoma
   paraganglioma.
b. occur bilaterally in _____%.   5%

240. True or False. A 40-year-old female   G7 p.679:160mm
complaints of a painless mass in her
right upper neck and has deviation of
the tongue to the right. The following
is the most likely source of her mass:
a. carotid bifurcation   true (Paragangliomas present
                                            with mass in neck and CN XI
                                            and CN XII nerve palsy.)
b. superior vagal ganglion   false
c. inferior vagal ganglion   false
d. hypoglossal nerve neuroma   false
e. auricular branch of vagus   false

241. Regarding carotid body tumors,   high   G7 p.680:25 mm
treatment carries a _____
complication rate.

242. Complete the following about glomus   G7 p.680:50mm
jugulare tumors:
a. They arise from _____ _____.   glomus bodies
b. Are they vascular or avascular?   vascular
c. Receives branches from the _____   external carotid artery

   _____ _____
  i.   a_____ p_____   ascending pharyngeal
  ii. p_____ a_____   posterior auricular
  iii. o_____   occipital
  iv. i _____ m_____   internal maxillary
d. _____ portion of the _____   petrous portion of the
   _____ _____   internal carotid artery

21

243. Characterize glomus jugulare tumors.   G7 p.680:88mm
   a. female to male ratio   6:1
   b. Does it occur bilaterally?   no
   c. presenting symptoms
       i.   h_____ l_____   hearing loss
       ii. p_____ t_____   pulsatile tinnitus
   d. clinical exam abnormalities
       i.   h_____ l_____ and   hearing loss and vertigo CN
            v_____   VIII
       ii. t_____ p_____ t_____   loss of taste posterior third of
                                              tongue CN IX
       iii. v_____ c_____ p_____   vocal cord paralysis CN X
       iv. t _____ and SCM w_____   trapezius and
                                              sternocleidomastoid (SCM)
                                              CN XI weakness
       v.   t_____ a_____ and CN   tongue atrophy CN XII and
            _____ i_____ to mass and   ipsilateral to mass and side
            s_____ of the hearing loss

244. During surgical excision of a   G7 p.680:170mm
     paraganglioma the patient is noted to
     have abrupt onset of hypotension and
     respiratory distress. This is most likely
     related to
   a. intracranial pressure (ICP) changes   no
   b. vasovagal response   no
   c. inadvertent compression of airway   no
   d. tumor manipulation   yes
   e. due to r_____ of h_____ or   release of histamine or
       b_____   bradykinin

245. Describe glomus jugulare differential   G7 p.681:15 mm
     diagnosis.
   a. Distinguish from _____ _____ in   vestibular schwannoma
       the CPA
   b. True or False. By CT enhancement   false (Both enhance.)
   c. True or False. By presence of cystic   true (VS may have cystic
       component   component.)
   d. True or False. By angiography   true (GJ [glomus jugulare] is
                                               very vascular.)
   e. What else will be learned by   whether the transverse sinus
       angiography?   is occluded

246. Complete the following about glomus   G7 p.681:120mm
     jugulare:
   a. What chemical should be tested for?   vanillylmandelic acid (VMA)
   b. If elevated, indicative of secretion of catecholamines
       _____
   c. similar to _____   pheochromocytoma
   d. Treat medically with _____ and   alpha and β blockers
       _____
   e. New clinical marker is _____ (NMN)   normetanephrine   G7 p.679:90mm

21

■ Ependymoma

247. Complete the following about ependymoma: G7 p.682:165mm

a. Incidence among intracranial tumors in adults is _____%.   5 to 6%

b. Incidence among pediatric brain tumors is _____%.   9%

c. It occurs in children _____%.   70%

d. Incidence among spinal cord gliomas is _____%.   60%

e. Drop metastases occur in _____% of patients.   11%

f. What is the pathology of the distinctive type that occurs in the filum terminale?   myxopapillary   G7 p.683:190mm

248. Characterize intracranial ependymomas.   G7 p.683:160mm

a. usually occur in the _____ _____   fourth ventricle

b. dangerous to remove because they invade the _____   floor of the fourth ventricle

c. specifically they invade the _____   obex

d. current operative mortality _____%   5 to 8%

e. Is mortality higher in adults or in children?   children

249. Answer the following about postop ependymoma: G7 p.684:123mm

a. What must we do?   LP

b. When? _____ weeks postop   2

c. What should be sent to lab?   10cc CSF

d. If positive follow with _____   radiation   G7 p.684:140mm

e. True or False. Ependymoma is sensitive to radiation.   true

f. Name the tumor that is more sensitive.   medulloblastoma

250. True or False. Regarding primary brain tumors: G6 p.471:180mm

a. Calcifications, although uncommon in medulloblastomas, may be seen ~20% of the time.   false (< 10%)

b. The "banana sign" in the fourth ventricle refers to the medulloblastoma rather than to ependymomas.   true

c. Ependymomas rank second only to medulloblastomas in radiosensitivity.   true

d. Medulloblastomas arise from the roof of the fourth ventricle, the fastigium.   true

e. Ependymomas arise from the floor of the fourth ventricle, the obex.   true

251. What is the most common glioma of the spinal cord below the midthoracic region?   ependymoma   G7 p.685:100mm

21

■ Embryonal Tumors

252. **Complete the following about embryonal tumors:** G7 p.685:135mm

a. PNET stands for
   i.   P_____   Primitive
   ii. N_____   Neuro
   iii. E_____   Ectodermal
   iv. T_____   Tumors

b. These tumors include
   i.   P_____   Pineoblastoma
   ii. N_____   Neuroblastoma
   iii. E_____   Esthesioneuroblastoma
   iv. R_____   Retinoblastoma
   v.   M_____   Medulloblastoma

c.
   i.   They are _____ indistinguishable   histologically
   ii. but genetically _____.   distinct

d. Medulloblastomas are different. They contain G7 p.685:140mm
   i.   Beta _____   catenin
   ii. APC _____   mutations
   iii. And some originate from the   external granular
        _____ _____
   iv. layer of the _____.   cerebellum

253. **Embryonal tumors** G7 p.685:178mm

a. require entire _____ _____   spinal axis
   evaluation.

b.
   i.   Cranial radiotherapy is avoided   3
        before _____ years of age
   ii. to avoid i_____ impairment   intellectual
   iii. and growth r_____.   retardation

254. **Complete the following about supratentorial PNET (sPNETs):** G7 p.686:25mm

a. They occur in children under _____   5
   years of age.

b. They occur _____ in adults.   rarely

c. Histologically, they are _____ to identical
   medulloblastoma.

d.
   i.   They are _____ aggressive than   more
        medulloblastomas.
   ii. Survival is _____ and they   shorter
   iii. respond to therapy _____.   poorly

255. True or False. Regarding medulloblastoma: G7 p.686:55mm

a. It accounts for 15 to 20% of all intracranial tumors in children.
true

b. It is the most common malignant pediatric brain tumor.
true

c. There is a standardized chemotherapy, including lomustine (CCNU) and vincristine.
false (There is no standardized regimen; CCNU and vincristine are usually reserved for recurrences.) G7 p.687:115mm

d. Patients with residual medulloblastoma postresection and dissemination are a poor risk, with only a 35 to 50% chance of being disease free at 5 years.
true

256. Complete the following about medulloblastoma: G7 p.686:95mm

a. The clinical history is _____,
brief

b. typically only _____ to _____ weeks.
6 to 12

c. Their location of origin predisoses to _____.
hydrocephalus

d. They present with
    i. h_____
    headache
    ii. n_____
    nausea
    iii. a_____ and
    ataxia
    iv. seeding of the axis has occurred in _____ to _____ %.
    10 to 35%

257. True or false. Radiologically medulloblastomas are G7 p.686:135mm

a. cystic
false

b. solid
true

c. enhancing
true

d. on non-contrast CT they are hyperdense
true

258. Complete the following about medulloblastoma location: G7 p.686:157mm

a. Most are in the _____.
midline

b. Laterally situated tumors are more common in _____.
adults

259. Complete the following about drop mets to the spine with medulloblastoma: G7 p.686:157mm

a. The test that should be done is _____ _____ _____.
MRI with contrast

b.
    i. This study should be done _____
    preop
    ii. or within _____ to _____ weeks postop.
    2 to 3

260. Regarding the molecular biology of medulloblastoma, in 35 to 40% there is deletion of _____.
17p
G7 p.687:40mm

21

21

261. **True or False. Regarding epidermoid and dermoid brain tumors:**   G7 p.688:143mm

a. Epidermoid tumors tend to occur laterally, whereas dermoid tumors are more common near the midline.   true

b. Epidermoid tumors are associated with other congenital anomalies in up to 50% of cases.   false (Dermoid tumors are associated with other congenital anomalies in over 50%.)

c. Epidermoid cysts, also known as cholesteatomas, are often confused with cholesterol granuloma.   true   G7 p.689:62mm

262. **True or False. Regarding primary brain tumors:**   G7 p.690:50mm

a. Cholesterol granulomas usually involve vestibular or cochlear dysfunction.   true

b. Both epidermoid cysts and cholesterol granulomas have a pearly white gross appearance.   false (Cholesterol granulomas are brown.)

c. Mollaret meningitis is a rare variant of aseptic meningitis that may be seen in some patients with epidermoid cysts.   true   G7 p.690:85mm

263. **Complete the following about imaging of epidermoids:**   G7 p.690:122mm

a. On T1W1 they mimic _____.   CSF
b. On T2W1 they are _____ _____.   high signal
c. With contrast they _____ _____.   don't enhance
d.
   i. They pass from the _____ _____   posterior fossa
   ii. through the _____   incisura
   iii. into the _____ _____.   middle fossa
e.
   i. The best test to differentiate them from CSF is _____   DWI
   ii. where they show _____ _____   intense signal
   iii. because of _____ _____.   restricted diffusion

■ Pineal Region Tumors

264. **True or False. Regarding pineal region tumors:**   G7 p.691:130mm

a. The absence of the BBB in the pineal gland makes this area a susceptible site for hematogenous metastasis.   true

b. Nongerminomas include
   i. embryonal carcinoma   true
   ii. choriocarcinoma   true
   iii. teratoma   true
   iv. medulloblastomas   false

c. Germ cell tumors rarely give rise to tumor markers.   false

265. Complete the following about germ cell tumors: G7 p.692:50mm
a. In the CNS they arise in the _____. midline
b. In males they are most likely in the _____ region. pineal
c. In females they are most likely in the _____ region. suprasellar
d. Are germ cell tumors benign or malignant? malignant
e. They spread via the _____. CSF

266. True or False. Regarding germ cell tumors: G7 p.693:90mm
a. Germ cell tumors and pineal cell tumors occur primarily in childhood and young adults (< 40 years old). true
b. Clinical features of pineal region tumors may include hydrocephalus and Parinaud syndrome. true
c. Optimal management strategy for pineal region tumors has yet to be determined. true

267. True or False. Germinomas are very sensitive to radiation but not to chemotherapy. false (They are sensitive to both.) G7 p.694:165mm

268. Complete the following about surgery for pineal tumors: G7 p.695:78mm
a.
  i. The most common approach is the _____ _____. infratentorial supracerebellar
  ii. This cannot be used if the _____ is steep. tentorium
b.
  i. Another common approach is the _____ occipital transtentorial
  ii. which is best for lesions _____ at centered
  iii. or _____ to the tentorial edge superior
  iv. or _____ the vein of Galen. above

Choroid Plexus Tumors

269. True or False. Regarding brain tumors: G7 p.696:22mm
a. Choroid plexus tumors largely occur in patients less than 2 years old. true
b. Choroid plexus tumors do not grow with any particular rapidity. false (They sometimes grow rapidly.)

270. True or False. Regarding choroid plexus tumors:

a. They are usually located in: *G7 p.696:30mm*
   i.   adults _____   infratentorially
   ii. children _____   supratentorially
b. Hydrocephalus with choroid plexus   true   *G7 p.696:60mm*
   tumors may result from overproduction
   of CSF, although tumor removal does
   not always cure the problem.

271. CT or MRI usually demonstrates a mass   *G7 p.696:75mm*

a. located _____   intraventricularly
b. which is contrast _____.   enhancing
c. It has a _____ shape   multi-lobulated
d. with projecting _____   fronds
e. and commonly h_____.   hydrocephalus

272. True or False. Regarding primary CNS melanomas: *G7 p. 697:45mm*

a. Primary CNS melanoma does not arise   false
   from melanocytes in the leptomeninges.
b. The peak age for primary CNS melanoma   true
   is in the fourth decade.

■ Pediatric Brain Tumors

273. Complete the following about pediatric brain tumors: *G7 p.696:77mm*

a. What is the second most common   brain tumor
   childhood cancer?
b. What is the first?   leukemia
c. Brain tumor incidence in children is   2 to 5 cases/100,000
   _____.

274. Of all brain tumors in the age group 2 to 16, _____% are infratentorial.   42%   *G7 p.697:102mm*

275. True or False. The most common supratentorial tumors in children are   *G7 p.697:137mm*

a. astrocytoma   true
b. pinealoma, teratoma, choroid plexus   true
   tumors, craniopharyngioma
c. medulloblastoma   false

276. True or False. Regarding pediatric brain tumors: *G7 p.697:170mm*

a. 50% of brain tumors in neonates are of   false (90%)
   neuroectodermal origin
b. Many of the brain tumors in infants   true
   < 1 year old escape diagnosis until they
   are quite large due to the plasticity of
   the infant's skull.
c. Astrocytomas are the most common   true
   supratentorial tumors in pediatrics as in
   adulthood.

277. What are the most common
symptoms of intracranial tumor in
children?

   Hint: tumors
   a. t _____   throwing
   b. u_____   up
   c. m_____   macrocrania
   d. o_____   oral intake poor
   e. r_____   regression in milestones
   f. s_____   seizures

■ Skull Tumors

278. **The most common primary bone
tumor of the calvarium**

   a. is the _____.   osteoma
   b. It usually involves only the _____
      _____.   outer table

   c. At surgery you can leave the inner table
      _____.   intact

279. **True or False. Regarding skull tumors:**

   a. Hemangiomas comprise 15% of skull   false (7%)
      tumors.
   b. 50% of hemangiomas on skull x-ray show   true
      a circular lucency with a honeycomb or
      trabecular pattern.

280. **Characterize skull tumor x-rays.**

   a. The margin of an epidermoid is   edges distinct
      _____.   (epidermoid = ED well
                                            defined—sclerotic)
   b. The margin of an eosinophilic granuloma   edges graded (eosinophilic
      is _____.   granuloma = EG
                                            nonsclerotic—beveled edges)

281. **Complete the following about skull
tumors:**

   a. True or False. Eosinophilic granuloma is   true
      generally a condition of youth.
   b. True or False. Eosinophilic granulomas   false
      cause a usually nontender enlarging skull
      mass.
   c. True or False. The CT appearance of   true
      eosinophilic granulomas includes a soft
      mass within an area of bone destruction
      having a central density.
   d. On skull x-ray of eosinophilic granuloma   graded (beveled) = EG
      the edges are _____.

282.   True or False. Regarding skull tumors: G7 p.700:115mm

a. Hyperostosis frontalis interna (HFI) is a benign, irregular thickening of the inner table of the frontal bone that is rarely expressed bilaterally.   false (It is almost always bilateral.)

b. HFI has also been called a metabolic craniopathy.   true

c. HFI has been associated with Morgagni syndrome.   true

283.   Answer the following about fibrous dysplasia: G7 p.701:89 mm

a. True or False. It is benign.   true

b. True or False. It is inheritable.   false

c. True or False. It can cause cranial nerve deficits.   true (especially hearing)

d. True or False. It may be tender to touch.   true

e. True or False. Alkaline phosphatase is invariably elevated.   false (only in 33% of patients)

f. Appearance on x-ray is that of _____ _____.   ground glass   G7 p.701:187 mm

g. It can be treated with _____.   calcitonin   G7 p.270:823mm

■ Cerebral Metastases

284.   Complete the following about cerebral metastases: G7 p.702:48mm

a. The most common brain tumor is the _____.   metastasis

b. It will be multiple in _____% on MRI.   70%

c. Need biopsy for solitary lesion because _____% will not be a metastasis.   11%

285.   Complete the following about brain tumors: G7 p.702:72mm

a. Metastatic brain tumors represent _____% of all brain tumors that occur.   50%

b. How often is the brain metastases the only site of spread?   9%

c. Which primary CNS tumors spread via the CSF?

   i. g_____   glioma

   ii. e_____   ependymoma

   iii. P_____   PNET

   iv. p_____   pineal tumors

d. Where do metastases occur?

   i. g _____-w_____ j_____   gray-white junction

   ii. t_____ p_____ and o_____ l_____ junction.   temporal parietal and occipital lobe junction

   iii. c_____ _____%   cerebellum 16%

286. **Regarding a metastatic tumor at the time of neurological diagnosis, how many of the cerebral metastases are considered solitary as studied by**
   G7 p.702:105mm
   a. CT? _____%
   b. MR? _____%

   50% seem to be solitary
   only 30% seem to be solitary
   (The rest are multiple because MR is more sensitive and identifies more than one metastasis.)

287. **Complete the following about cerebral metastases:**
   G7 p.703:65mm
   a. Where do brain metastases come from? Hint: lubrim
      i. lu_____   lung
      ii. b_____   breast
      iii. r_____   renal
      iv. i_____   intestinal tract
      v. m_____   melanoma
   b. Percent from each of the above primary sites
      i. _____%   44%
      ii. _____%   10%
      iii. _____%   7%
      iv. _____%   8%
      v. _____%   3%
   c. At autopsy what percent of these tumors has metastasized to the brain?
      i. lung _____%   21%
      ii. breast _____%   9%
      iii. renal _____%   11%
      iv. GI _____%   3%
      v. melanoma _____% 40%
   d. Which tumor is most likely to be found as a metastasis to the brain?

   small cell lung cancer (SCLC)

288. **Complete the following about small cell lung cancer (SCLC):**
   G7 p.703:175mm
   a. aka _____ _____ cancer   oat cell
   b. Strongly associated with _____   cigarette smoking
      _____
   c. Reaction to radiation is _____   very sensitive   G7 p.704:40mm
      _____

289. **Most common type of nonsmall cell lung cancer is _____.**

   adenocarcinoma   G7 p.704:80mm

21

290. **True or False. Protocol for newly diagnosed lung lesion plus single brain lesion. You should**   G7 p.704:125mm

  a. remove the solitary brain lesion   false

  b. biopsy the brain lesion   false

  c. biopsy the lung lesion   true

     i. because if it is _____   SCLC

    ii. you will treat with _____   radiation

291. **The most common source of cerebral metastatic disease comes from the _____.**   lungs (SCLC)   G7 p.703:160mm

292. **Complete the following about metastatic melanoma:**   G7 p.704:160mm

  a. Longevity after detected in the brain is _____ days.   113 days

  b. Unless it is a single melanoma metastasis, then patient may live _____ years.   3 years

  c. True or False. Melanoma is responsive to chemotherapy and radiation.   false (very poor response)

293. **Complete the following about melanoma treatment:**   G7 p.705:85mm

  a. With chemotherapy for melanoma, the gold standard is _____.   dacarbazine

  b. Immunotherapy for melanoma that is as effective as chemotherapy is a vaccine: _____.   Melacine   G7 p.705:115mm

  c. Prognosis   G7 p.705:165mm

     i. Median survival is _____ months   18

    ii. 5 year survival is _____%   20%

294. **True or False. Regarding cerebral metastases:**

  a. The primary site for a brain metastasis can always be identified.   false (never identified in 14% of patients)   G7 p.704:150mm

  b. Renal cell carcinoma frequently presents as isolated cerebral metastases.   false (It has usually spread widely before invading the CNS.)   G7 p.705:183mm

295. **Characterize metastatic brain tumor presentation.**   G7 p.706:52mm

  a. headache in _____%   50%

  b. seizures _____%   15%

  c. hemorrhage occurs in   G7 p.706:80mm

     i. m_____ m_____   metastatic melanoma

    ii. c_____   choriocarcinoma

    iii. r_____ c_____ c_____   renal cell carcinoma

21

296. **Answer the following about the workup of a solitary brain lesion:** G7 p.706:128mm

a. In a patient who has no history of cancer, negative chest x-ray, and negative intravenous pyelogram (IVP), what percent will be
   i. metastases — 7%
   ii. primary brain tumors — 87%
   iii. nonneoplastic — 6%
b. If the patient has a history of cancer, what percent will be metastatic? — 93%
c. Most commonly _____ — adenocarcinoma G7 p.707:61mm
d. But the primary may remain occult in _____% — 88%

297. **Complete the following about cerebral metastases:** G7 p.707:90mm

a. True or False. A patient with known cancer of the breast 2 years earlier develops a seizure and MRI shows a brain lesion. You may consider this a metastasis from the breast and treat her with radiation and chemotherapy. — false (7 to 11% of patients with a history of cancer and an abnormal CT or MRI scan will not have a metastasis.)

b. What should be advised? — biopsy (You should do a biopsy to identify glioblastoma, low-grade glioma, abscess, etc.)

c. With optimal treatment what is the prognosis for patients with brain metastases? — 26 to 32 weeks

298. **True or False. Most important factor in prognosis is:** G7 p.707:130mm

a. tumor type — false
b. time since diagnosis — false
c. Karnofsky performance score — true
d. better prognosis with a score > _____ — 70 G7 p.707:140mm

299. **Tumors considered radioresistant are** G7 p.707:140mm
Hint: last m(a)rc

a. l_____ _____ — (NSCLC) nonsmall cell lung cancer
b. a_____ — adenocarcinoma
c. s_____ — sarcoma
d. t_____ — thyroid
e. m_____ — malignant melanoma
f. (a)
g. r_____ _____ — renal cell
h. c_____ — colon

21

300. **Tumors considered radiosensitive are**   G7 p.708:115mm
Hint: gllemmS
a. g_____ c_____ t_____   germ cell tumors
b. l_____   lymphoma
c. le_____   leukemia
d. m_____ m_____   multiple myeloma
e. S_____   SCLC

301. **Complete the following about cerebral**   G7 p.708:132mm
metastases:
a. After the usual dose of radiation therapy
for cerebral metastases what percent of
patients develop dementia at
  i.   1 year _____%   11%
  ii. 2 years _____%   50%
b. The standard dose is
  i.   _____ Gy in   30
  ii. _____ fractions over   10
  iii. _____ weeks   2

302. **True or False. The results of operating**   true   G7 p.709:100mm
on multiple metastases are similar to
the results of operating on a single
metastasis, if all of the lesions are
resected completely.

303. **Characterize outcomes of treatment**   G7 p.710:60mm
for cerebral metastases survival.
a. untreated patients _____   1 month
b. steroids _____   2 months
c. steroids plus radiation _____   3 to 6 months
d. steroids plus radiation plus surgery   8 months
_____
e. if systemic disease _____   20% live 1 year
f. if no systemic disease _____   80% live 1 year

304. **Which patient lives longer: one who**   control rates are similar   G7 p.710:155mm
has a metastasis and is treated with
radiosurgery plus whole brain
radiation or one who has a metastases
and is treated with surgery plus whole
brain radiation?

305. **Which patient lives longer: one who**   survival is similar   G7 p.710:155mm
has multiple metastases that were
totally removed or one who has a
single metastases that was totally
removed?

■ Carcinomatous Meningitis

306. **Complete the following about**   G7 p.711:45 mm
carcinomatous meningitis:

a. Symptoms
   i. h_____   headache
   ii. m_____ c_____ n_____   multiple cranial nerve
       d_____   dysfunction
b. CSF is eventually abnormal in _____% 95%
   of patients.
c. What size sample of CSF is needed?   at least 10 cc of CSF
d. Survival
   i. without treatment is _____   2 months
   ii. with treatment is _____   5 to 8 months

■ Foramen Magnum Tumors

307. **Foramen magnum tumors present**   G7 p.712:45mm
with

a. n_____ p_____   neck pain
b. w_____   weakness
   i. which begins in the _____   ipsilateral
      hand/arm
   ii. then progresses to the _____   ipsilateral
       lower extremity
   iii. then progresses to the _____ LE contralateral
   iv. and finally to the _____ hand contralateral
       and arm
c. this is called _____ _____   rotating paralysis   G7 p.712:60mm
d. sensory loss if present is _____ to the contralateral to the mass
   _____
e. eyes may show d_____-b_____   down-beat nystagmus
   n_____

■ Idiopathic Intracranial Hypertension

308. **Complete the following about**   G7 p.713:73mm
idiopathic intracranial hypertension:

a. Also known as p_____ c_____   pseudotumor cerebri
b. Diagnostic criteria
   i. CSF pressure above _____   above 20 to 25 cm H_2O
   ii. CSF composition   normal protein, glucose, and
                                          cell count
   iii. symptoms and signs   of increased pressure
   iv. radiologic studies   normal CT and MRI
c. Severe visual defects occur in   4 to 12%
   _____%.
d. Best test to follow vision is _____. perimetry

309. Characterize pseudotumor cerebri.

G7 p.713:100mm

a. gender preponderance _____   female 2 to 8:1
b. size of patient _____   more frequent with obesity
c. childbearing years _____   more frequent
d. Can this condition recur?   yes
e. What is the most serious consequence of this condition?   visual loss
f. How long does it take for visual changes to occur?   occurs in 4 to 12% unrelated to duration of symptoms
g. How should the vision be followed?   by perimetry

310. List pseudotumor cerebri diagnostic criteria.

G7 p.714:13mm

Hint: rinc
a. Radiology studies are _____.   normal
b. Intracranial pressure is _____.   high
c. Neurological exam is _____.   normal
d. Composition of CSF is _____.   normal

311. Describe pseudotumor cerebri treatment.

G7 p.717:90mm

a. Withdraw patient from o_____ c_____ and o_____ m_____.   oral contraceptives and other medications
b. Use medications such as
   i. D_____   Diamox
   ii. L_____   Lasix
   iii. d_____   dexamethasone
c. Procedures to consider include
   i. s_____ L_____   serial LPs
   ii. l_____-p_____ s_____   lumbo-peritoneal shunt
   iii. o_____ s_____ f_____   optic sheath fenestration

312. True or False. Regarding pseudotumor cerebri, the following are frequently used methods in the surgical treatment of pseudotumor cerebri:

G7 p.718:28mm

a. lumbar puncture   true
b. lumboperitoneal shunt   true
c. ventriculoperitoneal shunt   true
d. decompression of optic sheath   true

■ Empty Sella Syndrome

313. Matching. Match the type of empty sella origin with its clinical characteristics/features.

G7 p.719:95mm

Characteristic:
① visual deterioration; ② obese women; ③ treat surgically; ④ headache, dizziness, seizures; ⑤ surgery not indicated; ⑥ postsurgical
Origin:
a. primary origin (idiopathic)   ②, ④, ⑤
b. secondary origin (post surgical)   ①, ③, ⑥

314. **Complete the following about empty sella syndrome:**

G7 p.719:125mm

a. True or False. May have elevated prolactin.

true

b. If so how can you differentiate from prolactinoma by endocrine testing?

TRH stimulation

c. if prolactinoma

no PRL rise

d. if empty sella

normal PRL rise

■ Tumor Markers

315. **True or False. This tumor marker usually indicates astroglial origin.**

G7 p.720:38mm

21

a. glial fibrillary acid protein (GFAP)

true (GFAP is rarely found outside the CNS. Thus the presence of GFAP in a tumor found in the CNS is usually taken as good evidence for glial origin of the tumor.)

b. S-100 protein

false

c. cytokeratin

false

d. neuron specific enolase (NSE)

false

e. human chorionic gonadotropin (HCG)

false

316. **True or False. This tumor marker may be helpful in differentiating metastatic tumor from primary CNS tumors.**

G7 p.720:85mm

a. GFAP

true (indicates astroglial origin)

b. S-100 protein

true (similar to GFAP, may arise from Schwann cells and be positive in melanomas, head trauma, and Creutzfeldt-Jakob)

c. cytokeratin

true (may help distinguish metastatic tumors, stains epithelial cells)

d. NSE

true (metastatic small cell tumors to the brain staining positive due to lung)

e. HCG

true (high levels indicate cerebral metastases from uterine or testicular choriocarcinoma)

f. α-fetoprotein

true (cancer of ovary, stomach, lung, colon, pancreas)

g. carcinoembryonic antigen (CEA)

true

h. CSF-CEA

true, (leptomeningeal spread of lung cancer, breast, bladder cancer, malignant melanoma)

317. Complete the following about tumor marker MIB-I: G7 p.720:100mm

a. A high number indicates _____ _____.   mitotic activity

b. It correlates with degree of _____.   malignancy

c. It is used for
   i.   a_____   astrocytoma
   ii. m_____   meningioma
   iii. b_____ c_____   breast cancer
   iv. l_____   lymphoma

318. True or False. Which tumor marker do you also use in head trauma?   G7 p.721:175mm

a. GFAP   false

b. S-100 protein   true (S-100 protein levels rise after head trauma.)

c. CEA   false

d. HCG   false

e. cytokeratin   false

■ Neurocutaneous Disorders

319. True or False. The following are neurocutaneous disorders: G7 p.722:45mm

a. Sturge-Weber syndrome   true

b. neurofibromatosis   true

c. tuberous sclerosis   true

d. von Hippel-Lindau disease   true

e. Foix-Alajouanine syndrome   false (Foix-Alajouanine syndrome, acute or subacute neurologic deterioration in a patient with a spinal arteriovenous malformation without evidence of hemorrhage)

320. True or False. Features for neurofibromatosis 1 include   G7 p.723:35mm

a. more than six café au lait spots   true

b. peripheral neurofibromatosis (NF)   true

c. gene is on chromosome 17q 11.2   true

d. optic glioma   true

e. bilateral acoustic neuroma   false (almost never bilateral; bilateral are the hallmark of neurofibromatosis 2)

321. Complete the following about genetics of NF-1:   G7 p.723:145mm

a. It is a_____ d_____.   autosomal dominant

b. After age 5 it has _____% penetrance.   100%

c. It is on chromosome _____   17q11.2

d. which codes for _____.   neurofibromin

322. **True or False. When comparing NF1 with NF2, the following is in both:**

G7 p.724:70mm

a. Antigenetic nerve growth factor is increased.

false (Antigenetic nerve growth factor does not occur with NF1 only with NF2.)

b. Skin nodules, dermal neurofibromas — true

c. Multiple intradural spinal tumors are common. — true

d. Autosomal dominant inheritance — true

G7 p.724:140mm

e. Malignant tumors that have increased frequency — true

323. **Complete the following about neurofibromatosis 2:**

G7 p.724:110mm

a. Despite its name it has no _____. — neurofibromas

b.

   i.   NF2 is due to a _____ — mutation

   ii. on chromosome _____ — 22q 12.2

   iii. which results in inactivation of s_____. — Schwannomin

c. It is associated with bilateral (2) v_____ s_____. — vestibular schwannoma

G7 p.724:110mm

d. Most NF2 patients will become _____. — deaf

e. Pregnancy may _____ the growth of eight nerve tumors. — accelerate

■ Tuberous Sclerosis

324. **Complete the following about tuberous sclerosis:**

G7 p.725:28mm

a. List the key clinical features of tuberous sclerosis.
Hint: sam

   i.   s_____ — seizures

   ii. a_____ s_____ — adenoma sebaceum

   iii. m_____ r_____ — mental retardation

b. CNS finding is typically a s_____ n_____—a h_____. — subependymal nodule—a hamartoma

c. Common neoplasm is a s_____ g_____ c_____ a_____. — subependymal giant cell astrocytoma

d. CT shows i_____ s_____ c_____. — intracerebral subependymal calcifications (usually subependymal)

325. **True or False. The clinical triad of tuberous sclerosis includes**

G7 p.725:28mm

a. seizures — true

b. mental retardation — true

c. sebaceous adenomas — true

d. port-wine facial nevus — false

21

326. True or False. Regarding tuberous sclerosis:

G7 p.725:140mm

a. In infants the earliest finding is of ash leaf macules. — true

b. Myoclonus found in children is often replaced by partial complex seizures in adults. — true

c. Facial adenomas are present at birth. — false (Facial adenomas are not present at birth but occur by age 4 years in 91% of patients.)

d. Retinal hamartomas are present. — true in ~50% of patients

327. List the key features of Sturge-Weber syndrome.
Hint: abc

G7 p.726:85mm

a. a_____ — atrophy: localized cerebral cortical atrophy and calcification

b. b_____ _____ — birth mark: ipsilateral port-wine facial nevus (usually in distribution of trigeminal nerve)

c. c_____ — calcification: plain skull films classically show "tram tracking"

328. True or False. The port-wine facial nevus associated with Sturge-Weber syndrome is

G7 p.726:118 mm

a. ipsilateral to the seizures — false (It is contralateral.)

b. in the distribution of the third division of the trigeminal nerve — false (in distribution of the first division)

c. contralateral to the "tram tracking" on plain x-rays — false (Nevus is ipsilateral to "tram tracks.")

d. rarely bilateral — true

■ Spine and Spinal Cord Tumors

329. Compartment locations of spinal tumors and their incidence are

G7 p.728:57mm

a. extradural _____% — tumor (55%)
b. intradural _____% — extramedullary (40%)
c. intramedullary _____% — spinal cord tumor (5%)

330. Osteoblastic tumors indicate

G7 p.728:107mm

a. in men likely _____ — prostate metastasis
b. in women likely _____ — breast cancer metastasis

331. One cause of vertebra plana is e_____ g_____. — eosinophlic granuloma

G7 p.729:28mm

332. **True or False. The most common extradural spinal tumor causing vertebral osteolytic defect on x-ray is**

G7 p.729:28mm

a. giant cell tumors — false
b. aneurysmal bone cyst — false
c. osteoblastoma — false
d. eosinophilic granuloma — true

333. **True or False. The following spinal tumors are usually primary in the spine:**

G7 p.729:45mm

a. Ewing sarcoma — false (Aggressive malignant tumor with a peak incidence during second decade of life. Spine metastases are more common.)
b. chordoma — true
c. chondrosarcoma — true
d. vertebral hemangioma — true
e. osteogenic sarcoma — true

334. **Characterize spinal meningiomas.**

G7 p.729:155mm

a. Peak age is _____. — 40s
b. The female:male ratio is _____ : _____. — 4:1
c. Main symptom is _____. — pain
d. Main sign preop is d_____ w_____. — difficulty walking

335. **Characterize spinal lymphoma.**

G7 p730 :65mm

a. It occurs in patients who have _____-_____ lymphoma. — non-Hodgkins
b. Incidence in these patients is from 1 to _____%. — 10%

336. **True or False. The two most common intramedullary spinal cord tumors are**

G7 p.730:122mm

a. teratoma — false
b. astrocytoma — true
c. ependymoma — true
d. dermoid — false
e. malignant glioblastoma — false

337. **True or False. The following is an intramedullary spinal cord tumor:**

G7 p.730:122mm

a. dermoid — true
b. teratoma — true
c. lipoma — true

21

	d.	neuroma	true (very rarely intramedullary)
	e.	meningioma	false (Meningiomas are usually intradural but may be partially or wholly extradural and are always extramedullary. 15% of spinal meningiomas are extradural. The other examples are miscellaneous intramedullary tumors.)

338. Considering epidermoid tumors, they are   G7 p.731:80mm
- a. most common in _____ or _____   conus or filum
- b. usually m_____   myxopapillary
- c. must image the _____ _____   entire neuraxis
- d. most are e_____   encapsulated
- e.
  - i. treatment is _____ _____   total excision
  - ii. by dividing the _____   filum

339. Characterize astrocytoma of the cord.   G7 p.731:160mm
- a. It occurs at all _____.   levels
- b. Most common is _____.   thoracic
- c. _____% are cystic.   38%
- d. Fluid has high _____.   protein

340. Lipoma is usually associated with _____.   dysraphism   G7 p.732:15mm

341. Characterize hemangioblastoma.   G7 p.732:50mm
- a.
  - i. It is usually associated with _____ _____-_____   von Hippel-Lindau
  - ii. in _____%.   33%
- b. Surgically treat it like an _____.   AVM

342. True or False. The tumor least common as an intramedullary spinal cord tumor is   G7 p.732:70mm
- a. astrocytoma   false
- b. ependymoma   false
- c. dermoid   false
- d. lipoma   false
- e. metastatic tumor   true (Most spinal metastases are extradural; only a few hundred case reports of intramedullary spinal cord tumor metastases exist, accounting for only 3.4% of symptomatic metastatic spinal cord lesions.)

21

343. **Complete the following about metastases intraparenchymal:**   G7 p.732:70mm
a. Rare—only a few _____ cases   hundred
b. Primarily from
   i.   S_____   SCLC
   ii.   b_____   breast
   iii. m_____ _____   malignant melanoma
   iv. l_____   lymphoma
   v. c_____   colon

344. **Complete the following about intramedullary spinal cord tumors:**   G7 p.732:100mm
a. The pain pattern suggestive of spinal cord tumor is pain _____ _____.   upon recumbency
b. Children present most commonly with _____ _____.   gait disturbance   G7 p.732:117mm

21

345. **Complete the following about spine and spinal cord tumors:**   G7 p.733:65mm
a. Spinal fluid that clots is called _____.   Froin syndrome
b. Clotting is due to _____.   fibrinogen

346. **True or False. With intraoperative spinal cord monitoring, a proof of improved outcome has been established for**   G7 p.734:15mm
a. SSEP   false
b. MEP   false

347. **Complete the following about prognosis of spinal cord tumors:**   G7 p.734:115mm
a. Better results in patients with _____   lesser deficits
b. Ependymoma
   i.   Improved outcome with _____   total removal
   ii. Myxopapillary tumors do _____   better
   iii. If symptoms less than _____ years   2
c. Astrocytoma
   i.   True or False. There is a cleavage plane.   false
   ii. Functional results _____ than ependymoma   poorer
   iii. Recurrence rate at 5 years is _____%   50%

348. **Complete the following about spinal schwannomas:**   G7 p.734:165mm
a. Slow growing _____ tumors   benign
b. 75% arise from the _____ roots   dorsal (sensory)
c. Early symptoms are often _____   radicular
d. Most are _____   intradural   G7 p.735:165mm
e. Dumbbell
  i. Have a _____   waist
  ii. Usually at the _____   dura
  iii. Sometimes these are classified as   I
       type _____
  iv. Sometimes at the _____   foramen
  v. These are classified as type   II
     _____
f. Nerve sacrifice is usually _____   not required   G7 p.736:13mm
   _____ because the involved fascicles
   are often _____ _____

349. **Complete the following about bone tumors of the spine:**   G7 p.736:50mm
a. Osteolytic metastases (Hint: bl^{2}emp^2):
  i. b_____   breast
  ii. l_____   lung
  iii. l_____   lymphoma
  iv. e_____   eosinophilic granuloma
  v. m_____   multiple myeloma
  vi. p_____   prostate
  vii. p_____   plasmacytoma
b. Osteolytic metastases   G7 p.736:75mm
  i. b_____   breast
  ii. p_____   prostate

350. **True or False. Regarding osteoid osteomas:**   G7 p.737:15mm
a. They are benign lesions presenting less   true
   than 1 cm in size.
b. Osteoid osteomas often degenerate into   false
   osteoblastomas.
c. Osteoid osteomas occur more   false
   commonly in the pedicle than
   osteoblastomas.
d. They are expansile destructive lesions.   false (Osteoblastomas are
                                               expansile destructive lesions)

351. **Osteoid osteoma. The diagnosis is**   G7 p.737:35mm
a. osteoid osteoma if it is less than   1 cm
   _____ _____ in size.
b. osteoblastoma if it is more than   1 cm
   _____ _____ in size.
c. They are histologically _____.   identical

21

352. True or False. The distributions of benign osteoblastomas in the spine are

G7 p. 737:50mm

a. 10% cervical, 50% thoracic, 40% lumbar   false
b. 25% cervical, 35% thoracic, 35% lumbar   true
c. 50% cervical, 10% thoracic, 40% lumbar   false
d. 35% cervical, 25% thoracic, 35% lumbar   false

353. Benign osteoblastoma and osteoid osteoma usually

G7 p.737:125mm

a. have the symptom of n_____ p_____   night pain
b. which is relieved by a_____.   aspirin

354. The most common primary

G7 p.738:20mm

a. bone cancer is _____.   osteosarcoma
b.
  i. Spinal form occurs in the _____ region   lumbosacral
  ii. in males in their _____.   40s
c. Biopsy needle tract _____ the area.   contaminates
d. Survival is _____ months.   10

355. True or False. Vertebral hemangiomas

G7 p.738:75mm

a. are rare tumors   false (occurs in 9 to 12% of the population)
b. may be malignant   false (never found to be malignant)
c. are often symptomatic   false (rarely symptomatic)
d. are radiosensitive   true (used for the uncommon painful lesion that can't be treated by excision or vertebroplasty)
e. x-rays show _____ _____   vertical striations
f. or _____ appearance   honeycomb

G7 p.738:170mm

356. Complete the following about multiple myeloma (MM):

G7 p. 740:40mm

a. If a single lesion is found it is called p_____.   plasmacytoma
b. In 70 to 80% this will progress to

G7 p. 742:15mm

  i. m_____ m_____ in   multiple myeloma
  ii. _____ years.   10
c. A urine test for MM is done to identify

G7 p. 741:30mm

  i. _____ _____ _____   kappa Bence-Jones protein
  ii. found in _____% of cases.   75%
d. The most definitive test is b_____ m_____ b_____.   bone marrow biopsy

G7 p. 741:90mm

357. Giant cell tumors

G7 p. 742:38mm

a. are considered in the same category as a_____ b_____ c_____.   aneurysmal bone cysts
b. The recommended treatment is i_____ c_____.   intratumoral curettage
c. Consider preop e_____.   embolization

21

358. Complete the following regarding spinal epidural metastasis:

G7 p.742:110mm

a. It occurs in _____% of all cancer patients.

10%

b. It most commonly arises from

   i. l_____ b_____ g_____ and

lung breast gastrointestinal

   ii. p_____ m_____ l_____.

prostate myeloma lymphoma

c. It is thought to reach the spine by the B_____ p_____.

Batson plexus

d. The site of metastasis is p_____ to the length of the segment of spine.

proportional

e. First symptom is usually

   i. p_____ which is

pain

   ii. worse in r_____.

recumbency

359. Complete the following regarding spinal epidural metastasis:

G7 p.743:114mm

a. Outcome depends on p_____ n_____ s_____.

presenting neurologic status

b. Treatment for patient with new symptoms consists of

   i. d_____

decadron

   ii. s_____

surgery

   iii. r_____

radiation

c. Indication for surgery is

   i. greater than _____% block

80%

   ii. r_____ p_____

rapid progression

360. Complete the following about MRI scans in spinal epidural metastasis:

a. They detect multiple sites of cord compression in _____%.

20%

G7 p.744:130mm

b. They are _____ on T1.

hypointense

G7 p.744:150mm

c. They are _____ on T2.

hyperintense

361. What is the treatment for SEM?

G7 p. 747:65mm

a. Chemotherapy is _____.

ineffective

b. Vertebroplasty/kyphoplasty reduces pain by _____%.

84%

G7 p. 747:150mm

c. Radiation treatment

G7 p. 748:28mm

   i. How soon after diagnosis?

within 24 hours

   ii. After surgery?

within 2 weeks

d. Preop embolization

G7 p. 748:60mm

   i. Appropriate for _____ _____ tumors

highly vascular

   ii. such as r_____ _____

renal cell

   iii. t_____

thyroid

   iv. h_____

hepatocellular

362. Characterize surgical treatment.

G7 p.748:78mm

a. Laminectomy is a _____ treatment

poor

b. because it _____ the spine.

destabilizes

c. It is better to do surgery _____

anteriorly

d. and add _____.

instrumentation

22

Radiation Therapy

■ Conventional External Beam Radiation

1. **What are the four "R's" of external beam radiation?**   G7 p.770:105mm
   a. rep_____   repair
   b. reo_____   reoxygenation
   c. repop_____   repopulation
   d. red_____   redistribution

2. **Complete the following about cranial radiation:**   G7 p.770:177mm
   a. After surgery most surgerons wait _____ to _____ days.   7 to 10
   b. Tumors that melt away with XRT are
      i.   l_____   lymphomas
      ii. g_____ c_____   germ cell

3. **True or False. Regarding radiation necrosis (RN):**   G7 p.771:20mm
   a. RN is easy to differentiate from tumor recurrence.   false
   b. Best test to differentiate is   G7 p.771:150mm
      i.   MR spectroscopy if mass is pure tumor   true
      ii. MR spectroscopy if mass is pure necrosis   true
      iii. MR spectroscopy if mass is mixed   false (unreliable)
      iv. SPECT (poor man's pet scan)   true   G7 p.772:30mm
   c. Treatment   G7 p.772:45mm
      i.   Most RN will respond to steroids.   true
      ii. Mass effect dictates advisability of surgery whether RN or recurrent tumor.   true

4. **Spinal radiation**   G7 p.722:115mm
   a. can produce _____.   myelopathy
   b. can increase risk of developing spinal _____ _____.   cavernous malformation

5. **Complete the following about radiation myelopathy (RM):**   G7 p.772:180mm

    a. Most important factor is rate of radiation _____.   application

    b. Second is total _____ _____.   radiation dose

6. **Is stereotactic radiosurgery (SRS) useful for:**   G7 p.774:135mm

    a. venous angiomas?   no

    b. cavernous angiomas?   no

■ Stereotactic Radiosurgery

7. **Complete the following about stereotactic radiosurgery:**   G7 p.775:17mm

    a. For most cases what is the optimal treatment for vestibular schwannoma?   surgery

    b. What alternative is available?   SRS

    c. When would the alternative for the patient be considered?

        i. p_____ m_____ c_____   poor medical condition

        ii. o_____ a_____ g_____   older age group

8. **Answer the following about stereotactic radiosurgery:**   G7 p.776:157mm

    a. Accuracy is never better than _____.   0.6 mm

    b. If embolization is used what precaution is advised before SRS?   wait 30 days between procedures

    c. What dose is optimal for an arteriovenous malformation (AVM)?   10 to 15 Gy to periphery of AVM

    d. What dose is optimal for tumors?   10 to 15 Gy with tumor in the 80% isodose line

    e. What dose is optimal for metastatic tumors?   15 Gy to center of tumor in the 80% isodose line

9. **Complete the following regarding the results, in percent, of SRS obliteration of:**   G7 p.777:110mm

    a. AVM

        i. AVM at 1 year _____   46 to 61%

        ii. AVM at 2 years _____   86%

        iii. under 2 cm _____   94%

        iv. over 2.5 cm _____   50%

    b. acoustic tumor

        i. decreased in size _____   44%

        ii. stabilized in size _____   42%

        iii. increased in size _____   14%

    c. local metastatic control _____   88%

10. **What is advised if, after SRS, an AVM persists after 2 to 3 years?**   may re-treat with SRS   G7 p.777:160mm

22

11. **Is there any difference in outcome with SRS by radio-resistant versus radio-sensitive tumors?**   no   G7 p.778:45mm

12. **Which has a better response, supra- or infratentorial metastases?**   supratentorial   G7 p.778:60mm

13. **Which premedication is given before SRS?**   steroids and phenobarbital   G7 p.778:100mm

14. **During the latency period is there a higher incidence of hemorrhage from AVM?**   no, approximately 3 to 4% per year   G7 p.778:118mm

■ Interstitial Brachytherapy

15. **Answer the following about interstitial brachytherapy:**   G7 p.779:60mm
    a. How much radiation is given?   60 Gy
    b. To what area?   a volume that extends 1 cm beyond the contrast-enhancing tumor
    c. At what rate?   40 to 50 c Gy/h
    d. For how many days?   6
    e. What is the radiation amount that will cause tumor growth to stop?   30 c Gy/h
    f. With this protocol what percent of patients develop symptomatic radiation necrosis?   40%

22

23

Stereotactic Surgery

■ **Stereotactic Surgery**

1. **True or False. Indications for stereotactic surgery include**

   G7 p.782:125mm

   a. biopsy of multiple lesions — true

   b. brachytherapy implants — true (catheter placement for brachytherapy)

   c. treatment of chronic pain — true (electrode placement for pain, seizures)

   d. gamma knife radiosurgery — true (lesion generation for trigeminal pain)

   e. biopsy of a deep cerebral lesion — true

   f. hematoma evacuation — true (evacuation of intracerebral hemorrhage, cystic fluid)

   g. localization of lesion for open craniotomy — true

2. **True or False. Stereotactic biopsy contraindications include**

   G7 p.783:65mm

   a. coagulopathy — true

   b. multiple lesions — false (Multiple lesions are an indication for stereotactic biopsy.)

   c. brain stem lesions — false (A brain stem lesion is an indication for stereotactic biopsy.)

   d. inability to tolerate general anesthesia — false (can usually tolerate local anesthesia)

   e. thrombocytopenia — true (Platelets below 50,000 are an absolute contraindication to biopsy.)

   f. inability to cooperate for biopsy — false (may do stereotactic biopsy under general anesthesia)

3. True or False. The yield rate for stereotactic biopsy is G7 p.783:90mm

a. higher for enhancing lesions than for nonenhancing

true

b. lower for enhancing lesions than nonenhancing

false

c. enhancing and nonenhancing lesions have equal yield rates

false

d. yield rates range from 82 to 99%

true

4. True or False. The most common complication of stereotactic surgery is G7 p.783:107mm

a. hemorrhage

true (Most are too small to be clinically significant. The hemorrhage rate is higher in AIDS and in central nervous system lymphoma.)

b. infection

false

c. inability to localize lesion

false

d. inability to provide sufficient tissue quality/quantity for biopsy

false

5. Answer the following regarding stereotactic biopsy: G7 p.783:113mm

23

a. True or False. The risk for major complication due to stereotactic biopsy is higher in patients with multifocal high-grade gliomas than in patients with AIDS.

false

b. Relative risk for patients that are

i. immune compromised _____ to _____ %

0 to 12%

ii. nonimmune compromised _____ to _____%

0 to 3%

iii. or have glioma _____%

3%

24

Peripheral Nerves

■ Peripheral Nerves

1. **True or False. The peripheral nervous system includes**
   G7 p.786:35 mm
   a. spinal nerves — true
   b. all cranial nerves — false
   c. cranial nerves III-XII — true
   d. cervical, brachial, lumbosacral plexus — true

2. **True or False. Upper motor neuron paralysis includes**
   G7 p.786:135mm
   a. clonus — true
   b. hyperactive reflexes — true
   c. muscle spasms — true
   d. atrophy — false
   e. fasciculations — false
   (Choices d and e are characteristic of lower motor neuron paralysis.)

3. **List the 11 muscles of the shoulder and their nerves and roots.**
   G7 p.787:40mm
   Hint: pqrst (tssrppldbb)
   a. muscle, t_____ — trapezius
       i. nerve, s_____ a_____ — CN X1 spinal accessory
       ii. roots, _____ — C3,4
   b. muscle, s_____ a_____ — serratus anterior
       i. nerve, l_____ t_____ — long thoracic
       ii. roots, _____ — C5,6,7
   c. muscle, s_____ — supraspinatus
       i. nerve, s_____ — suprascapular
       ii. roots, _____ — C4,5,6
   d. muscle, i_____ — infraspinatus
       i. nerve, s_____ — suprascapular
       ii. roots, _____ — C5,6
   e. muscle, r_____ — rhomboids
       i. nerve, d_____ s_____ — dorsal scapular
       ii. roots, _____ — C4,5

f. muscle, p_____ m_____
    i.   nerve, a_____ t_____

    ii. roots, _____
g. muscle, p_____ m_____
    i.   nerve, a_____ t_____

    ii. roots, _____
h. muscle, l_____ d_____
    i.   nerve, t_____
    ii. roots, _____
i. muscle, d_____
    i.   nerve, a_____
    ii. roots, _____
j. muscle, b_____
    i.   nerve, m_____
    ii. roots, _____
k. muscle, b_____
    i.   nerve, m_____
    ii. roots, _____

pectoralis minor
anterior thoracic (med) aka
pectoral nerve
C7,8
pectoralis major (lat.
anterior thoracic anterior
thoracic med) aka pectoral
nerve
C4,5,6,7,8
latissimus dorsi
thoracodorsal
C5,6,7,8
deltoid
axillary
C5,6
brachialis
musculocutaneous
C5,6
biceps
musculocutaneous
C5,6

**4. List 11 muscles of the shoulder and
arm, their nerve, and their action.**

G7 p.787:40mm

24

a. muscle, t_____
    i.   nerve, _____
    ii. action, _____ _____
b. muscle, s_____ _____
    i.   nerve, _____ _____
    ii. action, _____ _____
         _____
c. muscle, s_____
    i.   nerve, _____
    ii. action, _____ _____
         _____
d. muscle, _____
    i.   nerve, _____
    ii. action, _____ _____
         _____
e. muscle, r_____
    i.   nerve, _____ _____
    ii. action, _____ _____
f. muscle, p_____ m_____
    i.   nerve, _____ _____
         _____
    ii. action, _____ _____
g. muscle, p_____ m_____
    i.   nerve, _____ _____
         _____ _____ _____
    ii. action, _____ _____
         _____ _____ _____
         _____

trapezius
CNX1
shrug shoulders
serratus anterior
long thoracic
forward shoulder thrust

supraspinatus
suprascapular
abduct arm 90 degrees

infraspinatus
suprascapular
backhand tennis shot

rhomboids
dorsal scapular
abduct scapulae
pectoralis minor
pectoral nerve medial

adduction arm
pectoralis major
pectoral nerve lateral and
medial
adduction arm and push arm
forward

h. muscle, l_____ d_____   latissimus dorsi
   i.   nerve, _____   thoracodorsal
   ii. action, _____ _____,   adduct arm, ladder climb,
       _____ _____, _____   cough
i. muscle, d_____   deltoid
   i.   nerve, _____   axillary
   ii. action, _____ _____ _____   abduct arm > 90 degrees
j. muscle, b_____   brachialis
   i.   nerve, _____   musculocutaneous
   ii. action, _____ _____   flex forearm
k. muscle, b_____   biceps
   i.   nerve, _____   musculocutaneous
   ii. action, _____ and _____   flex and supinate forearm
       _____

5. True or False. The suprascapular nerve innervates which of the following?   G7 p.787:75mm

a. teres major   false—subscapular nerve (C5-C7)
b. teres minor   false—axillary nerve (C4-C5)
c. infraspinatus   true
d. supraspinatus   true

6. The suprascapular nerve contains roots from _____, _____, and _____.   C4, C5, C6   G7 p.787:75mm

7. Describe the latissimus dorsi muscle.   G7 p.787:82mm

a. function
   i.   l_____ _____   ladder climbing
   ii. c_____   cough
   iii. a_____   adductor—together with pectoralis
b. nerve   thoracodorsal nerve
c. cord   posterior cord
d. roots   C6,7,8

8. True or False. The deltoid muscle   G7 p.787:90mm

a. abducts arm 0 to 90 degrees   false (The arm is abducted 0 to 90 degrees by the supraspinatous muscle.)
b. abduct arm > 90 degrees   true
c. is innervated by the axillary nerve   true
d. rotates the arm out   false (Arm is rotated out by the infraspinatus muscle.)

9. True or False. The abductor pollicis longus   G7 p.788:60mm

a. is innervated by the median nerve   false
b. is innervated by the radial nerve   true
c. is innervated by the ulnar nerve   false
d. is innervated by the posterior interosseous nerve   true (The posterior interosseus nerve is a continuation of the radial nerve in the forearm.)

10. **True or False. The median nerve is responsible for the following movements of the thumb:**
    a. adduction
    b. abduction
    c. extension
    d. flexion
    e. opposition

    false (served by ulnar nerve)
    true
    false (served by radial nerve)
    true
    true

11. **Complete the following about the movements of the thumb:**
    a. Actions of nerves to the thumb
        i. median nerve, Hint: FAO
            F—action, f_____
            muscle, f_____ p_____
            b_____ and l_____
            root, _____
            A—action, a_____
            muscle, a_____ p_____
            b_____
            root, _____
            O—action, o_____
            muscle, o_____ p_____
            root, _____
        ii. ulnar nerve
            action, a_____
            muscle, a_____ p_____
            root, _____ _____
        iii. radial nerve
            action, e_____
            muscle, e_____ p_____
            b_____ and l_____
            root, C_____ and C_____

    flexion
    flexor pollicis brevis and
    longus
    C8, T1, median
    abduction
    abductor pollicis brevis

    C8, T1, median
    opposition
    opponens pollicis
    C8, T1

    adduction
    adductor pollicis
    C8, T1

    extension
    extensor pollicis brevis and
    longus
    C7, C8

    b. Plane of movement for the thumb
        i. extension is _____
        ii. flexion is _____
        iii. adduction is _____
        iv. abduction is _____
        v. opposition is _____

    plane of palm
    plane of palm
    perpendicular to palm
    perpendicular from palm
    across the palm

12. **Complete the following about peripheral nerves of the leg:**
    Hint: fosis pdstp (*follow our sign. it says "please don't spoil the plants"*)
    a. f_____
    b. o_____
    c. s_____
    d. i_____
    e. s_____
    f. p_____
    g. d_____
    h. s_____
    i. t_____
    j. p_____

    femoral
    obturator
    superior gluteal
    inferior gluteal
    sciatic (trunk)
    peroneal (trunk)
    deep peroneal
    superficial peroneal
    tibial
    pudendal

24

13. Name the nerves of the lower extremities and the roots that form them.

G7 p.788:145mm

a. f_____   femoral, 1,2,3
b. o_____   obturator, 2,3
c. s_____   superior gluteal, 4, 5, S1
d. i_____   inferior gluteal, 5, S1, S2
e. s_____   sciatic, 5, S1, S2
f. p_____   peroneal, 4, 5, S1
g. d_____   deep peroneal, 4, 5
h. s_____   superficial peroneal, 5, S1
i. t_____   tibial, 4, 5, S1, S2, S3
j. p_____   pudendal, S2, S3, S4

14. Name the nerves of the lower extremities and the muscles and function of the muscles they serve.

G7 p.788:155mm

a. nerve, f_____   femoral
   i. muscle, i_____, q_____   iliopsoas, quadriceps femoris,
     f_____, s_____   sartorius
   ii. function, f_____ h_____   flex hip
b. nerve, o_____   obturator
   i. muscle, a_____   adductor
   ii. function, a_____ t_____   adduct thigh
c. nerve, s_____ g_____   superior gluteal
   i. muscle, g_____ m_____   gluteus medius
   ii. function, a_____ t_____   abduct thigh
d. nerve, i_____ g_____   inferior gluteal
   i. muscle, g_____ m_____   gluteus maximus
   ii. function, f_____ l_____   flex leg
e. nerve, s_____ t_____   sciatic trunk
   i. muscle, b_____ s_____   biceps femoris, semi
     s_____   tendenosis, semi
                   membranosis
   ii. function, e_____ t_____   extend thigh
f. nerve, d_____ p_____   deep peroneal
   i. muscle, t_____ a_____,   tibialis anterior, extensor
     e_____ h_____ l_____   hallucis longus (EHL)
   ii. function, g_____ t_____   great toe extension, foot
     e_____, f_____ d_____   dorsiflexion
g. nerve, s_____ p_____   superficial peroneal
   i. muscle, p_____ l_____   peroneus longus
   ii. function, p_____ f_____   plantar flexion foot and toes
     f_____ and t_____
h. nerve, t_____   tibial
   i. muscle, p_____ t_____,   posterior tibial,
     g_____, s_____, f_____   gastrocnemius, soleus, flexor
     h_____ l_____   hallucis longus (FHL)
   ii. function, p_____ f_____   plantar flex foot and toes
     f_____ and t_____
i. nerve, p_____   pudendal
   i. muscle, p_____, s_____   perineal, sphincters
   ii. function, v_____ c_____ of   voluntary contraction of
     p_____ f_____   pelvic floor

24

15. **True or False. The gluteus maximus muscle**   G7 p.789:37mm

   a. abducts thigh — true (The gluteus maximus abducts thigh in a prone position.)

   b. adducts thigh — false (thigh—adduction — the obturator externus muscle and pectineus muscle)

   c. medially rotates thigh — false (thigh—medial rotation — the gluteus medius and minimus muscle)

   d. externally rotates thigh — false (thigh—external rotation — the obturator externus muscle)

   e. is innervated by superior gluteal nerve — false (The gluteus maximus is innervated by the inferior gluteal nerve.)

16. **True or False. The tibialis anterior muscle is responsible for foot**   G7 p.789:60mm

   a. dorsiflexion — true

   b. plantar flexion — false (plantar flexion—soleus muscle, gastrocnemius muscle)

   c. eversion — false (eversion—peroneus longus and brevis muscles)

   d. inversion — false (inversion—posterior tibialis muscle)

17. **Complete the following about the function of peripheral nerves:**   G7 p.789:65mm

   a. The function of extension of the great toe is served by

      i. muscle, _____ _____ _____ — extensor hallucis longus

      ii. root, _____ — L5

   b. The function of foot dorsiflexion is served by

      i. muscle, _____ _____ — tibialis anterior

      ii. root, _____ — L4

   c. Which is the best L5 muscle? (Hint: The letter E is the fifth letter in the alphabet.) — extensor hallucis longus   G7 p.789:140mm

18. **True or False. The extensor hallucis longus muscle**   G7 p.789:65mm

   a. is the best L5 muscle — true

   b. extends great toe — true

   c. dorsiflexes foot — true

   d. is innervated by the deep peroneal nerve — true

19. **Complete the following regarding timing of surgical repair of nerves:**   G7 p.790:55mm

   a. If the nerve must regenerate a long distance, repair should be done _____. — early

   b. After _____ months most muscles cannot recover. — 24

24

Brachial Plexus

20. **True or False. The brachial plexus is formed by the dorsal rami of C5-T1.**

false (It is formed by the ventral rami of C5-T1. The dorsal rami innervate the paraspinal muscles.)

G7 p.790:90mm

21. **Draw a diagram of the brachial plexus.**

G7 p.790:90mm

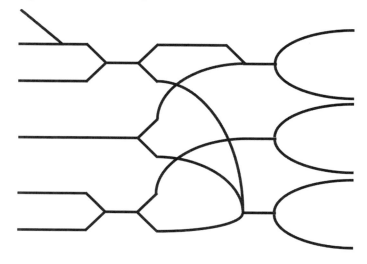

Fig. 24.1

24

22. **On your diagram of the brachial plexus, label the following:**
① roots C4-T1; ② organization RTDCN (roots, trunks, divisions, chords, nerves); ③ names of trunks—SMI (superior, middle, inferior); ④ add names of cords—LMP (lateral, medial, posterior)

G7 p.790:90 mm

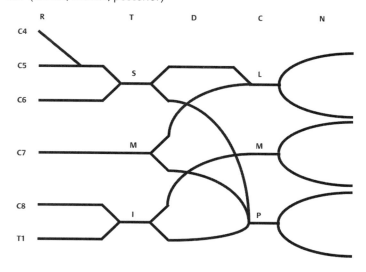

Fig. 24.2

23. Add the nerves to the basic outline of
     the brachial plexus nerves: 16. (Hint:
     Donald says somewhat loudly,
     "Mickey Mouse, you are right to so
     sincerely love Minnie Mouse madly.")

G7 p.790:92mm

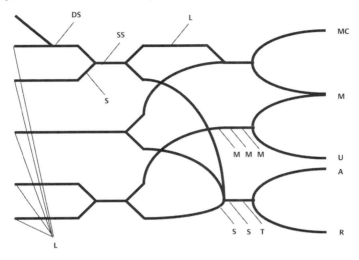

Fig. 24.3

24. Draw the complete brachial plexus.

G7 p.790:93mm

24

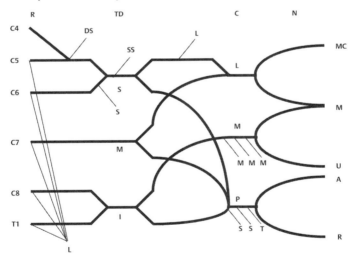

Fig. 24.4

25. **Draw the left brachial plexus—outline.**   G7 p.790:94 mm

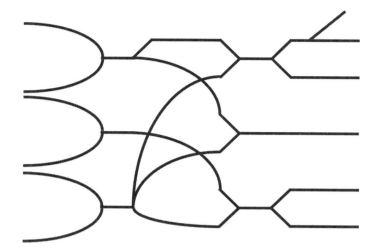

Fig. 24.5

26. **Draw the left brachial plexus and add details requested in questions 21 through 23.**   G7 p.790:95mm

24

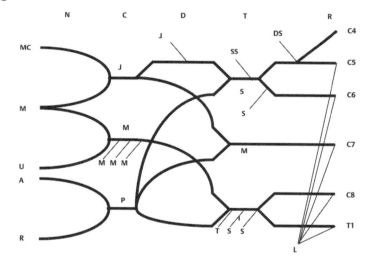

Fig. 24.6

27. **Complete the following about the brachial plexus:**   G7 p.790:100mm
     a. Name the roots (6).   C4, C5, C6, C7, C8, T1
     b. Name the segments (5). (Hint: Run to do Cindy's needs.)   roots. trunks, divisions, chords, nerves

c. Name the nerves (16). (Hint: Donald says somewhat loudly, "Mickey Mouse, you are right to so sincerely love Minnie Mouse madly.")

dorsal scapular
suprascapular
subclavius
lateral pectoral
musculocutaneous
median
ulnar
axillary
radial
thoracodorsal
subscapular upper
subscapular lower
long thoracic
medial pectoral
medial brachial cutaneous
medial antebrachial cutaneous

d. Name the trunks (3).
e. Name the cords (3).

superior, middle, inferior, lateral, medial, posterior

28. **Trace, using the brachial plexus diagram, the theoretically possible root contribution to each nerve and then compare with the actual root contribution in each nerve.**

G7 p.790:100mm
Fig. 24-1

24

a. nerve, d _____ s_____
   i. theoretical, _____
   ii. actual, _____
b. nerve, s_____
   i. theoretical, _____
   ii. actual, _____
c. nerve, s_____
   i. theoretical, _____
   ii. actual, _____
d. nerve, l_____ p_____
   i. theoretical, _____
   ii. actual, _____
e. nerve, m_____
   i. theoretical, _____
   ii. actual, _____
f. nerve, m_____
   i. theoretical, _____
   ii. actual, _____
g. nerve, u_____
   i. theoretical, _____
   ii. actual, _____
h. nerve, a_____
   i. theoretical, _____
   ii. actual, _____
i. nerve, r_____
   i. theoretical, _____
   ii. actual, _____
j. nerve, t_____
   i. theoretical, _____
   ii. actual, _____

dorsal scapular
C4,5
C4,5
suprascapular
C4,5,6
C4,5,6
subclavius
C6
C6
lateral pectoral
C4,5,6,7
C4,5,6,7
musculocutaneous
C5,6,7
C5,6,7
median
C5,6,7, T1
C5,6,7, T1
ulnar
C8, T1
C7,8, T1
axillary
C4,5,6,7,8, T1
C4,5,6,7,8, T1
radial
C4,5,6,7,8, T1
C4,5,6
thoracodorsal
C5,6,7,8, T1
C6,7,8

k. nerve, s_____ u_____   subscapular upper
    i.   theoretical, _____   C5,6,7,8, T1
    ii. actual, _____   C5,6,7
l. nerve, s_____ l_____   subscapular lower
    i.   theoretical, _____   C5,6,7,8, T1
    ii. actual, _____   C5,6,7
m. nerve, l_____ t_____   long thoracic
    i.   theoretical, _____   C5,6,7
    ii. actual, _____   C5,6,7
n. nerve, m_____ t_____   medial thoracic (pectoral)
    i.   theoretical, _____   C8, T1
    ii. actual, _____   not listed
o. nerve, m_____ b_____   medial brachial
    i.   theoretical, _____   C8, T1
    ii. actual, _____   not listed
p. nerve, m_____ a_____   medial antebrachial
    i.   theoretical, _____   C8, T1
    ii. actual, _____   not listed

29. **List the brachial plexus nerves (except**   G7 p.790:100mm
    for median ulnar and radial), the   Table 24-4
    muscles they serve, the roots that are
    in that nerve, and the action of the
    muscles.
    a. nerve, d_____ s_____   dorsal scapular
        i.   muscle,_____ _____   levator scapulae
        ii. root, _____   C3,4,5
        iii. action, _____ _____   elevate scapulae
    b. nerve, d_____ s_____   dorsal scapular
        i.   muscle, _____   rhomboids
        ii. root, _____   C4,5
        iii. action, _____ _____   adduct and elevate scapula
        _____ _____
    c. nerve, s_____   suprascapular
        i.   muscle, _____   supraspinatus
        ii. root, _____   C4,5,6
        iii. action, _____ _____   adduct arm 0 to 90 degrees
        _____ _____ _____
    d. nerve, s_____   supraspinatus
        i.   muscle, _____   infraspinatus
        ii. root, _____   C5,6
        iii. action, _____ _____ _____ rotate arm out
    e. nerve, m_____   musculocutaneous
        i.   muscle, _____ _____   biceps brachii
        ii. root, _____   C5,6
        iii. action, _____ _____   flex and supinate forearm
        _____ _____
    f. nerve, m_____   musculocutaneous
        i.   muscle, _____   coracobrachialis
        ii. root, _____   C5,6,7
        iii. action, _____ _____   flex and adduct forearm
        _____ _____

24

g. nerve, m_____   musculocutaneous
   i.   muscle, _____   brachialis
   ii. root, _____   C5,6
   iii. action, _____ _____   flex forearm
h. nerve, a_____   axillary
   i.   muscle, _____   deltoid
   ii. root, _____   C5,6
   iii. action, _____ _____ _____   abduct arm > 90 degrees
i. nerve, s_____   subscapularis
   i.   muscle, _____ _____   teres major
   ii. root, _____   C5,6,7
   iii. action, _____ _____   adduct arm
j. nerve, t_____   thoracodorsal
   i.   muscle, _____ _____   latissimus dorsi
   ii. root, _____   C5,6,7,8
   iii. action, _____ _____,   adduct arm, ladder, cough
       _____, _____

k. nerve, a_____   axillary
   i.   muscle, _____ _____   teres minor
   ii. root, _____   C4,5
   iii. action, _____ _____   rotation lateral
l. nerve, l_____ t_____   long thoracic
   i.   muscle, _____ _____   serratus anterior
   ii. root, _____   C5,6,7
   iii. action, _____ _____   forward shoulder thrust
       _____

30. Considering the brachial plexus and radial nerve, list the branches of the radial nerve cascade in proper sequence and the function of the muscles.

G7 p.791:30mm

24

Hint: rest in peace, retbes in peeeeeae

a. r_____   radial
b. e_____   extensor
c. t_____   triceps
d. b_____   brachioradialis
e. e_____   extensor carpi radialis
f. s_____   supinator
g. i_____   i
h. n_____   n posterior interosseus nerve
i. p_____   p
j. e_____   extensor carpi ulnaris
k. e_____   extensor digitorum
                      communis
l. e_____   extensor digiti minimi
m. e_____   extensor pollicis brevis
n. e_____   extensor pollicis longus
o. a_____   abductor pollicis longus
p. e_____   extensor indicis

31. **True or False. The radial nerve is** G7 p.791:29mm
formed by
  a. C5-T1   false
  b. C5-C8   true
  c. C6-T1   false
  d. C5-C7   false

32. **True or False. Regarding the radial** G7 p.791:29mm
nerve, it
  a. is formed by C5-C8   true
  b. innervates triceps   true
  c. innervates supinator   true
  d. innervates brachioradialis   true
  e. continues into forearm as posterior   true
      interosseus nerve

33. **What is innervated by the axillary** G7 p.791:105mm
nerve?
  a. t_____ m_____   teres minor
  b. d_____   deltoid

34. **Regarding the brachial plexus and** G7 p.791:120mm
median nerve, list the 11 branches of
the median nerve cascade in proper
sequence.
  a. p_____   pronator teres
  b. f_____   flexor carpi radialis
  c. p_____   palmaris longus
  d. f_____   flexor digitorum superficialis
  e. f_____   flexor digitorum profundus
  f. f_____   flexor pollicis longus
  g. p_____   pronator quadratus
  h. f_____   flexor pollicis brevis
  i. a_____   abductor pollicis brevis
  j. o_____   opponens pollicis
  k. l_____   lumbricales 1 and 2

35. **Regarding the brachial plexus and** G7 p.791:120mm
median nerve, list the 11 branches of
the median nerve cascade and the
function of the muscles.
  a.
    i. p_____ t_____   pronator teres
    ii. function: f_____ p_____   forearm pronator
  b.
    i. f_____ _____ _____   flexor carpi radialis
    ii. function: r_____ f_____ of   radial flexion of hand
       h_____
  c.
    i. p_____ _____   palmaris longus
    ii. function: h_____ f_____   hand flexion
  d.
    i. f_____ _____ _____   flexor digitorum superficialis
    ii. function: f_____ m_____   flex middle phalanx, fingers 2
       p_____, fingers _____ to   to 5
       _____

24

e.
   i.   f_____ _____ _____   flexor digitorum profundus
   ii. function: f_____ d_____   flex distal phalanx, fingers 2
       p_____, fingers _____ to   to 3
       _____

f.
   i.   f_____ p_____ l_____   flexor pollicis longus
   ii. function: f_____ d_____   flex distal phalanx of thumb
       p_____ of t_____

g.
   i.   p_____ _____   pronator quadratus
   ii. function: p_____ f_____   pronates forearm

h.
   i.   f_____ p_____ b_____   flexor pollicis brevis
   ii. function: f_____ p_____   flexes procimal phalanx of
       p_____ of t_____   thumb

i.
   i.   a_____ _____ _____   abductor pollicis brevis
   ii. function: a_____ t_____   abducts thumb metacarpal
       m_____

j.
   i.   o_____ _____   opponens pollicis
   ii. function: op_____ t_____   opposes thumb metacarpal
       m_____

k.
   i.   l_____ 1 and 2   lumbricales
   ii. function: e_____ 2 d_____   extend 2 distal phalanges of
       p_____ of _____ 2 and 3   fingers 4 and 5

36. **Which muscles in the hand are
innervated by the median nerve?**
    Hint: loaf

   a. l_____   lumbricals 1 and 2
   b. o_____   opponens pollicis
   c. a_____   abductor pollicis brevis
   d. f_____   flexor pollicis brevis

G7 p.791:150mm

37. **Which muscles are served by the
anterior interosseous nerve?**

   a. f_____ d_____ p_____   flexor digitorum profundus
   b. f_____ p_____ l_____   flexor pollicis longus
   c. p_____ q_____   pronator quadratus

G7 p.791 :170mm

38. **Regarding the brachial plexus and
ulnar nerve, list the muscles served by
the ulnar nerve cascade in proper
order and the function of the muscles.**
    Hint: *"Ffaf*ner *I Love Hi*m"

   a.
       i.   f_____ c_____ u_____   flexor carpis ulnaris
       ii. function: u_____ f_____ of   ulnar flexion of hand
          h_____

G7 p.792:25mm

24

b.
   i.   f_____ _____ _____   flexor digitorum profundus
   ii. function: f_____ d_____   flex distal phalanx of fingers 4
       p_____ of f_____ _____   and 5
       and _____

c.
   i.   a_____ p_____   adductor pollicis
   ii. function: t_____ a_____   thumb adductor

d.
   i.   f_____ _____ _____   flexor pollicis brevis
   ii. function: f_____ p_____   flex proximal phalanx of
       p_____ of t_____   thumb

e.
   i.   i_____   interossei
   ii. function: dorsal a_____   abducts
   iii. function: palmar a_____   abducts flex proximal
       f_____ p_____ p_____ at phalanges at metacarpo
       m_____ joints   phalangeal joints

f.
   i.   l_____   lumbricales
   ii. function: e_____ t_____   extends two distal phalanges
       d_____ p_____ of _____ of 3 and 4 at interphalangeal
       _____ and _____ at   joints
       i_____ j_____

g. h_____   hypothenar abductor digiti
                          minimi, flexor digiti minimi
                          opponens
   i.   function: a_____ l_____   abduction little finger
       f_____
   ii. function: f_____ l_____   flex little finger
       f_____

24

39. Study Chart.

G7 p.791:20mm

Radial	Ulnar	Median
RETBES in PE5AE	FFAF ILH	PFPF3PFAOL
RETBES in PEEEEEAE		

Radial	Ulnar	Median
radial	flexor carpi ulnaris	pronator teres
extensor		
triceps	flexor digitorum profundus	flexor carpi radialis
brachioradialis	adductor pollicis	almaris longus
extensor carpi radialis	flexor pollicis brevis	flexor digitorum superficialis
supinator	interossei	flexor digitorum profundus
i	lumbricales	flexor pollicis longus AIN
n } PIN	hypothenar	pronator quadratus
p		flexor pollicis brevis
extensor carpi ulnaris		abductor pollicis brevis
extensor digitorum		opponens pollicis
extensor digiti minimi		lumbricales
extensor pollicis brevis		
extensor pollicis longus		
abductor pollicis longus		
extensor indicis		

40. Which muscles in the arm are innervated by the ulnar nerve?   none   G7 p.792:30mm

41. **Regarding the following additional (2) nerves of the brachial plexus, number the roots and name the muscles and their actions:**

G7 p.792:60mm
also
G7 p.792:110mm

  a. nerve, musculocutaneous

     i. roots, _____   C5,6,7

     ii. muscles, ① b_____,   ① biceps,
       ② c_____, ③ b_____   ② coracobrachialis,
                         ③ brachialis

     iii. action, ① f_____ f_____ and ① flex forearm and supinates
       s_____

     iv. ② f_____ f_____ and   ② flex forearm and adducts
       a_____

     v. ③ f_____ f_____   ③ flex forearm

  b. nerve, axillary

     i. roots, _____   C4,5,6

     ii. muscles, ① d_____,   ① deltoid, ② teres minor
       ② t_____ m_____

     iii. action, ① a_____ a_____ ① abduct arm 30 to 90
       _____ to _____ degrees   degrees

     iv. ② l_____ a_____ r_____ ② lateral arm rotation

42. **Complete the following about anatomic variants with Martin-Gruber anastomosis:**

G7 p.792:135mm

  a. Connections between the _____ and _____ nerves   median; ulnar

  b. In the _____   forearm

  c. Found in _____% of cadavers   23%

24

▪ Peripheral Neuropathies

43. **List the etiology.**
   Hint: dang the rapist

G7 p.793:65mm

  a. d_____   diabetes
  b. a_____   alcohol
  c. n_____   nutritional, B_{12}
  d. g_____   Guillain-Barré
  e. t_____   traumatic
  f. h_____   hereditary
  g. e_____   entrapment
  h. r_____   renal, radiation
  i. a_____   amyloid
  j. p_____   porphyria, paraneoplastic
  k. i_____   infectious, Hanson
  l. s_____   sarcoidosis
  m. t_____   toxins, heavy metals

44. Complete the following regarding peripheral neuropathy:

G7 p.793:130mm

a. The most common peripheral neuropathy that is an inherited disorder is C_____-M_____-T_____ s_____.
Charcot-Marie-Tooth syndrome

b. The percent of patients with diabetes mellitus who develop diabetic neuropathy is _____%.
50%

45. Which syndrome is associated with pure sensory neuropathy?
paraneoplastic syndrome (also seen with pyridoxine therapy)

G7 p.794:75mm

46. True or False. Alcohol neuropathy includes

G7 p.794:100mm

a. motor neuropathy — false
b. sensory neuropathy — true
c. absent Achilles reflex — true
d. intense pain — false

47. Brachial neuritis

G7 p.794:78mm

a. aka P_____ t_____ syndrome — Parsonage tumor
b. aka i_____ brachial plexus neuropathy — idiopathic
c. Etiology: _____ — unclear
d. Prognosis: _____ — good
e. Predominant symptom: _____ — pain
f. Followed by: _____ in _____% — weakness, 96%
g. Confined to shoulder girdle in _____% — 50%

48. True or False. The most important study in the diagnosis of lumbosacral plexus neuropathy is

G7 p.796:45mm

a. magnetic resonance imaging (MRI) — false
b. computed tomography (CT) — false
c. electromyography (EMG) — true (EMG in lumbosacral neuropathy—rule out diabetic neuropathy!)
d. erythrocyte sedimentation rate (ESR) — false

49. EMG in lumbosacral neuropathy shows what in regards to:

G7 p.796:45mm

a. fibrillation potentials _____ — increased
b. motor unit potentials in number _____ — decreased
c. motor unit potentials in amplitude _____ — increased
d. motor unit potentials in duration _____ — increased
e. motor unit potentials that are _____ — polyphasic
f. have changes involving at least _____ segments — 2
g. _____ the paraspinal muscles is highly _____ — sparing, diagnostic

24

50. **Complete the following about diabetic neuropathy:**

G7 p.796:65mm

a. Diabetic patients show neuropathy or EMG changes _____%.

50

b. The first symptom of diabetes may be _____.

neuropathy

c. Neuropathy might be reduced by control of blood _____.

sugar

51. **Complete the following about drug-induced neuropathy:**
   Hint: CDEF

G7 p.797:145mm

a. C_____

Chemotherapy drugs

b. D_____

Dilantin

c. E_____

Elavil

d. F_____

Flagyl

52. **True or False. Femoral neuropathy includes**

G7 p.798:25mm

a. weakness of quadriceps and iliopsoas

true

b. patellar reflex—reduced

true

c. femoral stretch—positive

true

d. sensation over lateral calf reduced

false (Femoral neuropathy includes ↓ sensation over anterior thigh and medial calf.)

53. **Answer the following regarding femoral neuropathy:**

G7 p.798:35mm

a. Name the muscle responsible for
   i. knee extension

quadriceps femoris

   ii. hip flexion

iliopsoas

b. To distinguish L4 radiculopathy from femoral neuropathy, L4 radiculopathy would not involve the _____.

iliopsoas

c. Femoral neuropathy is caused by
   i. d_____

diabetes

   ii. c_____

compression

54. **True or False. The most frequent cause of femoral neuropathy is**

G7 p.798:75mm

a. intraabdominal tumor

false

b. retroperitoneal hematoma

false

c. diabetes

true (Diabetes is the most frequent cause. All options can cause femoral neuropathy.)

d. entrapment due to inguinal hernia

false

e. trauma

false

24

55. **True or False. Regarding AIDS neuropathy:** G7 p.798:110mm
    a. It usually presents as proximal symmetric polyneuropathy. false (It is a distal symmetric polyneuropathy.)
    b. Only HIV+ patients do not develop it. true
    c. It never includes sensory elements. false (usually includes numbness and tingling)
    d. It has infectious etiology. true
    e. It may be caused by lymphomatous invasion of the meninges or nerves. true

56. **Complete the following about monoclonal gammopathy:** G7 p.799:28mm
    a. Include entities such as
       i. m_____ myeloma
       ii. Waldenström _____ macroglobulinemia
    b. Responsible for _____% of neuropathies 10%

57. **Complete the following about perioperative neuropathies ulnar:** G7 p.799:126mm
    a. Avoid elbow flexion of greater than _____ degrees. 110
    b. It tightens the _____ _____ retinaculum. cubital tunnel

58. **Complete the following about lower extremity neuropathy:** G7 p.799:172mm
    a.
       i. Common peroneal in _____% 81%
       ii. risk is _____ position lithotomy
    b. femoral neuropathy where there is hemorrhage in the _____ muscle psoas G7 p.800:27mm
    c. meralgia paresthetica G7 p.800:40mm
       i. tends to occur _____ bilaterally
       ii. in young slender _____ males
       iii. positioned _____ prone
       iv. in operations lasting _____ hours 6 to 10
       v. recovers in approximately _____ _____ 6 months

59. **What is the management of lower extremity neuropathy?** G7 p.800:53mm
    a. Call neurologist if not better in _____ days. 5
    b. Do EMG not earlier than _____ weeks. 3

60. **Complete the following about amyloid neuropathy:** G7 p.800:82mm
    a. Amyloid can be deposited in _____ _____. peripheral nerves
    b. It produces a _____ neuropathy. Sensory
    c. It can produce pressure on nerves, i.e., _____ _____. carpal tunnel

61. **Complete the following about post-cardiac catheterization neuropathy:** G7 p.800:145mm
   a. It involves the _____ nerve. femoral
   b. It usually involves _____. hematomas

62. **Describe the anatomy of the peripheral nerve.** G7 p.801:53mm
   a. Which connective tissue membrane surrounds individual axons? endoneurium surrounds individual axons
   b. Which surrounds groups of axons (i.e., fascicles)? perineurium bundles axons (covered by endoneurium) into fascicles
   c. Which surrounds groups of fascicles (i.e., nerves)? epineurium groups fascicles (covered by perineurium) into nerve trunk

63. **Complete the following regarding injury and regeneration of nerve:** G7 p.801:75mm
   a. The regeneration rate = _____ 1 mm/day (i.e., 1 inch per month)
   b. Sunderland system
      i. first-degree anatomy _____ preserved; conduction block, compression, or ischemia
      ii. second-degree axon _____ connective tissue is _____ injured; endo-, peri-, epineurium intact (endoneurium provided tube for regeneration)
      iii. third-degree axon and endoneurium d_____ axon and endoneurium disrupted (grossly normal appearance, recovery related to extent of intrafascicular fibrosis)

64. **Complete the following about the peripheral neuropathies:** G7 p.801:75 mm
   a. fourth-degree axon endoperi _____ interruption of all elements but epineurium is intact, nerve is indurated and enlarged G7 p. 802:82mm
   b. fifth-degree axon endoperi and epineurium is completely t_____ completely transected
   c. sixth-degree mixed _____ through _____ degree injuries mixed first through fourth G7 p.802:105mm

65. **Complete the following about the peripheral neuropathies:** G7 p.801:110mm
   a. Nerve regeneration occurs at the rate of _____ mm/day. 1 mm/day G7 p.802:62mm
   b. Nerve regeneration occurs at the rate of _____ inch(es)/month. 1 inch/month

24

c. Describe injury classification of peripheral nerves and regeneration prognosis.

two classifications: Seddon and Sunderland

   i. axon compressed

first-degree = Seddon neuropraxia; conduction block from compression or ischemia; anatomy preserved

   ii. axon injured

second-degree = Seddon axonotmesis; injury to axon with Wallerian degeneration; endoneurium/perineurium/epineurium intact; endoneurium provides "tube" to optimize successful reinnervation of target muscle

   iii. axon and endoneurium disrupted

third-degree = axon and endoneurium disrupted; recovery inversely related to interfascicular fibrosis; gross normal appearance

   iv. axon, endoneurium and perineurium disrupted

fourth-degree = interruption axon, endoneurium, perineurium; gross reveals indurated enlarged nerve

   v. axon endo-, peri-, and epineurium disrupted

fifth-degree = Seddon neurotmesis; complete transection of axon, endo-, peri-, epineurium

66. **What are etiologies of brachial plexus injuries?**
Hint: cpt

    G7 p.801:130 mm

a. c_____   compression
b. p_____   penetration
c. t_____   traction

67. **Complete the following about traction (stretch) injuries of the brachial plexus selectively:**

    G7 p.801:138mm

a. spare the
   i. _____ _____   medial cord
   ii. _____ _____   median nerve
b. injure the
   i. _____ _____   posterior cord
   ii. _____ _____   lateral cord

68. Complete the following about the peripheral neuropathies:

G7 p.801:150 mm

a. What nerve injury cannot be repaired?

proximal to dorsal root ganglion (i.e., preganglionic)

b. What is the evidence for such an injury? Hint: prEHms

pain
rhomboids
EMG
Horner
meningocele
scapula

69. List the characteristics of Erb and Klumpke brachial plexus injury.

G7 p.802:130mm

a. e_____   extended
b. r_____   rotated
c. p(b)_____   pronated
d. k(cl)_____   claw
e. l_____   lower roots C8 T1
f. u_____   ulnar type claw plus
g. m_____   median type claw
h. p_____   palsy

70. Describe upper and lower brachial plexus injury.

G7 p.802:135mm

a. upper brachial plexus injury
   i.   D_____-E_____ palsy   Duchenne-Erb palsy
   ii. u_____ p_____ C_____,   upper plexus C5, C6
        C_____
   iii. f_____ s_____ h_____   forceful separation humeral
        h_____ from s_____   head from shoulder
   iv. d_____ or m_____   commonly dystocia or
        c_____   motorcycle crash
   v.   i_____ r_____ a_____   internally rotated arm with
        with e_____ e_____   extended elbow
   vi. b_____ t_____   bellhop's tip, hand not
                                              affected

b. lower brachial plexus injury
   i.   K_____ P_____   Klumpke palsy
   ii. l_____ p_____ C_____,   lower plexus C8, T1
        T_____
   iii. s_____ p_____ of a_____ sudden pull of abducted arm
        a_____ i_____   in
   iv. f_____ or P_____ t_____ fall or Pancoast tumor
        s_____   syndrome
   v.   c_____ h_____ with   claw hand with
        w_____/w_____ of   weakness/wasting of small
        s_____ h_____ m_____   hand muscles
   vi. s_____ h_____   simian hand

24

71. Complete the following about brachial plexus birth injuries:

G7 p.802:135mm

a.
    i.   most common is _____   upper
    ii. consisting of C5-C6_____% and   50%
    iii. C5, C6-C7 _____%   25%
    iv. lower C8-T1 _____%   2%
b. combined is _____%   20%
c. bilateral _____%   4%
d. spontaneous recovery is _____%   90%

72. Characterize upper brachial plexus injury—Erb palsy.

G7 p.802:140mm

a. roots involved _____   C5 (ABCDE) fifth letter of alphabet, Erb palsy mainly C5 and also C6, C7

b. position of upper extremity (Hint: erp)
    i.   e_____   extended
    ii. r_____   rotated
    iii. p_____   pronated
    iv. looks like _____ _____ _____   bellhop's tip position

c. Weak muscles and their roots
    i.   d_____   deltoid
        roots, _____   C5, C6
    ii. b_____   biceps
        roots, _____   C5, C6
    iii. r_____   rhomboids
        roots, _____   C4, C5
    iv. b_____   brachioradialis
        roots, _____   C5, C6
    v.   s_____   supraspinatus
        roots, _____   C4, C5, C6
    vi. i_____   infraspinatus
        roots, _____   C5, C6
d. mechanism _____ _____   shoulder separation
e. from:
    i.   b_____ i_____   birth injuries
    ii. m_____ a_____   motorcycle accidents

73. Characterize lower brachial plexus injury—Klumpke palsy.

G7 p.802:155mm

a. roots involved   C7, C8, T1
b. position of upper extremity (Hint: klump)
    i.   kl_____   claw hand (Simian hand)
    ii. u_____   ulnar claw
    iii. m_____   plus median claw
    iv. p_____   paralysis
c. weak muscles
    i.   upper extremity _____   small muscles of hand
    ii. face _____   Horner if T1 involved
d. mechanism: traction on _____ arm   abducted
e. from
    i.   f_____   falls
    ii. b_____   birth
    iii. P_____   Pancoast tumors

24

74. **Complete the following regarding birth injury of brachial plexus:**   G7 p.802:175mm
   a. incidence is _____   0.3 to 2/1000 births
      i. upper   50% C5, C6
      ii. upper plus C7   25% C5, C6, C7
   b. mixed   20%
   c. lower   2% C7, T1
   d. bilateral   4%

75. **True or False. The following are indications for early surgical exploration of the brachial plexus:**   G7 p.803:105mm
   a. any injury needs repair   false (most injuries maximal deficit at onset then improve)
   b. progressive deficit   true (progressive deficit likely vascular injury, explore immediately)
   c. clean sharp injury   true (clean, sharp, fresh lacerating injuries → explore acutely and repair end-to-end tension-free within 72 hours)
   d. gunshot wound (GSW) to brachial plexus   false (surgery is of little benefit)

76. **List medical etiologies of entrapment neuropathies.**   G7 p.804:85mm
   a. a_____   arthritis rheumatoid
   b. a_____   acromegaly
   c. a_____   amyloidosis
   d. p_____   polymyalgia rheumatica
   e. c_____   carcinomatosis
   f. d_____   diabetes
   g. g_____   gout
   h. h_____   hypothyroidism

77. **Name the two most common syndromes of median nerve entrapment.**   G7 p.806:60mm
   a. c_____ t_____ s_____   carpal tunnel syndrome
   b. p_____ t_____ s_____   pronator teres syndrome

78. **Describe carpal tunnel syndrome (CTS) anatomy.**   G7 p.806:72mm
   a. The median nerve passes under the _____ _____ _____.   transverse carpal ligament
   b. The motor branch either goes
      i. _____ or   under
      ii. _____ the ligament   pierces
   c. and serves the _____ muscles,   loaf
   d. which are
      i. l_____   limbricales 1 and 2
      ii. o_____   opponens pollicis
      iii. a_____   abductor pollicis
      iv. f_____   flexor pollicis brevis

24

79. Answer the following about carpal tunnel syndrome: G7 p.806:150mm
   a. The transverse carpal ligament extends   3 cm
      how far beyond the distal wrist crease?
   b. What is the name of the sensory nerve?   palmar cutaneous branch   G7 p.806:160mm
   c. It arises _____ cm proximal to the   5.5 cm
      wrist.
   d. It passes _____ the transverse carpal above   G7 p.806:172mm
      ligament
   e. and serves the _____ _____   thenar eminence
      sensation.

80. Complete the following about the median nerve: G7 p.806:177mm
   a. Describe the sensory distribution of the
      median nerve.
      i.   thumb: _____ aspect   palmar
      ii. fingers: _____, _____ and   index, middle, and half of ring
           half of _____
      iii. _____ eminence and adjacent   thenar
      iv. _____ palm   radial
   b. crosses _____ transverse carpal   above
      ligament

81. Describe main trunk median nerve compression.   G7 p.807:17mm
   a. above elbow due to _____ _____   Struthers ligament →
                                                supracondylar to medial
                                                epicondyle, mostly
                                                asymptomatic

   b. at elbow
      i.   b_____ a_____   bicipital aponeurosis
      ii. p_____ t_____   pronator teres
      iii. s_____ b_____   sublimis bridge
   c. Honeymoon paralysis is due to _____   direct compression
      _____.
   d. Benediction hand is due to weakness of   flexor digitorum profundus   G7 p.807:30mm
      _____ _____ _____ I and II.

82. Characterize pronator teres syndrome (PTS).   G7 p.807:60mm
   a. It compresses the _____ nerve   median
   b. where it dives between the two heads of   pronator teres
      the _____ _____.
   c. Symptoms are
      i.   pain in the _____   palm
      ii. weakness in the _____   grip
      iii. paresthesias in the _____ and   thumb and index finger
           _____.
      iv. It differs from CTS in that there is no nocturnal pain in pronator
           _____,   teres syndrome
      v.   but there is _____ in PTS   pain in the palm
      vi. because the _____ branch is   median palmar cutaneous
           compressed in PTS.

83. **Describe pronator teres syndrome.**   G7 p.807:60mm
a.
   i.   caused by repeated _____   pronation
   ii. with a _____ _____   tight fist
b.
   i.   due to _____ _____ where it   nerve entrapment
      dives between
   ii. two heads of the _____   pronator teres
      _____.
c. Symptoms are
   i.   a_____   ache
   ii. p_____ in p_____   pain in palm
   iii. w_____ g_____   weak grip
d. Distinguished from carpal tunnel
    syndrome by
   i.   no n_____ e_____   nocturnal exacerbation

84. **What are the key features of anterior**   G7 p.807:95mm
interosseous neuropathy?
a.
   i.   loss of f_____   flexion
   ii. of the d_____ p_____   distal phalanges
   iii. of the t_____   thumb
   iv. and i_____ f_____   index finger
b. due to
   i.   weakness of the f_____   flexor digitorum profundus
      d_____ p_____ and the
   ii. f_____ p_____ l_____   flexor pollicis longus
c. no loss of _____   sensation (anterior
                              interosseous is pure motor)
d. patient can't _____   make "OK" sign
e. treatment
   i.   e_____   no identifiable cause—
                              expectant; management 8 to
                              12 weeks
   ii. e_____   if no improvement or if
                              progression proceed with
                              surgical exploration

24

85. **Answer the following about the**   G7 p.807:100mm
anterior interosseous nerve:
a. If injured a person can't do what with the   make an "O"
    thumb and index finger?
b. There is weakness of the
   i.   f_____ d_____ p_____   flexor digitorum profundus
      and
   ii. f_____ p_____ l_____   flexor pollicis longus
c. Is part of what nerve?   median
d. Syndrome may be caused by _____   constricting
    ligament.
e. Is there any sensory loss?   no sensory loss

86. Describe the epidemiology of carpal tunnel syndrome.   G7 p.808:78mm

a. What is the most common median nerve entrapment neuropathy?   carpal tunnel syndrome

b. It is due to _____.   compression of the median nerve

c. Where?   distal to wrist crease
d. Age _____   middle-aged patient
e. Male/female ratio _____   4:1
f. Bilateral _____%   bilateral > 50%
g. Worse in _____   dominant hand
h. Phalen sign is performed by _____ of the wrist   forced flexion   G7 p.808:85mm
i. and is positive in _____%.   80%

87. What is double-crush syndrome?   G7 p.809:130mm

a. It involves two sites.
   i. _____   cervical radiculopathy
   ii. _____   median/ulnar neuropathy
b. It is exacerbated by _____.   neck movement
c. Pathophysiology
   i. postulated that _____ compression   cervical
   ii. compromises _____ _____   axoplasmic flow
   iii. predisposing _____ _____ _____ injury   nerve to distal

88. Answer the following about carpal tunnel syndrome: G7 p.810:25mm

a. What is the most sensitive electrodiagnostic test for carpal tunnel syndrome?   sensory latency nerve conduction velocity (NCV)

b. Which should be faster, median sensory conduction velocity or ulnar sensory conduction velocity?   median

c. By how much?   4 m/s faster

89. Complete the following about carpal tunnel syndrome: G7 p.810:165mm

a. Describe treatment.
   i. sp_____   splint
   ii. st_____   steroids
   iii. su_____   surgery
b. Incision should be slightly to the _____ side of the interthenar crease   ulnar
c. to avoid
   i. p_____ c_____ b_____ and/or   palmar cutaneous branch   G7 p.812:43mm
   ii. a_____ r_____ t_____ m_____ b_____.   anomalous recurrent thenar motor branch   G7 p.812:70mm

24

90. Complete the following about the ulnar nerve: G7 p.812:155mm

a. Name the roots.
ulnar components C7, C8, T1

b. Motor findings of entrapment? (Hint: abcWF)   G7 p.813:17mm

   i. a_____
interossei wasting; atrophy, particularly thumb web space

   ii. b_____
benediction hand

   iii. c_____
claw deformity

   iv. W_____
Wartenberg sign: abducted little finger   G7 p.813:22mm

   v. F_____
Froment thumb sign   G7 p.813:27mm

c.

   i. pain and tingling in _____ _____
little finger

   ii. and _____ _____ _____ _____
ulnar half ring finger

91. Answer the following about ulnar nerve entrapment: G7 p.813:17mm

a. What occurs to interossei?
atrophy

b. Little finger weak on

   i. _____ is called
adduction

   ii. W_____ s_____.
Wartenberg sign (little finger held in abduction)

c. Holding a piece of paper requires modification because of a weak

   i. _____ _____ and is called
adductor pollicis

   ii. _____ _____ _____ _____.
Froment prehensile thumb sign

d. Waving goodbye demonstrates a c_____ d_____
claw deformity of the hand

   i. also known as m_____ en g_____
main en griffe   G7 p.813:40mm

   ii. also known as b_____ h_____.
benediction hand

e. What other nerve injury can produce

   i. benediction hand?
median

   ii. upon what attempted action?
making a fist

92. Describe Wartenberg sign.   G7 p.813:22mm

a. It affects the _____.
little finger

b. What occurs to the _____?
little finger

c. It rests in _____
abduction

d. due to weakness of the t_____ p_____ i_____ m_____.
third palmar interosseous muscle

e. Which nerve is involved?
ulnar

93. Describe Froment sign.   G7 p.813:27mm

a. Test by having the patient g_____
grasp a piece of paper

b. using his t_____ and i_____ f_____.
thumb and index fingers

c. If the _____ nerve is weak what happens?
ulnar

24

d.   Thumb b_____ b_____   bends backward (i.e., flexing
                                                   the distal phalanx or
                                                   extending proximal phalanx
                                                   of the thumb)

e.   Because ulnar innervated _____   adductor pollicis
     _____ is weak

f.   Therefore the body substitutes for it the   stronger flexor pollicis longus
     _____ _____ _____
     _____,

g.   which is innervated by the _____   anterior interosseous nerve,
     _____ _____ of the _____   median
     nerve.

94.   Describe ulnar nerve entrapment.   G7 p.813:70mm
a.   Injury above elbow due to
     i.   i_____ to m_____   injury to medial cord
           c_____
     ii.   kinking at the a_____ of   arcade of Struthers
           S_____   aponeurotic band
b.   Entrapment at the e_____   elbow   G7 p.813:90 mm
     i.   aka t_____ u_____   "tardy ulnar palsy" (delayed
           p_____   presentation—initial case 12
                                                years > from injury to elbow—
                                                elbow dislocation/lateral
                                                condyle fracture; nerve is
                                                superficial, fixed and crosses
                                                joint)
     ii.   NCV is less than _____ m/s   48 m/s
     iii. or a difference between the 2 slides 10 m/s
           of greater than _____ m/s
c.   Entrapment in the f_____   forearm
d.   Entrapment in the   wrist/hand
     w_____/h_____

95.   What are surgical treatment options   G7 p.814:150mm
     for ulnar compression at the elbow?
a.   de_____ without _____   simple nerve decompression
                                                without transposition
b.   de_____ with _____   nerve decompression with
                                                transposition
c.   medial _____   epicondylectomy
d.   Results in %   G7 p.815:125mm
     i.   excellent _____%   60%
     ii.   fair _____%   25%
     iii. poor _____%   15%
e.   True or False. What responds better?
     i.   pain and sensory loss   true
     ii.   weakness and atrophy   false

96.   Answer the following about   G7 p.815:155mm
     entrapement in the forearm—cubital
     tunnel syndrome:
a.   Involves which nerve?   ulnar
b.   Due to which muscle?   flexor carpi ulnaris

c. The mechanism is compression between the

    i.   m _____ e_____ and the
    ii. o _____ p_____

(Just distal to the elbow, the ulnar nerve passes from the groove between the) medial epicondyle and the olecranon process to enter the two heads of the flexor carpi ulnaris under the fascial band connecting the two heads (the cubital tunnel)

d. results in a _____ W_____,
    F_____, c_____

atrophy of the interrossei, Wartenberg sign, Froment prehensile thumb sign, claw deformity of the hand (main en griffe)

97. **Characteristics of the cubital tunnel syndrome are**

    G7 p.815:155mm

  a. c_____
  b. c_____
  c. u_____
  d. b_____
  e. i_____
  f. t_____

  g. t_____

  h. a_____
  i. l(el)_____ e_____

claw deformity
(flexor) carpi ulnaris
ulnar nerve
band is tight
interossei atrophied
thumb sign Froment prehensile
two heads of flexor carpi ulnaris
atrophy of interossei
elbow epicondyle

98. **Describe the borders of the Guyon canal.**

    G7 p.816:25mm

  a. roof
    i.   p _____ f_____
    ii. p _____ b_____ m_____
  b. floor
    i.   f_____ r_____ of the
        p_____
    ii. p_____ l_____
  c. Below the floor is the t_____
    c_____ l_____.
  d. It contains only the _____ nerve and artery.

palmar fascia
palmar brevis muscle

flexor retinaculum of the palm
pisohamate ligament
transverse carpal ligament

ulnar (At the middle of the canal the nerve divides into deep and superficial branches. Superficial branch is mostly sensory [except for the branch to palmar brevis] and supplies hypothenar eminence and ulnar half of ring finger. The deep [muscular] branch innervates hypothenar muscles, lumbricals 3, 4, and interossei.)

24

99. **Describe the types of ulnar nerve lesions in Guyon canal type—location of compression—weakness-sensory deficit.**
G7 p.816:70mm

a. type I
  i.   location of compression — just proximal to or within Guyon canal
  ii. weakness — all intrinsic muscles innervated by ulnar nerve
  iii. sensory deficit — palmar ulnar distribution (palmar ulnar distribution: the hypothenar eminence and ulnar half of ring finger both on the palmar surface only)

b. type, II
  i.   location of compression — along deep branch
  ii. weakness — muscles innervated by deep branch (depending on location may spare hypothenar muscles)
  iii. sensory deficit — none

c. type III
  i.   location of compression — distal end of Guyon canal
  ii. weakness — none
  iii. sensory deficit — palmar ulnar distribution (the hypothenar eminence and ulnar half of ring finger both on the palmar surface only)

100. **Complete the following regarding radial nerve injuries:**
G7 p.816:145mm

a. Sensation loss in the web space of the thumb indicates injury in the _____. — hand

b. Pain at the lateral epicondyle indicates compression of the _____ _____ _____ _____ _____. — supinator tunnel at the elbow

c.
  i.   Finger drop indicates injury to the _____ — PIN
  ii. resulting from entrapment at the a_____ of F_____. — arcade of Frohse

d.
  i.   Wrist drop indicates injury to _____-_____ _____ — mid-upper arm
  ii. where the nerve is in the _____ _____. — spiral groove

e. Triceps plus all distal muscle weakness indicates injury at the _____ — axilla

f. above plus weakness of the deltoid and latissimus dorsi indicates injury to the _____ — posterior cord

g. above plus winging of the scapula on the forward shoulder thrust indicates injury to the _____. — roots

24

101. **Differentiate radial nerve injury from brachial plexus posterior cord injury.** G7 p.816:145mm

a. Check the function of the _____ and

b. _____ muscles.

deltoid

latissimus dorsi radial nerve arises from posterior divisions of the three trunks of the brachial plexus to form the posterior cord. Sparing of deltoid (axillary) and latissimus dorsi (thoracodorsal) localizes injury to radial nerve and not the more proximal portion of the posterior cord.

102. **Differentiate axilla and mid-upper arm radial nerve compression.** G7 p.816:175mm

a. Check the function of the _____ muscle.

b. Wrist drop plus weak triceps implicates injury at _____.

c. Wrist drop but normal triceps implicates injury at _____.

triceps

axilla; crutch misuse, weak triceps and distal, radial innervated muscles

mid-upper arm; sites: spiral groove, intermuscular septum; improper arm positioning with; intoxication "Saturday night palsy"; iatrogenic surgical positioning; callus old humeral fracture; wrist drop-normal triceps; DDX (lead poisoning)

24

103. **Describe mid-upper or forearm radial nerve compression.** G7 p.817:38mm

a. Radial nerve compression mid-upper arm produces

 i. w_____ (w_____ d_____) and

 ii. _____ _____

 iii. because it compresses _____ and _____ _____ _____.

weakness (wrist drop)

wrist numbness

PIN and superficial (sensory) radial nerve (finger drop)

b. Injury to the posterior interosseous nerve (PIN) produces G7 p.817:75mm

 i. _____ of fingers

 ii. but no weakness of _____

 iii. because it compresses _____ and not the s_____ r_____ n_____.

weakness

numbness

PIN (motor) and not the superficial radial nerve (sensory)

c. Injury at the supinator tunnel produces G7 p.817:105mm

 i. _____ but no

 ii. _____ and no

 iii. _____.

pain

weakness

numbness

104. **Complete the following about peripheral neuropathies:**   G7 p.817:80mm
    a. PIN refers to the _____ _____ _____   posterior interosseous nerve
    b. a continuation of the _____ nerve,   radial
    c. which serves the
        i.   e_____ of the f_____ and the   extensors of the fingers
        ii. a_____ p_____ l_____   abductor pollicis longus

105. **Complete the following about the radial nerve and wrist weakness:**   G7 p.817:55mm
    a. Failure of wrist extension (wrist drop) indicates _____ radial nerve injury.   proximal
    b. Failure of finger extension (finger drop) indicates _____ injury.   PIN

106. **Describe forearm/hand radial nerve compression management.**   G7 p.817:95mm
    a. posterior interosseous syndrome _____ _____ and _____ _____ _____   Surgical exploration if no improvement after 4 to 8 weeks expectant management. Lyse constrictions and arcade of Frohse.
    b. supinator tunnel syndrome _____ _____ and _____ _____ _____   Responds to nerve decompression. Lyse constrictions and extensor carpi radialis brevis.
    c. hand injury
        i.   Clinically you find _____ _____ _____ _____   small area of sensory loss dorsal
        ii. at the _____ _____ _____ of _____   web space of thumb
        iii. often caused by _____.   handcuffs
        iv. Symptoms are mild so _____ _____ _____ _____.   no surgery is needed

107. **Describe the suprascapular nerve.**   G7 p.818:35mm
    a. Formed from roots _____   C5, C6
    b. Entrapped at _____ _____ _____   transverse scapular ligament (TSL) (History: antecedent frozen shoulder or trauma)
    c. Sensory symptoms _____ _____ _____ _____ _____   referred, poorly localized shoulder pain. Nerve innervates joint capsule, no cutaneous representation.
    d. Motor symptoms
        i.   atrophy of _____ and _____   infraspinatus and supraspinatus
        ii. weakness of a _____ _____ _____ _____ from 0 to _____ degrees   supraspinatus upper extremity abduction; 30
        iii. weak _____ tennis shot   backhand
    e. Is EMG helpful?   yes, to distinguish from rotation cuff injury

f. Treatment _____   surgery; if fails to improve cut
                                      TSL
g. Differentiate from C5 cervical   rhomboid and deltoid (will
    radiculopathy and upper brachial plexus   show weakness in
    lesion by testing _____ and   C5 radiculopathy)
    _____.

108. Define meralgia paresthetica.   G7 p.818:150 mm
  a. hyperpathia located at the l _____   lateral upper thigh (burning
      u_____ t _____   pain with hyperpathia)
  b. entrapment of the l _____ f_____   lateral femoral cutaneous
      c_____ nerve
  c. True or False. It contains motor and   false (pure sensory L2, L3)
      sensory fibers.

109. Complete the following about   G7 p.820:95mm
     peripheral neuropathies:
  a. Which is the most common nerve to   the common peroneal nerve
      develop acute compression palsy?
  b. At what location?   fibular head
  c. It results in impairment of
      i.   motor function: _____ _____   foot drop
      ii. sensory loss: _____ of _____ dorsum of foot

110. Matching. Match the following: G7 p.820:114mm
     Nerve also known as:
     ① musculocutaneous
     ② medial popliteal
     ③ lateral popliteal
     ④ anterior tibial
  a. tibial L4-5, S2-3   ②
  b. common peroneal L4-5, S1   ③
  c. deep peroneal L4-5, S1   ④
  d. superficial peroneal L5, S1   ①

111. Matching. Match the nerve with the   G7 p.820:114mm
     function it serves.
     Nerve functions:
     ① plantar flexors and inversion
     ② origin of deep and superficial peroneal
     ③ dorsiflexors superation toe extensors
     ④ plantar flexors and eversion
  a. tibial   ①
  b. common peroneal   ②
  c. deep peroneal   ③
  d. superficial peroneal   ④

112. Matching. Match the following nerve   G7 p.820:114 mm
     and its area of isolated sensory loss:
     Nerve area of isolated sensory loss:
     ① lateral aspect of calf and dorsum of
     foot
     ② space between great and second top
  a. deep peroneal   ②
  b. superficial peroneal   ①

24

113. **Matching. Match the nerve with its characteristics.**
     G7 p.820:119mm
     Characteristic:
     ① passes behind the fibular head; ② is the most common nerve to develop acute compression palsy; ③ serves the foot extensors; ④ serves the foot evertors; ⑤ space between great toe and second toe; ⑥ dorsum of foot
     Nerve:
     a. common peroneal   ①, ②
     b. deep peroneal   ③, ⑤
     c. superficial peroneal   ④, ⑥

114. **True or False. Loss of pinprick sensation to the web space between the great toe and first toe can occur with**
     G7 p.820:134mm
     a. superficial peroneal nerve compression   false (sensory loss lateral leg and dorsum of foot)
     b. deep peroneal compression   true
     c. S1 nerve root compression   false (sensory loss to lateral foot and little toe)
     d. none of the above   false

115. **True or False. Entrapment of the common peroneal nerve at the fibular head may result in:**
     G7 p.785:107mm
     a. weak soleus muscle   false (innervated by the tibial nerve)
     b. foot drop   true
     c. weak biceps femoris muscle   false (biceps femoris innervated by sciatic proximal to take off of common peroneal)   G7 p.1195:70mm
     d. sensory impairment in the lateral calf and dorsum of foot   true (foot drop and sensory impairment in lateral calf and dorsum foot)

116. **True or False. A foot drop may result from**
     G7 p.821:27mm
     a. parasagittal meningioma   true   G7 p.1196:60mm
     b. deep peroneal nerve palsy   true   G7 p.1195:180mm
     c. L5 radiculopathy (occasionally L4)   true (L5 is more commonly the cause of foot drop.)   G7 p.1195:180mm
     d. superficial peroneal nerve palsy   false (There is weakness of foot eversion but not foot drop.)   G7 p.820:140mm
     e. common peroneal nerve palsy   true   G7 p.821:16mm

117. **True or False. Peroneal nerve palsy may result from**
     G7 p.821:55mm
     a. diabetes mellitus   true
     b. clipping injury in a football player   true
     c. venous thrombosis   true
     d. leprosy (Hansen disease)   true

118. True or False. The posterior tibial nerve may be

G7 p.822:62mm

a. found in the tarsal tunnel — true
b. found posterior and inferior to the medial malleolus — true
c. trapped at the retinacular ligament — true
d. classically responsible for nocturnal pain and paresthesia at the heel — false (Heel is spared. Paresthesias are in the toes and sole of the foot.)

119. Matching. Match the following nerves with their functions and alternate names:

G7 p.820:114mm

Function and alternate name:
① also known as musculocutaneous;
② also known as medial popliteal;
③ also known as lateral popliteal; ④ also known as anterior tibial; ⑤ serves plantar flexors of foot plus inversion;
⑥ origin of deep plus sup P; ⑦ foot dorsiflexors supination and toe extensors; ⑧ foot plantar flex and eversion; ⑨ space between great and second toe; ⑩ lateral aspect of the calf and dorsum of foot
Nerve:

a. tibial L4, 5, S2, S3 — ②, ⑤
b. common peroneal — ③, ⑥
c. deep peroneal L4, 5, S1 — ④, ⑦ , ⑨
d. superficial peroneal L5, S1 — ①, ⑧ , ⑩

■ Thoracic Outlet Syndrome

120. True or False. Clinical presentation of the thoracic outlet syndrome may include

G7 p.822:155mm

a. pallor and ischemia of hand and fingers — true
b. arm swelling and edema — true
c. brachial plexus lower trunk dysfunction — true
d. brachial plexus medial cord dysfunction — true

121. True or False. Regarding the thoracic outlet syndrome, conservative treatment may be as effective as the surgical treatment. — true

G7 p.823:130mm

24

25

Neuro-ophthalmology

■ Nystagmus

1. **Complete the following about nystagmus:**   G7 p.828:50mm
   a. What is nystagmus? i_____   involuntary rhythmic
      r_____ o_____ of the eyes   oscillation
   b. What is the most common form?   jerk nystagmus
   c. How is its directionality defined?   fast component
   d. What is the abnormal component?   slow component
   e. What is vertical nystagmus indicative of?
      i.   p_____ f_____ p_____   posterior fossa pathology
      ii. s_____   sedatives
      iii. a_____ d_____   antiepileptic drugs

2. **Seesaw nystagmus occurs with a**   diencephalon   G7 p.828:68mm
   lesion in the _____.

3. **Nystagmus retractorius occurs with a**   upper midbrain tegmentum; G7 p.828:83mm
   lesion in the _____ _____   pinealoma
   _____; for example p_____.

4. **Ocular bobbing occurs with a lesion in** pontine tegmentum   G7 p.828:135mm
   the _____ _____.

5. **Matching. Match the form of**   G7 p.828:70mm
   nystagmus and the location of the
   lesion.
   Form:
   ① seesaw nystagmus; ② convergence
   nystagmus; ③ nystagmus retractorius;
   ④ downbeat nystagmus; ⑤ upbeat
   nystagmus; ⑥ abducting nystagmus;
   ⑦ ocular bobbing
   Location:
   a. diencephalon   ①
   b. upper midbrain tegmentum   ②
   c. midbrain tectum   ③
   d. pons medial longitudinal fasciculus (MLF)   ⑥, ⑦
   e. medulla   ⑤
   f. post-fossa—cervicomedullary junction   ④

6. **Name the location of the lesion in nystagmus.**
   G7 p.828:70mm
   a. seesaw nystagmus   diencephalon
   b. nystagmus retractorius   upper midbrain
                                  tegmentum/pineal region
   c. downbeat nystagmus   cervicomedullary junction
                                  (foramen magnum)
   d. upbeat nystagmus   medulla
   e. ocular bobbing   pons

■ Papilledema

7. **Complete the following about papilledema:**
   G7 p.828:165mm
   a. What is papilledema caused by?   Thought to be caused by
                                         axoplasmic stasis. Theory:
                                         ① Increase intracranial
                                         pressure (ICP) transmitted to
                                         the optic disk via
                                         subarachnoid (SA) space.
                                         Retinal venous pulsations
                                         obliterated. ② Retinal
                                         arterial: venous pressure ratio
                                         < 1.5:1.
   b. How long does it take to develop? 24 to 48 hours
   c. What is the earliest it is seen?   6 hours
   d. Does it cause visual blurring?   no (unless severe and
                                         prolonged)
   e. Does it cause visual field distortion? no (unless severe and
                                         prolonged)
   f. Differentiate from optic neuritis.
      i. funduscopy _____ _____   may look alike
         _____
      ii. visual lost more with _____ optic neuritis
         _____
      iii. pain on palpation more with   optic neuritis
         _____ _____

8. **What is the differential diagnosis for unilateral papilledema?**
   G7 p.829:30mm
   Hint: Fiom
   a. F_____-_____   Foster-Kennedy
   b. i_____   inflammation
   c. o_____ _____   optic glioma
   d. m_____ _____   multiple sclerosis

25

■ Pupillary Diameter

9. **Complete the following concerning the pupillodilator nerve fibers:**   G7 p.829:180mm
   a. first-order sympathetic nerve fibers
      i.   origin, p_____ h_____   posterolateral hypothalamus
      ii. destination, i_____ cell column   intermediolateral
           (_____ to _____)   (C8 to T2)
      iii. neurotransmitter, a_____   acetylcholine (ACh)
   b. second-order sympathetic nerve fibers
      i.   origin, i_____ cell column   intermediolateral
      ii. destination, s_____ c_____   superior cervical ganglion
           g_____
   c. third-order sympathetic nerve fibers
      i.   origin, s_____ c_____   superior cervical ganglion
           g_____
      ii. destination, p_____ m_____   pupillodilator muscle (long
           of the eye, l_____ g_____,   ciliary nerves), lacrimal gland,
           M_____ m_____   Müller muscle
      iii. neurotransmitter, n_____   norepinephrine

10. **How are pupillodilator muscles arranged?**   radially   G7 p.829:180mm

11. **Describe the anatomy of sympathetic outflow to the eye.**   G7 p.829:180mm
    Hint: hilsc
    a. h_____   hypothalamus
    b. i_____ _____ _____   intermediolateral cell column
    c. l_____ _____ _____   lateral horn cells

25

d. c_____ _____

ciliary ganglion
Sympathetic summary: first order: posterolateral (a) hypothalamus → descend in midbrain tegmentum uncrossed to pons, medulla, spinal cord (SC) to the (b) intermediolateral cell columns, C8-T2 (ciliospinal center of Budge). → synapse with (c) lateral horn cells acetylcholine (ACh) and give off second-order neurons (a) (preganglionics). Second order: enter sympathetic chain → (b) superior cervical ganglion. Third order: (a) (postganglionics): go up with common (b) carotid artery (CCA) those that mediate sweat to face go up external carotid artery (ECA), the rest go up internal carotid artery (ICA). Some pass: = (d) V1 → ciliary ganglion → (e) pupillodilator norepinephrine (NE)= ICA → (f) ophthalmic artery → (g) lacrimal gland and the Müller muscle.

12. **The pupilloconstrictor (parasympathetic) are muscles arranged c_____ as a s_____.**

concentric as a sphincter   G7 p.830:55mm

13. **Describe the parasympathetic outflow to the eyes.**
Hint: Ect
a. E_____
b. c_____
c. t_____

G7 p.830:75mm

Edinger-Westphal
ciliary ganglion
third nerve
Parasympathetics summary: Preganglionics arise in the *Edinger-Westphal* nucleus at the level of the superior colliculus synapse in the ciliary ganglion. Postganglionics travel on the *third* nerve to (e) innervate sphincter pupillae and ciliary muscle (thickens lens causing accommodation via relaxation).

25

14. Describe the pupillary light reflex.

G7 p.830-:75mm

Hint: ropEtcs

a. r_____   retina
b. o_____   optic nerve
c. p_____   pretectal
d. E_____   Edinger-Westphal
e. t_____   third nerve
f. c_____   ciliary ganglion
g. s_____   sphincter light reflex

Summary: Mediated by (a) rods and cones of retina. Transmit via axons to (b) optic nerve (ON). Bypass lateral geniculate body (unlike vision) synapse in (c) pretectal nuclear complex. Connect to both (d) Edinger-Westphal nuclei. Preganglionics travel in (e) third nerve to (f) ciliary ganglion, etc. Cornea rods and cones (retina) axons optic nerve bypass lateral geniculate body pretectal nuclear complex Edinger-Westphal nuclei (both preganglionics) to ciliary ganglion. Postganglionics via third nerve to pupillary sphincter. Ciliary muscles thicken (relax) causing accommodation.

25

15. Complete the following about Argyll Robertson pupil:

G7 p.830:140mm

Hint: ALRP = Argyll Robertson pupil = absent light response pupil

a. Key feature is _____ _____ _____ _____ or ALRP.   absent light response pupil

b. It occurs in _____.   syphilis

c. Near light dissociation means the pupil constricts when focusing on an object _____   near

d. but the pupil does not react to _____.   light

16. In which condition do you have light-near dissociation, that is, an Argyll Robertson pupil?   syphilis

G7 p.830:140mm

17. **Complete the following about Argyll Robertson pupil:**

   a. Light-near dissociation refers to pupillary _____

      constriction

   b. on convergence and _____ of papillary constriction to shining of the light into the eye

      absence

   c. classically described in _____

      syphilis

   d. also known as _____ _____ _____

      Argyll Robertson pupil

   Hint: prostitutes principle, "They accommodate but don't react."

G7 p.830:135mm

■ Alterations in Pupillary Diameter

18. **Does afferent pupillary defect cause anisocoria?**

      no

G7 p.831:25mm

19. **Complete the following about anisocoria:**

   a. Unequal pupils with an affarent pupillary defect (Marcus-Gunn) means there are _____ _____.

      two lesions

   b. Physiologic anisocoria occurs in _____% of people.

      20%

   c. The difference is usually _____ mm.

      0.4

   d. Sudden onset of anisocoria is usually due to _____.

      drugs

   e. Sympathomimetics cause _____ to _____ mm of dilation and

      1 to 2

   f.

     i. parasympatholytics cause _____ mm of dilation and the

       8

     ii. eye _____ _____ react to light.

       does not

G7 p.831 :25mm

20. **Complete the following about Horner syndrome:**

   a. The abnormal pupil is _____.

      smaller

   b. Ptosis is on the side of the _____ pupil.

      small

G7 p.831:100mm

21. **With third nerve palsy, if there is ptosis it will be on the side of the _____ pupil.**

      large

G7 p.831:110mm

22. **Complete the following about oculomotor neuropathy:**

   a. Example is _____

      diabetes

   b. Usually _____ the pupil

      spares

   c. Usually resolves in _____ _____

      8 weeks

G7 p.831:116mm

25

23. Complete the following about third nerve compression:

G7 p.831:121mm

a. Example is _____   aneurysm
b. Most common is _____   P-comm
c. Occasionally _____ _____   basilar bifurcation
   aneurysm
d. Usually _____ _____ _____   does not spare
   the pupil

24. What is the differential diagnosis of anisocoria?

G7 p.831:38mm

Hint: u tAp Hat

a. u_____   uncal herniation (also has mental status changes)

b. t_____   trauma (traumatic iridoplegia mydriasis or miosis)

c. A_____   Adie pupil (iris palsy—impaired postganglionic parasympathetics)

d. p_____   physiologic (less than 1 mm difference—20% of population)

e. H_____   Horner syndrome (impaired sympathetics to pupillodilator muscle)

f. a_____   aneurysm (posterior communicating, basilar)

g. t_____   third nerve palsy (pupil sparing-diabetes mellitus [DM 1], ETOH, cavernous aneurysm)

25. What is the differential diagnosis for Marcus-Gunn pupil?

G7 p.831:170mm

a. Location of lesion _____   ipsilateral to impaired direct reflex anterior to chiasm

   i. r_____—d_____ i_____   retina—detachment, infarction

   ii. n_____—m_____ s_____,   nerve—neuritis, multiple sclerosis (MS, viral)—trauma
       v_____, or t_____

b. In Marcus Gunn is/are the
   i. third nerve intact?   yes
   ii. parasympathetic nerves intact?   yes

26. Complete the following about Adie pupil:

G7 p.832:40mm

a. An Adie pupil is an _____ palsy resulting   iris

b. in a _____ pupil, due to   dilated
c. impaired _____ _____.   postganglionic parasympathetics

d. Clinically, patients exhibit _____-_____ _____.   light-near dissociation

e. Typically it occurs in a _____ in her _____.   woman; twenties

25

27. **The patient with an Adie pupil has a**   G7 p.832:45mm
   a. dilated or constricted pupil?   dilated
   b. due to impaired preganglionic fibers or postganglionic fibers?   postganglionic
   c. thought to be caused by a _____ _____   viral infection
   d. of the _____ _____   ciliary ganglion

■ Horner Syndrome

28. **Horner syndrome is caused by interruption of sympathetics to the eye and face anywhere along their path. Name specific causes that affect the following:**   G7 p.833:80mm
   a. first-order neurons (three causes)
      i. i _____   infarction from vascular occlusion (usually posterior inferior cerebellar artery)
      ii. s _____   syringobulbia
      iii. i _____ n _____   intraparenchymal neoplasm
   b. second-order neurons (three causes)
      i. l _____ s _____   lateral sympathectomies
      ii. s _____ c _____ t _____   significant chest trauma,
      iii. a _____ p _____ n _____ (P _____ t _____)   apical pulmonary neoplasms (Pancoast tumor)
   c. third-order neurons (five causes)
      i. n _____ t _____   neck trauma (e.g., carotid dissections)
      ii. c _____ v _____ d _____   carotid vascular disease
      iii. c _____ b _____ a _____   cervical bony abnormalities
      iv. m _____   migraine
      v. sk _____ -b _____ n _____   skull-base neoplasms

29. **The ptosis is due to paralysis of the _____ and _____ _____ muscles.**   superior and inferior tarsal   G7 p.833:80mm

30. **Is the ptosis complete or partial?**   partial   G7 p.833:80mm

31. **Enophthalmos is due to paralysis of M _____ muscle, which is or is not involved in Horner syndrome?**   Müller muscle; is involved   G7 p.833:89mm

32. **Trace the third-order neuron in the pupillodilation/sympathetic path. Neurons from the s _____ c _____ g _____ to the p _____ m _____ and M _____ m _____.**   superior cervical ganglion to the pupillodilator muscle and Müller muscle   G7 p.833:125mm

25

33. **True or False. Answer the following regarding Horner syndrome:**   G7 p.833:125mm

   a. In a patient with Horner syndrome and preserved sweating of the face, the lesion is located
      i. in the first-order neuron — false
      ii. in the second-order neuron — false
      iii. in the third-order neuron — true (Injured fibers on ICA produce Horner, intact sweat fibers to face on ECA.)

   b. This is compatible with a Pancoast tumor. — false (Pancoast tumor would affect the sympathetics between the spinal cord and superior cervical ganglion [i. e., second-order neurons]. The fibers to sweat glands would be damaged because they had not yet separated to travel with the ECA.)

34. **Complete the following about Horner syndrome:**   G7 p.833:160mm

   a. What medication is used if diagnosis of Horner syndrome is in doubt? — cocaine

   b. How does it work? — cocaine blocks norepinephrine (NE) reuptake

   c. Therefore in Horner syndrome the pupil will _____. — not dilate with cocaine (there is no NE release)

   d. In a normal patient the pupil will _____. — dilate normally

■ Extraocular Motor System

35. **Matching. From the list below identify the cranial nerve that innervates the muscle.**   G7 p.834:45mm

   Nerve:
   ① III; ② IV; ③ VI Hint: L6 SO4
   Muscle:
   a. medial rectus — ①
   b. inferior rectus — ①
   c. inferior oblique — ①
   d. superior rectus — ①
   e. superior oblique — ②
   f. lateral rectus — ③

36. **Complete the following regarding the frontal eye field:**   G7 p.834:52mm

   a. True or False. It moves eyes laterally to the opposite side. — true

   b. It is located in the Brodmann area _____. — 8

   c. Its fibers go through the _____ of the _____ _____. — genu of the internal capsule

d. It sends fibers to the ipsilateral _____ _____ _____ _____ nucleus.

paramedian pontine reticular formation (PPRF)

e. It sends fibers to the ipsilateral _____ nucleus

sixth

f. and the contralateral _____ nucleus

third

g. via the _____ _____ _____.

medial longitudinal fasciculus (MLF)

h. The right paramedian pontine reticular formation (PPRF) controls lateral eye movements to the _____.

right

37. Complete the following about the extraocular motor system:

G7 p.834:90mm

a. Injury to the medial longitudinal fasciculus (MLF) is called _____.

internuclear ophthalmoplegia (INO)

b. Convergence is _____ _____.

not impaired

c. If the right MLF is injured the right eye will not _____ _____.

move medially (adduct)

d. The left eye on looking laterally shows
  i. w_____ _____ a_____
  ii. n_____ or adduction.

weakness on abduction

nystagmus

e. The most common cause of MLF malfunction is _____ _____.

multiple sclerosis (MS)

38. Name three causes of non-pupil-sparing oculomotor palsy.
Hint: tau

G7 p.835:40mm

a. t_____

tumor

b. a_____

aneurysm (posterior communicating artery, basilar tip)

c. u_____

uncal herniation

39. Name seven causes of pupil-sparing oculomotor palsy.
Hint: mEtDacc

G7 p.835:100mm

a. m_____

myasthenia gravis

b. E_____

ETOH

c. t_____

temporal arteritis

d. D_____

DM

e. a_____

atherosclerosis

f. c_____ _____ _____

chronic progressive ophthalmoplegia

g. c_____ _____ _____

cavernous sinus lesions

40. Complete the following about trochlear nerve palsy (IV):

G7 p.835:160mm

a.
  i. In relation to the aqueduct the trochlear nucleus lies _____

ventral

  ii. At the level of the _____ _____

inferior colliculi

b.
  i. The axons pass _____

dorsally

  ii. Decussate _____

internally

c. It innervates the _____ _____ muscle

superior oblique

d. The superior oblique muscle
   i. Which primarily depresses the _____ eye? — adducted
   ii. In primary gaze it moves the eye _____ and _____. — down and out

41. Complete the following about the unique features of the trochlear nerve: G7 p.835:172mm
a. Nucleus is on the _____ side of the — opposite
b. muscle it goes to: _____ _____ _____. — superior oblique muscle
c. It is the only nerve to decussate _____. — internally
d. It is the only nerve to exit _____ to the brain stem. — posterior
e. True or false. It passes through the annulus of Zinn. — false
f. Palsy results in eye deviation _____ and _____. — up and in   G7 p.836:18mm
g. Head is tilted to the _____ _____ the IV palsy. — side opposite
h. Diplopia is exacerbated when looking _____ (i.e., _____). — down; stairs

42. Name the causes of abducens palsy.   G7 p.836:45mm
Hint: abducens
a. a_____ — arteritis, aneurysms
b. b_____ — sixth nerve palsy
c. d_____ — diabetes, Dorello canal (Gradenigo syndrome)
d. u_____ — uncontrolled ICP, pseudotumor, trauma, tumor
e. c_____ — cavernous sinus lesions, clivus, chordoma, or fracture
f. e_____ — eye disease, thyroid, myasthenia gravis
g. n_____ — neoplasms
h. s_____ — sphenoid sinusitis (Gradenigo syndrome)

43. Matching. Match the syndrome with the nerves involved in multiple extraocular motor involvement.   G7 p.836:125mm
Syndrome:
① cavernous sinus; ② superior orbital fissure; ③ orbital apex
Nerves involved:
a. II — ③
b. III — ①, ②, ③
c. IV — ①, ②, ③
d. V^1 — ①, ②, ③
e. V^2 — ①
f. V^3 —
g. VI — ①, ②, ③

25

Tolosa-Hunt Syndrome

44. **Is the ophthalmoplegia painful or painless?**

painful

G7 p.837:175mm

45. **Which nerve(s) is/are involved?**

any nerve traversing the cavernous sinus

G7 p.837:175mm

46. **The pupil is usually _____.**

spared

G7 p.837:175mm

47. **How long do symptoms last?**

days to weeks

G7 p.837:175mm

48. **Can there be spontaneous remission?**

yes

G7 p.837:175mm

49. **Can there be recurrent attacks?**

yes

G7 p.837:175mm

50. **Is there systemic involvement?**

no

G7 p.837:175mm

51. **How is it treated?**

systemic steroids = 60 to 80 mg prednisone by mouth daily (slow taper)

G7 p.837:175mm

52. **The disease is thought to be a _____ _____.**

nonspecific inflammation

G7 p.837:175mm

53. **The inflammation is located at the _____ _____ _____.**

superior orbital fissure

G7 p.837:175mm

54. **Complete the following about Raeder paratrigeminal neuralgia:**

G7 p.838:50mm

a. Name two components.

   i. u_____ o_____ p_____

   unilateral oculosympathetic paresis (think Horner syndrome—anhidrosis ± ptosis)

   ii. h_____ t_____ n_____ i_____

   homolateral trigeminal nerve involvement (Horner syndrome and tic-like pain)

b. The pupil is _____.

   small

c. True or False. The pain is continuous.

   false (intermittent, tic-like)

d. The pain is located at the_____.

   trigeminal nerve V^1 (ophthalmic division) and sympathetics

55. **Complete the following regarding Gradenigo syndrome:**

G7 p.838:85mm

a. Name the classic triad.

   i. p_____ of_____

   palsy; abducens

   ii. p_____ where? _____

   pain; retro-orbital

   iii. d_____ e_____

   draining ear

b. Pain is located at the p_____ a_____.

   petrous apex

25

56. **Complete the following about Gradenigo syndrome:**   G7 p.838:85mm

a. What is Gradenigo syndrome?   apical petrositis
b. Involves _____ canal   Dorello
c. Features
    i.   G_____   Gradenigo
    ii. r_____ _____   retro-orbital pain
    iii. a_____ _____   apical petrositis—abducens palsy
    iv. d_____ _____   draining ear—Dorello canal
    v.   e_____ _____   ear draining
    vi. n_____ _____ _____ neuropathy of VI
    vii. i_____   inflammation
    viii. p_____   petrositis
    ix. o_____ p_____   orbital pain

■ Miscellaneous Neuro-ophthalmologic Signs

57. **Complete the following about ocular bobbing:**   G7 p.838:165mm

a. The eyes move _____.   downward
b. How many times per minute?   2 to 12
c. Ocular bobbing is associated with bilateral paralysis of _____ _____.   horizontal gaze
d. It is seen with destruction of the _____ _____.   pontine tegmentum

58. **Optic atrophy is due to a _____ lesion.**   compressive   G7 p.839:45mm

25

26

Neurotology

■ Dizziness and Vertigo

1. What is the definition of vertigo?

G7 p.840:78mm

a. sensation of _____   movement (usually spinning)
b. from
   i.   i_____ e_____ d_____ or   inner ear dysfunction or
   ii.   v_____ n_____ d_____   vestibular nerve dysfunction

2. True or False. Inner ear dysfunction presenting with vertigo includes the following:

G7 p.840:82mm

a. labyrinthitis   true
b. trauma, i.e., e_____ l_____   true (i.e., endolymphatic leak)
c. drugs, i.e., a_____   true (i.e., aminoglycosides)
d. acoustic neuroma   false (Acoustic neuroma does not cause inner ear dysfunction but may cause vertigo from compression of the vestibular nerve.)
e. vertebrobasilar insufficiency   true (Other causes of vertigo include inner ear causes: Meniere disease, benign/paroxysmal positional vertigo, syphilis.)

3. Complete the following regarding cupulolithiasis:

G7 p.840:90mm

a. What is cupulolithiasis? c_____ c_____ in s_____ c_____   calcium concretions in semicircular canal
b. It is also known as b_____ p_____ v_____.   benign (paroxysmal) positional vertigo
c. Symptoms are made manifest by _____ _____.   head turning
d. Patient is usually in _____.   bed
e. Is it self-limiting?   yes
f. For how long?   usually not for > 1 year
g. Is hearing affected?   no hearing loss

4. Describe indications and complications of selective vestibular neurectomy (SVN). G7 p.841:40mm

a. Indications
  i. M_____ d_____   Meniere disease
  ii. p_____ v_____ i_____   partial vestibular injury
b. Rationale?   In disabling cases of vertigo,
                                        refractory to
                                        medical/nondestructive
                                        surgical treatment. SVN
                                        preserves hearing; is 90%
                                        (Meniere disease) and 80%
                                        (vertiginous spells) effective.

c. Complications
  i. h_____ l_____   hearing loss (unusual)
  ii. o_____   oscillopsia (Dandy syndrome)
  iii. l_____ of b_____ in the   loss of balance in the dark
       d_____   with bilateral SVN

5. Answer the following about the vestibular nerve: G7 p.841:117mm

a. In which half of the eighth nerve   superior
   complex?
b. What color relative to the cochlear more gray
   nerve?
c. To preserve hearing what vessel must be artery of the auditory canal
   preserved?

6. True or False. CN VII can be differentiated from CN VIII at the internal auditory canal (IAC) by all of the following: G7 p.841:122mm

a. direct stimulation/recording   true
b. lies anterior/superior to VIII   true
c. transverse crest and Bill bar   true
d. darker color c/w CN VIII   false (CN VII is paler/whiter
                                         than CN VIII)
e. electromyographic (EMG) monitoring of true
   CN VII during manipulation

26

■ Meniere Disease

7. What is the clinical triad of Meniere disease? G7 p.842:33mm

a. v_____ v_____ a_____   violent vertigo attacks
b. t_____   tinnitus "escaping steam"
c. h_____ l_____   fluctuating *low*-frequency
                                        hearing loss

8. Meniere disease is also known as e_____ h_____. endolymphatic hydrops   G7 p.842:46mm

9. **True or False. Treatment of Meniere disease includes**
G7 p.843:23mm
   a. middle ear perfusion with gentamicin — true
   b. bilateral vestibular neurectomy — false (Bilateral ablative procedure is to be avoided.)
   c. salt restriction — true
   d. vestibular suppressants (e.g., Valium) — true
   e. endolymphatic shunting — true

■ Facial Nerve Palsy

10. **Segments of the facial nerve include**
    Hint: see my little tin man
G7 p.844:30mm
   a. c_____ — cisternal
   b. m_____ — meatal
   c. l_____ — labyrinthine
   d. t_____ — tympanic
   e. m_____ — mastoid

11. **Answer the following about supranuclear facial palsy:**
G7 p.844:55mm
   a. Which part of the face is involved? — lower only
   b. Emotional facial expression is _____. — intact
   c. The lesion is in the lowest part of the _____ _____. — precentral gyrus
   d. Part of the face is spared paralysis because the _____ _____ has _____ _____. — upper face; bilateral representation

12. **True or False. The following is correct regarding central facial palsy (supranuclear facial palsy):**
G7 p.844:55mm
   a. confined to lower face — true
   b. spares emotional facial expression — true
   c. lesion in most inferior opercular portion of precentral gyrus — true
   d. upper face has bilateral representation — true

26

13. **Complete the following regarding nuclear facial palsy:**
G7 p.844:80mm
   a. It causes paralysis of all _____ _____ _____ muscles. — ipsilateral CN VII innervated
   b. It plus sixth nerve palsy constitutes the _____-_____ syndrome. — Millard-Gubler
   c. It can be caused by a particular tumor called _____ — medulloblastoma
   d. especially when it _____ the _____ of the _____ _____. — invades the floor of the fourth ventricular
   e. True or False. Nuclear facial palsy is due to damage to the motor nucleus at the pontomedullary junction. — true

14. **True or False. Regarding CN VII anatomy:**

G7 p.844:100mm

a. enters superior-anterior portion of IAC — true
b. external genu is geniculate ganglion — true
c. GSPN first branch after the ganglion — true
d. exits at stylomastoid foramen — true

15. **Complete the following about the seventh nerve:**

G7 p.844:100mm

a. It exits the brain stem at the _____ _____. — pontomedullary junction

b. It enters the internal auditory canal at the _____ _____. — superoanterior portion

c. The geniculate ganglion is located in the _____ bone. — temporal

d. The first branch is the _____ _____ _____ _____ — greater superficial petrosal nerve

e. which goes to the _____ _____ — pterygopalatine ganglion
f. and innervates the _____ _____. — lacrimal gland—dry eye and nasal mucosa if injured

g. The next branch goes to the _____. — stapedius muscle—to ear—hyperacusis

h. The next branch is the _____ _____. — chorda tympani—taste

i. It then exits the s_____ f_____ — stylomastoid foramen
j. and sends branches to the _____. — face

16. **Name the facial nerve branches within the temporal bone and their function.**

G7 p.844:115mm

a. g_____ — greater superficial petrosal nerve (GSPN) to pterygopalatine ganglion, innervates nasal and palatine mucosa and lacrimal gland

b. s_____ — branch to stapedius muscle, volume regulation

c. c_____ — chorda tympani, taste sensation from anterior two thirds of tongue

d. fibers to s_____ g_____ — salivary glands, submandibular, sublingual

e. The nerve travels on to _____ _____. — facial muscles

17. **Name the facial nerve branches to the facial muscles cranial to caudal.**

G7 p.844:135mm

a. t_____ — temporal
b. z_____ — zygomatic
c. b_____ — buccal
d. m_____ — mandibular
e. c_____ — cervical

26

18. **Name the three most common causes** | G7 p.844:155mm
    of facial nerve palsy.
    a. B_____   Bell palsy
    b. h_____   herpes zoster oticus
    c. t_____   trauma/basal skull fracture

19. **Study Chart. Provide the differential** | G7 p.844:155mm
    diagnosis for facial nerve palsy.   facial nerve palsy
                                              acoustic tumor
                                              Bell—birth
                                              congenital
                                              diabetes
                                              fracture
                                              Guillain-Barré
                                              herpes zoster
                                              Klippel-Feil
                                              Lyme disease
                                              meningioma
                                              neoplasm
                                              otitis media
                                              parotid surgery
                                              sarcoid
                                              trauma

20. **Describe seventh nerve palsy.** | G7 p.845:80mm
    a. The most common cause of facial palsy   Bell palsy
       is _____ _____.
    b. Etiology: _____   unknown
    c. Probable etiology: v_____ i_____   viral inflammatory
       d_____ p_____   demyelinating polyneuritis
    d. It is caused by the _____ _____   herpes simplex
       virus.
    e. It progresses _____ _____   distally to proximally
       _____.
    f. Meaning
       i.   first   facial movements weak
       ii. then   loss of taste and salivation
       iii. and then   hyperacusis
       iv. and then   decreased tearing
    g. Percent that recover completely is   75 to 80%; 10%
       _____%; partially _____%.
    h. Manage with _____ and _____.   EMG and steroids

21. **Answer the following regarding Bell** | G7 p.845115mm
    palsy:
    a. What often precedes Bell palsy?   a viral syndrome
    b. What is the usual sequence of clinical
       findings? List in order:
       ① decreased tearing; ② hyperacusis;   ③, ④, ②, ①
       ③ facial muscle weakness; ④ loss of
       taste
    c. What treatment is recommended?   steroids

26

22. **What are the considerations for facial nerve injury surgical repair?**

G7 p.846:180mm

  a. if known to be interrupted _____   reanastomose early
  b. if known to be in continuity _____   several months of observation

  c. role of electrical testing _____   serial electrical testing after 1 week

---

■ Hearing Loss

23. **Describe the following about hearing loss:**

G7 p.848:40mm

  a. conductive
       i.   speech   normal or low volume
       ii. Rinne   air less than bone = negative (i.e., abnormal)
       iii. Weber lateralizes to _____ _____ side   poor hearing

  b. sensorineural
       i.   speech   loud
       ii. Rinne   air more than bone = positive (i.e., normal)
       iii. Weber lateralizes to _____ _____ side   good hearing

27

Head Trauma

■ Concussion

G7 p.850:42mm

1. True or False. The determination of concussion requires

a. loss of consciousness from closed head injury

false

b. brain swelling on computed tomography (CT) of the head

false

c. altered consciousness as a result of a closed head injury

true (The definition of concussion only requires altered consciousness after closed head injury. The other findings may be associated but are not definitive.)

d. nausea and vomiting after being hit in the head

false

G7 p.850:103mm

2. Complete the following about second impact syndrome:

a. List the known biochemical derangements caused by brain trauma-concussion. (Hint: acdefghi)

   i. a_____
   ii. c_____
   iii. d_____
   iv. e_____
   v. f_____
   vi. g_____
   vii. h_____
   viii. i_____

ATP:ADP ratio
calcium overloading
dysfunction of mitochondria
energy disturbances
fluxes of ions
glutamate release
hyperglycolysis
impaired oxidative metabolism
NAA: N-glutamate

b. can assess by measuring _____

c. restores after approximately _____ days

7 to 10

27

3. **Complete the following about concussion:**   G7 p.850:103mm
    a. In concussion what brain chemical changes in concentration?   glutamate
    b. Does it go up or down?   up
    c. What mechanism becomes impaired?   cerebral autoregulation
    d. It may predispose to m_____ c_____ e_____   malignant cerebral edema
    e. and make the patient susceptible to s_____ i_____ s_____.   second impact syndrome (SIS)

4. **True or False. The hyperglycolytic, hypermetabolic state associated with concussion can last for**   G7 p.850:108mm
    a. 0 hours (it doesn't occur)   false
    b. 2 to 4 hours   false
    c. 24 to 48 hours   false
    d. 5 to 7 days   false
    e. 7 to 10 days   true

5. **Complete the following for each grade of head injury as classified by the American Academy of Neurology (AAN) System:**   G7 p.850:175mm
    a. mild
        i.   loss of consciousness (LOC)   no
        ii. symptoms last for   less than 15 minutes
    b. moderate
        i.   LOC   no
        ii. symptoms last for   greater than 15 minutes
    c. severe
        i.   LOC   any
        ii. symptoms last for   even briefly

6. **True or False. The second impact syndrome (SIS)**   G7 p.851:15mm
    a. is rare   true
    b. requires two head injuries   true
    c. results from cerebral edema   true
    d. is responsible for the policy that "no symptomatic player plays"   true
    e. can have severe consequences   true

7. **Complete the following regarding SIS:**   G7 p.851:140mm
    a. SIS has a mortality of _____%.   50 to 100% (Second impact syndrome [SIS] mortality occurs in athletes who sustain a second head injury while still symptomatic from an earlier injury. They usually walk off the field, then deteriorate into a coma within minutes.)
    b. What treatment is effective for SIS?   none—condition may be refractory to all treatment

27

8. **True or False. When should a player return to the game after a mild concussion?** G7 p.851:88mm
   a. never (The player should leave the game.)   false
   b. only after resolution of symptoms   true
   c. only after CT shows no injury   false
   d. only after being able to walk or run without difficulty   false (A symptomatic patient should not return to competition.)

9. **With the indicated number and type of multiple concussions, when is a return to competition recommended?** G7 p.852:56mm
   a. 2 mild _____   1 week
   b. 2 moderate _____   1 month and CT
   c. 3 mild _____   consider season ending and CT
   d. 3 moderate _____   season ending
   e. 2 severe _____   season ending

10. **Answer the following about multiple sports related mild concussions:** G7 p.852:10mm
    a. How many mild concussions before an athlete should be told to discontinue for the season?   3
    b. What else should be done?   CT or MRI is recommended as well after 3 mild concussions

■ Neuroimaging

11. **Answer the following about head injury:** G7 p.853:155mm
    a. What percentage of patients with significant head injury (GCS ≤ 8) has spine injury?   4 to 5%
    b. Most injuries occur at levels _____.   C1-C3

12. **The criteria for diffuse head injury grades are the following:** G7 p.854:15mm
    a. Grade I
       i.   cisterns   open
       ii. shift   0
       iii. hemorrhage   0
       iv. mortality   10%
    b. Grade II
       i.   cisterns   open
       ii. shift   0 to 5 mm
       iii. hemorrhage   5 cc
       iv. mortality   14%
    c. Grade III
       i.   cisterns   compressed/absent
       ii. shift   0 to 5 mm
       iii. hemorrhage   > 25 cc
       iv. mortality   34%

27

d. Grade IV
    i.   cisterns   compressed/absent
    ii.   shift   > 5 mm
    iii. hemorrhage   > 25 cc
    iv.   mortality   56%

13. **True or False. Hypotension is rarely**   G7 p.854:55mm
     attributable to head injury except in
     the following circumstances:
     a. in extremis   true (terminal stages;
                                      dysfunction of the medulla)
     b. in infants   true (in infancy, where
                                      enough blood can be lost
                                      intracranially or into the
                                      subgaleal space to cause
                                      shock)
     c. massive scalp wounds   true (when enough blood has
                                      been lost from the scalp
                                      wounds to cause
                                      hypovolemia and
                                      hypotension)
     d. head injury and pelvic fracture   false (The head injury is
                                      incidental to the hypotension.
                                      Each fracture in the pelvis can
                                      be responsible for 1 L blood
                                      loss.)

14. **Complete the following:**   G7 p.854:55mm
     a. Delayed deterioration after head trauma   15%
         (i.e., talk and die) occurs in what percent
         of patients?
     b. List the usual causes.
         i.   i_____ h_____   intracranial hematoma (75%
                                      [epidural hematoma,
                                      subdural hematoma,
                                      traumatic contusions])
         ii.   e_____   edema
         iii. s_____   seizures
         iv.   h_____   hydrocephalus

15. **What are the two types of**   G7 p.852:165mm
     posttraumatic brain swelling?
     a. H_____   hyperemia
         i.   Blood volume is _____.   increased
         ii.   Autoregulation is _____.   lost
         iii. It is also known as _____.   malignant cerebral edema
         iv.   Mortality is close to _____%.   100%
     b. T_____ c_____ e_____   true cerebral edema
         i.   At autopsy _____ _____   brain seeps fluid
               _____.
         ii.   It combines both _____ plus   vasogenic plus cytotoxic
               _____ _____.   edema

16. **Complete the following about diffuse axonal injury (DAI):**   G7 p853 :35mm
   a. Due to r_____ acceleration/deceleration head injury   rotational
   b. Hemorrhagic foci occur in the
      i. c_____ c_____   corpus callosum
      ii. d_____ r_____ brain stem   dorsolateral rostral
   c.
      i. Consider if CT is essentially _____   normal
      ii. And loss of consciousness lasts more than _____ hours   6
      iii. Following h_____ i_____   head injury

■ Transfer of Trauma Patients

17. **Pretransfer assessments include**   G7 p.855:17mm
   a. A_____   ABG
   b. B_____   BP
   c. c_____   circulation Hgb Hct
   d. D_____   Dilantin levels
   e. e_____   electrolytes
   f. f_____   fever
   g. _____   spine x-rays

■ Neurosurgical Exam in Trauma

18. **Complete the following:**   G7 p.855:175mm
   a. Children who receive trauma to the back of their head can develop _____,   transient blindness
   b. which can last _____.   1 to 2 days

19. **Complete the following about examining a flaccid limb:**   G7 p.856:115mm
   a. Preserved reflexes indicates _____.   central nervous system injury
   b. Absent reflexes indicates _____.   root or nerve injury

20. **Complete the following:**   G7 p.857:140mm
   a. The percentage of patients with minor head injury who have findings on CT is _____%.   8 to 46%
   b. The most common finding is _____ _____.   hemorrhagic contusion

21. **A patient has a deteriorating neurological exam with a dilated pupil. The CT scanner is unavailable. The operating room (OR) is ready now. You decide to place a burr hole. On which side do you place the burr hole?**   ipsilateral to a blown pupil (This will be on the correct side in > 85% of epidurals and other extraaxial mass lesions.)   G7 p.858:32mm

27

22. Complete the following: G7 p.858:65mm

a. Comparing frontal and occipital skull   occipital
   fracture which is associated with a higher
   risk of intracranial injury?

b. Why?

   i.   Facial bones and _____ absorb   sinuses
        frontal impact.

   ii. Contrecoup against _____   frontotemporal bones
        _____ is more harmful.

   iii. Arms _____.   can't protect oneself with
                                                 outstretched arms as when
                                                 falling forward

■ Radiographic Evaluation

23. Extraaxial hematoma evacuation   greater than 1 cm thick   G7 p.858:115mm
(i.e., subdural or epidural) is indicated
when blood collection is _____.

24. True or False. The most common cause   G7 p.858:135mm
of subarachnoid hemorrhage is

a. aneurysm   false
b. trauma   true
c. dural arteriovenous fistulas   false
d. spontaneous   false

25. Intraventricular hemorrhage (IVH) is   G7 p.858:156mm
present in what percentage of severe
head injuries?

a. percent   10%
b. correlates with   poor outcome

26. Complete the following: G7 p.859:20mm

a. The term *diastasis* means _____.   separation
b. If diastasis of a suture occurs is it   yes
   considered a fracture?

27. Matching. After a head injury which   G7 p.859:40mm
test is appropriate for the following   Also
conditions?   G7 p.859:4135mm
                                                                            Also
                                                                            G7 p.860:18mm

Test:
① skull x-ray; ② CT scan; ③ MRI
Conditions:

a. GCS below 14   ②
b. CT unavailable   ①
c. search for DAI   ③
d. amnesia for injury   ②
e. signs of basal skull fracture   ②
f. inebriation   ②

27

■ ER Management Specifics

28. **Complete the following:**
G7 p.860:105mm
G7 p.860:118mm

a. What antiemetic is appropriate for the head injury patient? — Tigan

b. IV fluid consists of _____. — normal saline and 20 mEq KCl

c. The rate is _____. — 100 cc/hr

d. Do we run the patient dry? — no, that is obsolete

29. **True or False. Routine usage of paralytics in trauma patients may**
G7 p.860:170 mm

a. cause Guillain-Barré syndrome — false

b. lead to higher incidence of pneumonia and sepsis — true

c. cause syndrome of inappropriate antidiuretic hormone secretion (SIADH) — false

d. cause increased intensive care unit (ICU) stay — true

30. **Complete the following regarding hyperventilation:**
G7 p.861:105mm

a. It may exacerbate cerebral _____. — ischemia

b. True or False. It may be used prophylactically. — false

c. PCO_2 must never go below _____ mm Hg. — 30 mm Hg

d. Hyperventilation reduces _____. — cerebral blood flow

e. It does not necessarily reduce _____. — when $PCO_2 < 30$ mmHg

f. Hyperventilation may cause _____, — alkalosis

g. which increases protein binding of _____, — calcium

h. which can result in hypo_____ — calcemia

i. and show up clinically as _____. — tetany

31. **What conditions are associated with increased risk of posttraumatic seizures?**
Hint: a to i
G7 p.862:125mm

27

a. a_____ — alcohol abuse

b. b_____ — brain injury

c. c_____ — cortical contusion

d. d_____ — depressed skull fracture

e. e_____ — epidural hematoma

f. f_____ — fracture of skull

g. G_____ — Glasgow coma scale < 10

h. h_____ — hematoma

i. i_____ — injured brain

32. **True or False. The following conditions are associated with increased risk of posttraumatic seizures:**   G7 p.862:126mm
   a. acute subdural, epidural, or intracerebral hematoma   true
   b. open depressed skull fracture with parenchymal injury   true
   c. seizure within 24 hours after injury   true
   d. GCS < 10   true
   e. penetrating brain injury   true
   f. history of significant alcohol abuse   true
   g. cortical (hemorrhagic) contusion on CT   true

■ Head-Injured Patients with Associated Severe Systemic Injuries

33. **What is considered hypotension or hypoxia?**   G7 p.863:20mm
   a. blood pressure (BP) below _____   90 mm Hg
   b. PCO$_2$ below _____   60 mm Hg

34. **What chemical in the brain predisposes the head injury patient to disseminated intravascular coagulopathy (DIC)?**   thromboplastin   G7 p.863:60mm

35. **Complete the following:**   G7 p.863:125mm
   a. Visual system injury occurs in _____% of head injury patients.   5%
   b. Can hypopituitarism occur with head injury?   yes

36. **The optic nerve can be divided into four segments.**   G7 p.863:135mm
   a. Give the names and the length of each segment.
      i. segment 1 name _____, length _____   intraocular, 1 mm
      ii. segment 2 name _____, length _____   intraorbital, 25 to 30 mm
      iii. segment 3 name _____, length _____   intracanalicular, 10 mm
      iv. segment 4 name _____, length _____   intracranial, 10 mm
   b. Which segment is most commonly damaged with closed head injury?   intracanalicular segment

27

■ Exploratory Burr Holes

37. A unilateral blown pupil is on the same side of an epidural hematoma or other extraaxial mass lesion what percent of the time?

> 85%

G7 p.865:20mm

38. Complete the following regarding burr hole placement for dilated pupil:

G7 p.865:135mm

a. In cases where no CT scan can be done, list the placement for
   i.   burr hole #1   temporal ipsilateral
   ii. burr hole #2   temporal contralateral
   iii. burr hole #3   frontal ipsilateral
   iv. burr hole #4   parietal
   v.   burr hole #5   posterior fossa
b. How often were these positive?   56%
c. When positive the first burr hole was positive in _____%.   86%

■ Intracranial Pressure and Head Trauma

39. What is the relation between the intracranial pressure (ICP) and the cerebral perfusion pressure (CPP)?

G7 p.866:140mm

a. Formula

CPP = MAP* - ICP (cerebral perfusion pressure is the mean arterial pressure minus the intracranial pressure)

b. If your computer does not give you mean arterial pressure (MAP) how can you calculate it? (Hint: dds/3)

*MAP = 1 systolic plus 2 diastolic divided by 3

40. Answer the following:

G7 p.866:167mm

a. What is the normal CPP in adults?   > 50 mm Hg
b. What is the recommended CPP in head trauma?   > 60 mm Hg
c. If CPP is kept in good range is ICP above 20 mm Hg well tolerated?   no, it is detrimental

41. Complete the following:

G7 p.867:15mm

a. The modified _____ hypothesis states that   Monro-Kellie
b. the sum of the intracranial volumes of _____, _____, and _____   blood, brain, and CSF
c. and other components is _____.   constant
d. An increase in any one must be _____   offset
e. by an equal _____ in another   decrease
f. or else _____ will rise.   pressure
g. Pressure is _____ _____ throughout the intracranial cavity.   distributed evenly

27

42. **Complete the following:**   G7 p.868:50mm
    a. At what level of ICP do we treat   20 or greater
        intracranial (IC) hypertension (HTN)?
    b. What is the mortality rate for those   20%
        whose ICP is kept below 20 mm Hg?
    c. If ICP is higher mortality is _____.   also much higher

43. **What is considered a "deadly" ICP**   above 25 to 30 mm Hg   G7 p.868:80mm
    (i.e., likely to be fatal if not
    controlled)?

44. **CT finding may be correlated with a**   G7 p.868:84mm
    risk of intracranial hypertension.
    a. After a closed head injury, what % of   60%
        patients with abnormal CT will have
        intracranial hypertension?
    b. What % of patients with normal CT will   13%
        have intracranial hypertension?
    c. Give three risk factors for intracranial
        hypertension for patients with normal
        CT.
        i.   age above _____   40 years
        ii. blood pressure below _____   90 mm Hg
        iii. neurological status   decerebration/decortication
    d. With normal CT plus two risk factors   60%
        _____% will have ICP elevation.
    e. With normal CT plus only one risk factor   4%
        _____% will have ICP elevation.

■ ICP Monitoring

45. **Complete the following about ICP**   G7 p.868:130mm
    monitoring:
    a. One of the criteria for placement of an   8
        ICP monitor is a Glasgow coma scale
        (GCS) score below _____
    b. and a CT that is _____, or two of the abnormal
        following:
        i.   age above _____   40
        ii. systolic blood pressure (SBP) below   90
             _____
        iii. motor exam shows _____ or   decerebrate or decorticate
             _____ _____   posturing
    c. may discontinue monitor when ICP is   48 to 72 hours
        normal for _____ to _____ hours

46. **Complete the following about ICP**   G7 p.869:75mm
    monitoring:
    a. A criterion for discontinuing ICP   48 to 72 hours
        monitoring is normal ICP for _____ to
        _____ hours.
    b. Risk of hemorrhage from ICP monitor
        placement is
        i.   _____% requiring surgery and   0.5 to 2.5   G7 p.869:105mm
        ii. _____% incidental finding   1.4

27

47. **True or False. In regard to ICP monitoring, it is permissible to**   G7 p.869:145mm
 a. use antibiotics — true
 b. not use antibiotics — true
 c. place monitor in ICU — true
 d. place monitor in OR — true
 e. Patients who develop hemorrhage while ICP is being placed is 1.4%. — true

48. **Complete the following:**   G7 p.869:175mm
 a. Is the prophylactic change of external ventricular drain 5 days or less after insertion associated with a significant reduction in infection rates? — no
 b. Do we need to change the site every 5 days? — no

49. **Complete the following regarding conversion of mm Hg and cm H$_2$O:**   G7 p.870:160mm
 a. 1 mm Hg equals _____ cm of H$_2$O — 1.36 cm
 b. 1 cm H$_2$O equals _____ mm of Hg — 0.735 mm
 c. External auditory canal correlates with what intracranial structure? — foramen of Monro   G7 p.871:50mm

50. **Lundberg A waves are defined by**   G7 p.872:130mm
 a. ICP of _____ — > 50 mm Hg
 b. duration of _____ — 5 to 20 minutes
 c. plus _____ — increase in MAP

51. **Lundberg B waves are defined by**   G7 p.872:150mm
 a. ICP of _____ — 10 to 20 mm Hg
 b. duration of _____ — 30 seconds to 2 minutes
 c. varies with _____ — periodic respiration

52. **Regarding IVC problems, when open to drain, pressure reading from transducer is _____ _____.** — not meaningful   G7 p.873:150mm

53. **True or False. If an external ventricular catheter no longer functions, all of the following can be performed safely:**   G7 p.874:30mm
 a. lower drip nozzle — true
 b. verify clamps are open and air filter is dry — true
 c. flush distal tubing with saline — true
 d. flush IVC with up to 5 mL of saline under gentle pressure — false (Up to 1.5 mL of preservative-free saline can be used.)

54. **True or False. Possible causes of an ICP wave form that is dampened include all of the following:**   G7 p.874:65mm
 a. occlusion of the catheter proximal to the transducer — true
 b. catheter pulled out of ventricle — true
 c. collapsed ventricle — true
 d. air in the system — true
 e. intracranial hypertension — false

27

55. **What should happen to the ICP wave form in a patient with a decompressive craniectomy?** It should be dampened. G7 p.874:88mm

56. **Answer the following about arteriojugular venous oxygen content differences:** G7 p.874:145mm

   a. True or False. In head trauma the following arteriojugular venous difference in oxygen content ($AVDO_2$) difference indicates global cerebral ischemia and cerebral hyperemia, respectively:

   i. > 9 mL/dL, < 4 mL/dL true (With ischemia, the brain is oxygen starved, so more oxygen is extracted and the difference in O_2 between the arterial and venous blood is greater. The opposite is true in hyperemia.)

   ii. < 4 mL/dL, > 9 mL/dL false

   iii. > 12 mL/dL, < 6 mL/dL false

   iv. < 6 mL/dL, > 12 mL/dL false

   b. Another term for cerebral hyperemia is _____ _____. luxury perfusion

57. **Complete the following about brain tissue oxygen tension (pBtO$_2$):** G7 p.874:165mm

   a. Treatment threshold is pBtO$_2$ less than _____ mmHg. 15

   b. Death occurs with brief drop below _____ mm Hg. 6

   c.

   i. Level of less than _____ mm Hg 10

   ii. For more than _____ minutes increases the risk of bad outcome 30

   d. A probe should be placed in a patient with G7 p.874:182mm

   i. traumatic brain injury on the _____ _____ side least injured

   ii. subarachnoid hemorrhage near _____ vasospasm

   iii. intracerebral hemorrhage near the _____ hematoma

27

■ ICP Treatment Measures

58. **True or False. All of the following are general goals of ICP management:**   G7 p.877:18mm
   a. keep ICP < 20 mm Hg — true   G7 p.877:62mm
   b. keep CPP > 60 mm Hg (used to be > 70 mm Hg) — true   G7 p.877:125mm
   c. avoid SBP < 90 mm Hg — true
   d. avoid PO_2 < 60 mm Hg — true
   e. keep PCO_2 < 30 mm Hg — false (PCO_2 should be brought down below 30 mm Hg only in an acute ICP crisis and then only briefly.)

59. **True or False. The contraindications for administration of mannitol are the following:**   G7 p.877:100mm
   a. hypovolemia — true
   b. hypotension — true
   c. serum osmol > 320 — true
   d. cerebral infarction — false
   e. ICP < 20 mm Hg — true

60. **Complete the following about ICP treatment measures:**   G7 p.878:90mm
   a. Which antacid should be avoided if the patient is receiving phenytoin? — cimetidine
   b. Why? — drug—drug interaction
   c. What occurs? — dramatic elevation of drug concentration
   d. Due to? — inhibition of hepatic cytochrome oxidase
   e. The best choice may be _____. — sucralfate (Carafate)

61. **True or False. Fever should be controlled aggressively in the setting of elevated ICP.** — true   G7 p.878:100mm

27

62. **True or False. In traumatic brain injury, the following statements are correct:**   G7 p.878:120mm
   a. Pressors (e.g., dopamine) should be avoided because there is increased risk of hemorrhage. — false (The blood pressure should be maintained with pressors, if necessary.)
   b. The IV fluid of choice is isotonic saline + 20 mEq KCl/L. — true
   c. If mannitol is required the patient should be kept slightly hypovolemic to allow the serum osmolality to rise. — false (Hypovolemia decreases cerebral blood flow and may elevate ICP through autoregulatory cerebral vasodilation.)
   d. The patient's temperature is not important. — false

63. **Answer the following:**   G7 p.878:118mm
  a. Is it okay to use lactated Ringer solution   no
     for head injury patients?
  b. Why or why not?   it is hypotonic

64. **True or False. IV fluids in the head-**   G7 p.878:130mm
     injured patient
  a. should be sufficient to avoid   true
     hypotension.
  b. should be limited to "run the patient   false
     dry."
  c. Euvolemia should be maintained even if   true
     mannitol is required.

65. **True or False. The following can**   G7 p.879:14mm
     exacerbate intracranial hypertension:
  a. hyperglycemia   true (makes edema worse)
  b. hyperventilation   false
  c. hyperparathyroidism   false
  d. cholestasis   false

66. **Complete the following about the use**   G7 p.879:98mm
     of mannitol:
  a. Useful for intracranial   hypertension
  b.
     i. Usual dose advised is   0.25 to 1
         _____ gm/kg
     ii. Infused as a _____   bolus
     iii. Over _____ minutes   20
  c.
     i. This is followed by _____ gm/kg   0.25
     ii. Infused over _____ minutes   20
  d. If ICP remains over _____   20
  e. Must cease use if serum osmolarity rises   320
     above _____ mOsm/L

67. **True or False. Second-tier therapy for**   G7 p.880:15mm
     persistent intracranial hypertension
     includes all of the following:
  a. high-dose barbiturate therapy   true
  b. hyperventilation   true
  c. hypothermia   true
  d. decompressive craniectomy   true

68. **True or False. Hypothermia as a**   G7 p.880:25mm
     "second tier" therapy for persistent IC
     HTN may be associated with all of the
     following:
  a. decreased cardiac index   true
  b. thrombocytopenia   true
  c. elevated creatinine clearance   true
  d. seizures   false (Seizures are more apt
                                                  to occur with fever, not
                                                  hypothermia.)
  e. pancreatitis   true

27

69. **To treat refractory increased ICP a decompressive craniectomy**
G7 p.880:35mm
a. must be at least _____ cm in diameter   12 cm
b. should include a _____   duraplasty

70. **Complete the following:**
G7 p.880:65mm
a. True or False. In decompressive surgery for head injury, the following set of values describes the appropriate limits of temporal tip resection for the dominant and nondominant temporal lobes, respectively:
   i.   1 to 2 cm, 3 to 4 cm   false
   ii. 2 to 4 cm, 8 to 10 cm   false
   iii. 4 to 5 cm, 6 to 7 cm   true
   iv. 6 to 8 cm, 10 to 12 cm   false
   v. 0 cm, 4 to 5 cm   false
b. What other lobectomy may be performed?   frontal lobectomy
c. Are these very helpful?   they have shown no great therapeutic promise

71. **Complete the following about PCO_2:**
G7 p.881:82mm
a. Normocarbia is between _____ and _____ mm Hg.   35 to 40
b. Usual hyperventilation range is between _____ and _____ mm Hg.   30 to 35
c.
   i.   This will reduce ICP by _____ to _____%   25 to 30%
   ii. in about _____ seconds   30
   iii. and will last for _____ minutes.   5 to 20
d. A level of PCO_2 below _____ mm Hg risks ischemia.   30

72. **Complete the following about PCO_2 in the head-injured patient:**
G7 p.881:95mm
a. Normocarbia is considered to be _____ mm Hg.   35 to 40 mm Hg—use routinely
b. Hyperventilation to PCO_2 of _____ mm Hg.   30 to 35 mm Hg—brief use only

73. **True or False. When using mannitol it is best to**
G7 p.882:23mm
a. use intermittent bolus   true
b. use continuous infusion   false
c. use doses of 3g/kg   false
d. avoid hypotension below 90 systolic   true
e. maintain euvolemia   true
f. monitor serum osmolality   true
g. limit serum osmolality to below 320mOsm/L   true

27

74. **True or False. Mannitol lowers the ICP within a few minutes of administration by**

G7 p.882:47mm

a. decreasing the production of cerebrospinal fluid (CSF)

false

b. reducing the hematocrit and blood viscosity

true (The rapid effect of mannitol is not explained by an osmotic effect. Instead, mannitol increases the intravascular volume and lowers the hematocrit, thus lowering the blood viscosity. The brain responds to the increased blood flow through autoregulatory vasoconstriction, decreasing the volume of the intravascular blood compartment in the brain and lowering the ICP.)

c. causing an immediate diuresis and decrease in the intravascular volume

false

d. raising the serum osmolarity to establish an osmotic gradient between the blood and brain

false (Osmotic effect takes 15 to 30 minutes.)

75. **Mannitol works by two mechanisms.**

G7 p.882:69mm

a. Mechanism I

   i. This is a rapid mechanism that _____ _____ _____ by _____,

increases plasma volume by dilution

   ii. which improves _____

rheology

   iii. thereby improving _____ and _____ delivery,

CBF and O_2

   iv. which produces _____.

vasoconstriction

b. Mechanism II

   i. This is a slower _____ _____.

osmotic effect

   ii. Hypertonic plasma draws in _____ _____

edema fluid

   iii. from the _____,

brain

   iv. which takes _____ to _____ minutes to begin.

15 to 30

76. **The protocol for mannitol administration is**

G7 p.882:100mm

a. bolus

   i. dose _____ per kilogram

1 gram

   ii. infuse over _____ minutes

30 (rapidly)

   iii. onset _____ minutes

1 to 5

   iv. peaks _____ minutes

20 to 60

b. long term

   i. dose _____ per kilogram

0.25 to 0.50 gram

   ii. infuse over _____ minutes

30 to 60

77. **True or False.**   G7 p.882:115mm

  a. Administer mannitol best as a bolus.   true

  b. Administer mannitol best as a   false
     continuous drip.

  c. A continuous drip aggravates vasogenic   true
     edema.

  d. It is better to stop mannitol by tapering   true
     the dose.

  e. It is better to stop mannitol when it is no   false
     longer needed.

  f. Taper prevents rebound.   true   G7 p.882:128mm

78. **Three drugs used in the same patient**   G7 p.882:130mm
can produce a fatal syndrome.

  a. Name the three medications.
     (Hint: Dms)

     i.   D_____   Dilantin

     ii.   m_____   mannitol

     iii.   s_____   steroids

  b. Name the syndrome: h_____   hyperosmolar nonketotic
     n_____ s_____   state

79. **What is the mechanism of renal injury**   acute tubular necrosis   G7 p.882:143mm
associated with mannitol therapy for
high ICP (serum Osm > 320 mOsm/L)?

80. **True or False. Glucocorticoids have**   true (at least not at the doses   G7 p.883:97mm
little impact on cytotoxic cerebral   that have been tried)
edema due to head trauma.

81. **True or False. Steroids are not**   G7 p.883:107mm
recommended to treat patients with
traumatic brain injury because

  a. they work on vasogenic edema of   true
     tumors.

  b. they do not work on cytotoxic edema of   true
     traumatic brain injury (TBI).

  c. they have significant side effects.   true

  d. they increase the incidence of

     i.   coagulopathies   true

     ii.   hyperglycemia   true

     iii.   infection   true

     iv.   hypotension   false

■ High-Dose Barbiturate Therapy

82. **True or False. Theoretical benefits of**   G7 p.883:158mm
barbiturates in head injury include the
following:

  a. vasoconstriction in normal areas   true

  b. decreased metabolic demand   true

  c. free radical scavenging   true

  d. reduced intracellular calcium   true

  e. reduced extracellular calcium   false

  f. stabilized lysosomal activity   true

27

83.   True or False.

a.   When using pentobarbital for ICP control, the limiting factor is systemic hypertension.

false (Hypotension due to reduction of sympathetic tone is the limiting factor.)

b.   In those patients who respond mortality is lower.

true (Mortality in those who respond is 33%; mortality in those who do not respond is 75%.)

G7 p.883:180mm

84.   Complete the following about barbiturate coma:

a.   The goal is

i.   to reduce the cerebral metabolic rate of _____

$CMRO_2$

ii.   and cerebral b_____ f_____.

blood flow

b.   The protocol is pentobarbital IV

i.   A loading dose of _____ mg/kg

10

ii.   Over _____ minutes

30

iii.   Then _____ mg/hr for 3 doses

5

iv.   Then _____ mg/hr

1

G7 p.884:25mm

85.   The goals of barbiturate therapy are

a.   electroencephalogram (EEG) showing _____ _____.

burst suppression

b.   serum level of _____% pentobarbital.

3 to 5 mg%

G7 p.885:30mm

86.   Complete the following:

a.   If a patient is treated with pentobarbital coma how long does it take for baseline neurofunction to return?

2 days

b.   What decreased level of pentobarbital in the blood will permit a valid brain death assessment?

less than 10 µg/mL

G7 p.885:30mm

87.   Complete the following:

a.   The loading dose of thiopental is _____ mg/kg over _____,

5 mg/kg over 10 minutes

b.   followed with _____ mg/kg for _____.

5 mg/kg for 24 hours

G7 p.885:50mm

88.   Complete the following:

G7 p.885:87mm
Also
G7 p.25:25mm

a.   The most commonly reported side effect of propofol is _____.

hypotension—due to myocardial depression (rarely causes pancreatitis)

b.   It is used for neuroprotection in _____.

aneurysm surgery

27

■ Skull Fractures

89. **True or False. All of the following are indications for elevating a depressed skull fracture:** G7 p.885:165mm

a. fracture depressed full thickness of skull — true
b. deficit relating to underlying brain injury — true
c. open fracture — false (Depressed bone compressing sinus is not an indication for elevating that depressed fracture.)
d. dural laceration — true
e. depressed bone compressing sinus — false

90. **True or False. Regarding skull fracture:** G7 p.886:95mm

a. There is no evidence that elevating a depressed skull fracture will reduce the subsequent development of seizure. — true
b. CN VI palsy can occur after a clivus fracture. — true
c. Antibiotics should incontrovertibly be given in the case of basal skull fracture, especially with CSF fistula. — false (Giving antibiotics with skull fracture, even CSF leak, is controversial. Very limited data may suggest that the incidence of meningitis is not reduced and that resistant organisms may be selected by routine use of antibiotics.)
d. Intracranial passage of a nasogastric (NG) tube carries 64% mortality. — true
e. Recall that the SSS is often to the _____ of the sagittal suture. — right G7 p.887:128mm
f. Bone fragments that may have lacerated a sinus should be removed. — last G7 p.887:146mm

91. **True or False. CT is very sensitive in the detection of basal skull fractures.** — false (Plain x-ray and clinical exam are more sensitive.) G7 p.887:180mm

92. **Complete the following regarding basal skull fractures:** G7 p.888:20mm

a. True or False. Pneumocephalus may be seen on plain skull x-rays. — true
b. Postauricular ecchymosis is called _____. — Battle sign
c. True or False. Anosmia can be associated with temporal bone fractures. — false (with frontal bone fracture)
d. Sixth nerve palsy can occur with _____ fracture. — clival

93. **True or False. The following are clinical signs of basal skull fracture:** G7 p.888:30mm

a. CSF otorrhea or rhinorrhea — true
b. hemotympanum — true
c. depressed level of consciousness — false
d. Battle sign — true
e. injury to cranial nerve VII — true

27

94. True or False. The following cranial nerves can be injured in basal skull fractures: *G7 p.888:50mm*

a.	CN I	true
b.	CN II	true
c.	CN III	true
d.	CN IV	true
e.	CN V	true
f.	CN VI	true
g.	CN VII	true
h.	CN VIII	true
i.	CN IX	true
j.	CN X	true
k.	CN XI	true
l.	CN XII	true

95. True or False. Complications seen with basal skull fractures include   *G7 p.888:115mm*

a.	traumatic aneurysms	true
b.	carotid cavernous fistula	true
c.	meningitis	true
d.	facial palsy	true
e.	CSF fistula	true

96. True or False. Otorrhea and rhinorrhea are clinical indications for emergent treatment of basal skull fractures.   false (Only persistent CSF leaks from basal skull fractures warrant investigation and treatment.)   *G7 p.888:120mm*

97. Complete the following regarding basilar skull fracture involving the petrous part of the temporal bone: *G7 p.888:163mm*

a. longitudinal fracture
    i. incidence is _____%   70 to 90%
    ii. complication _____   leak of CSF
b. horizontal (transverse) fracture
    i. incidence is _____%   10 to 30%
    ii. complication _____   hearing loss = VII and VIII nerve injury

98. True or False. Regarding temporal bone fractures: *G7 p.888:165mm*

a.	The longitudinal fracture is more common.	true
b.	Transverse fractures spare the seventh and eighth nerves.	false
c.	Longitudinal fractures can disrupt the ossicular chain.	true
d.	Transverse fractures lie perpendicular to the external auditory canal (EAC).	true
e.	Longitudinal fractures can often be diagnosed on otoscopic examination.	true
f.	Longitudinal fractures can result in CSF leakage.	true

27

99. Complete the following: G7 p.888:166mm
  a. What are the two types of temporal bone fractures?
      i.   l_____   longitudinal
      ii. t_____   transverse (horizontal)
  b. Which is more common?   longitudinal fracture
     By what %?   90%
  c. Which damages hearing?   transverse fracture (horizontal)
  d. Which may injure the facial nerve?   transverse fracture
  e. CSF leak may occur with _____.   longitudinal fracture
  f. Mnemonic to recall these facts
      i.   Transverse _____   T = Gacial seventh
      ii. Horizontal _____   H = Hearing
      iii. Longitudinal _____   L = Leakage

100. True or False. Glucocorticoids have been proven to improve the functional outcome of traumatic facial nerve palsy.   false   G7 p.889:35mm

101. Complete the following about temporal bone fractures: G7 p.889:43mm
  a. True or False. They may result in immediate facial nerve palsy.   true
  b. How long until electromyography (EMG) reliably confirms nerve injury?   at least 72 hours
  c. Usually requires _____   surgery
  d. True or False. They may result in delayed facial nerve palsy.   true
  e. True or False. Delayed facial palsy is less likely to need surgery.   true

■ Clival Fractures

102. Complete the following about fractures of the clivus: G7 p.889:70mm
  a. True or False. They can produce
      i.   cranial nerve injuries   true
      ii. vascular injuries   true
      iii. CSF leakage   true
      iv. brain stem infarction   true
      v.   traumatic aneurysms   true
      vi. diabetes insipidus   true
  b. The nerves that may be injured are _____ through _____.   III; IV

27

■ Craniofacial Fractures

103. True or False. Indication for surgery for frontal sinus fractures are   G7 p.889:172mm
  a. anterior wall linear fracture   false
  b. posterior wall displaced fracture   true

104. **Matching. Match the type of LeFort fracture and structures involved.**
Type of fracture:
① LeFort I; ② LeFort II; ③ LeFort III
Structures involved:
a. maxilla — ①
b. inferior orbital rim — ②
c. orbital floor — ②, ③
d. nasofrontal suture — ②, ③
e. zygomatic arches — ③
f. zygomaticofrontal suture — ③
g. pterygoid plates — ③

G7 p.890:90mm

105. **True or False. The fracture producing craniofacial dislocation is known as:**
a. LeFort I — false
b. LeFort II — false
c. LeFort III — true
d. depressed fracture — false
e. Salter fracture — false

G7 p.890:90mm

106. **True or False. Congenital skull defects may result in pneumocephalus.** — true (especially if the defect includes the tegmen tympani)

G7 p.891:40mm

107. **Tension pneumocephalus might occur if**
a. n_____ o_____ anesthetic is used — nitrous oxide
b. c_____ air is trapped — cool
c. b_____ v_____ opening occurs — ball valve
d. g_____-p_____ organisms are present — gas-producing

G7 p.891:90mm

108. **True or False. The presence of intracranial air may produce a characteristic sign known as**
a. empty delta sign — false
b. Mt. Hashimoto sign — false
c. Dawson sign — false
d. Mt. Fuji sign — true
e. gas gap — false

G7 p.891:134mm

109. **What is the Mt. Fuji sign?** — pneumocephalus—the frontal poles surrounded by air

G7 p.891:134mm

110. **True or False. Pneumocephalus due to a gas-producing organism can be treated with antibiotics and the patient followed. The gas will be absorbed.** — true (Appropriate antibiotic therapy should be started. Tension pneumocephalus must be drained.)

G7 p.891:177mm

27

111. **Complete the following regarding growing skull fracture:**

G7 p. 892:65mm

a. It is called _____ _____ _____.

posttraumatic leptomeningeal cyst

b. It results from a combination of two injuries:
   i. s_____ f_____

skull fracture

   ii. d_____ t_____

dural tear

c. Why does it grow?

intact arachnoid pulsates

112. **Complete the following about pediatric skull fractures:**

G7 p.892:75mm

a. The development of a posttraumatic leptomeningeal cyst requires a widely separated skull fracture and a _____.

dural tear

b. The incidence in skull fracture is _____%.

0.05 to 0.6%

c. The mean age at injury is _____ and high index of suspicion up to age _____.

< 1 year; 3

d. It presents as a _____.

scalp mass

e. Treatment is mandatory _____.

dural closure

113. **Answer the following about a growing skull fracture:**

G7 p.892:80mm

a. It is also known as _____ _____.

leptomeningeal cyst

b. True or False. It is commonly seen within 2 weeks of injury.

false

c. 90% occur before age _____.

3

d. It may present as a _____.

scalp mass

e. It requires surgical repair of the _____.

dura

f. It occurs within _____ months of injury.

6

g. Screen linear fractures below age _____

3

h. by follow-up x-ray in _____ months.

2 to 4

■ Hemorrhagic Contusions

114. **True or False. Regarding delayed traumatic intracerebral hemorrhage (DTICH):**

G7 p.893:148mm

a. The patient typically has GCS ≤ 8.

true

b. Incidence is ≈ 10%.

true

c. Most DTICHs occur within 72 hours of trauma.

true

d. Some patients initially appear well and then deteriorate.

true

e. Coagulopathy contributes to DTICH.

true

27

115. **These factors contribute to formation of delayed traumatic intracerebral hemorrhage.**   G7 p.893:160mm
    a. systemic _____   coagulopathy
    b. hemorrhage into an area of _____   necrotic brain
       _____
    c. coalescence of extravasated _____   microhematomas

■ Epidural Hematoma

116. **Complete the following:**   G7 p.894:23mm
    a. Incidence of epidural hematoma is _____% of all head injuries.   1%
    b. Incidence of subdural hematoma is _____% of all head injuries.   2%
    c. Epidural hematoma male to female ratio is _____.   4:1
    d. Epidural hematoma arise from arterial bleeding in _____%.   85%
    e. Epidural hematoma patients develop a dilated pupil in _____%.   60%
    f. _____% are ipsilateral.   85%
    g. _____% had no loss of consciousness.   60%
    h. _____% had no lucid internal.   20%
    i. Mortality of epidural hematoma is _____.   20 to 55%

117. **True or False. Regarding epidural hematomas (EDHs):**   G7 p.894:23mm
    a. The source of bleeding is arterial 99% of the time.   false (The source of bleeding is arterial 85% of the time and most commonly from the middle meningeal artery.)
    b. Women are more commonly affected.   false (Men are more commonly affected—4:1—than women.)
    c. EDHs are rare before age 2.   true (EDHs are rare before age 2 years or greater than 60 years.)
    d. The anterior meningeal artery is the most common cause of the bleeding.   false (middle meningeal artery)

118. **True or False. Patients with epidural hematomas can present with an ipsilateral hemiparesis.**   true (There can be shift of the brainstem away from the mass causing compression of the opposite cerebral peduncle causing ipsilateral hemiparesis, also known as Kernohan notch phenomenon.)   G7 p.894:102mm

119. **What is Kernohan notch phenomenon?**

G7 p.894:102mm

a. compression of the _____

b. cerebral peduncle on the _____

c. which can produce ipsilateral _____

opposite tentorial notch hemiparesis to the intracranial mass lesion

120. **True or False. Concerning epidural hematomas:**

G7 p.894:110mm

a. A dilated pupil is not a good localizing sign as to the hematoma location.

false (It is a good sign.)

b. It occurs in more than 15% of head trauma admissions.

false (1%)

c. No initial loss of consciousness occurs in 60%.

true

d. No lucid interval occurs in 20%.

true

e. In pediatric head trauma, EDH should be suspected if there is a 10% drop in hematocrit after admission.

true

121. **True or False. A 5-year-old girl presents to the emergency room (ER) with a chief complaint of brief posttraumatic loss of consciousness after several hours of playing with her siblings. While she is being worked up in the ER, you get a call from your frantic intern who reports that the patient is now obtunded. You would expect the following signs and symptoms and would include the following statistics in your presumed diagnosis.**

G7 p.894:120mm

a. early bradycardia

false (Early bradycardia is included in the differential diagnosis of posttraumatic disorder described by Denny-Brown. Late bradycardia may be seen in your presumed diagnosis, epidural hematoma.)

b. Kernohan notch phenomenon

true (Ipsilateral hemiparesis has been described in EDH.)

c. 85% occurrence of associated ipsilateral pupillary dilation

true (60% of patients with EDH have a dilated pupil and 85% will be ipsilateral to the hematoma.)

d. a crescent-shaped high density lesion on CT

true (An EDH may resemble an SDH on CT; however, 84% of EDH cases have the "classic" CT appearance of a high-density biconvex lens-shaped mass.)

122. **What is the mortality rate of EDH?**

20 to 55%

G7 p.894:180mm

27

123. **Nonsurgical treatment is possible if**   G7 p.895:57mm
  a. size is less than _____ and   1 cm
  b. patient's symptoms are _____.   mild
  c. What may happen between days 5 and   increase in size of the
     16?   hematoma
  d. An epidural hematoma thicker than   1 cm
     _____ cm should have surgery.
  e. To document resolution repeat CT in   1 to 3
     _____ to _____ months.
  f. A volume of less than _____ cc   30   G7 p.895:117mm

124. **Complete the following about delayed**   G7 p.896:60mm
     epidural traumatic hematoma
     (DEPTH):
  a. It may occur in as many as _____% of   9 to 10%
     epidural hematomas.
  b. It may be related to increasing the   BP
     patient's _____
  c. or reducing the patients _____,   ICP
  d. especially following surgical removal of   epidural
     another _____.
  e. _____ is another predisposing factor.   Coagulopathy

125. **True or False. Regarding posterior**   G7 p.896:115mm
     fossa epidural hematoma:
  a. Nearly 85% will have an occipital skull   true
     fracture in adults.
  b. Dural sinus tears are common.   true
  c. Abnormal cerebellar signs are common.   false
  d. Overall mortality is over 25%.   true
  e. They represent ~5% of EDH.   true

■ Subdural Hematomas

126. **True or False. Regarding acute**   G7 p.896:160mm
     subdural hematoma (ASDH):
  a. There is more likely to be an underlying   true
     brain injury with an ASDH than with an
     EDH.
  b. On CT an ASDH typically appears   true
     crescentic in shape.
  c. One cause of the ASDH is the   true
     accumulation of blood around a
     parenchymal laceration.
  d. A "lucid interval" may be present.   true

127. **Complete the following about acute**   G7 p.897:25mm
     subdural hematomas:
  a. A patient on anticoagulation therapy has
     a greater chance of ASDH
     i.   if the patient is a male _____-   7
          fold.
     ii. if the patient is a female _____-   26
          fold.

27

b. How many days until the subdural membrane begins to form?

4

c. How long until acute blood on CT becomes isodense?

2 weeks

d. If CT after trauma is normal can we have a sense of security regarding that patient?

not entirely; delayed hematomas can occur

    i. DEPTH _____%

epidural 10%

G7 p.896:60mm

    ii. DASDH _____%

subdural 0.5%

G7 p.899:50 mm

128. Concerning treatment of acute subdural hematoma, you evacuate if the blood clot is

G7 p.897:90mm

a. _____ thick in adults

1 cm

b. _____ thick in pediatric patients

0.5 cm

c. by performing a _____

craniotomy

d. not a _____ _____

burr hole

129. Complete the following about subdural hematomas:

G7 p.898:40mm

a. True or False. Mortality from an acute subdural hematoma (ASDH) ranges from 50 to 90%.

true

b. Mortality is from the _____ _____ _____.

underlying brain injury and not from the extraaxial bleed

c. True or False. Mortality is higher in young people.

false (Mortality thought to be higher in aged patients.)

G7 p.898:47mm

d. Medication that increases mortality is _____.

anticoagulants

130. Complete the following about subdural hematomas:

G7 p.898:55mm

a. Is there a preferred time for SDH surgery?

yes

b. If so, when is it?

before 4 hours (patients operated within 4 hours of an acute SDH had a 30% mortality rate compared with 90% mortality if surgery was delayed > 4 hours.) Hint: 30 - 4 - 90 - more. Known as the "4-hour rule."

27

131. Give the statistics for acute subdural hematomas for the following:

G7 p.898:96mm

a. rate of seizures

9%

b. mortality in unhelmeted motorcyclists

100%

c. mortality in helmeted motorcyclists

33%

132. True or False. Acute subdural hematoma outcomes relate to the following factors:

G7 p.898:96mm

a. seizures

false

b. surgery later than 4 hours after injury

true

c. Glasgow coma scale

true (Lower number poor outcome.)

d. mechanism of injury — true (Motorcycle accidents are the worst.)

e. age — true (above 65 year olds 85% mortality)

f. postoperative ICP — true

g. if under 20 mm Hg 40% mortality — true

h. if above 45 mm Hg 100% mortality — true

133. Complete the following about interhemispheric subdural hematoma: G7 p.898:170mm

a. It is usually related to h_____ t_____. — head trauma

b. It may be due to a_____. — aneurysm

c. If symptomatic the falx syndrome consists of
Hint: psadlo

   i.   p_____ — paresis
   ii. s_____ — seizures
   iii. a_____ — ataxia
   iv. d_____ — dementia
   v.   l_____ difficulties — language
   vi. o_____ palsies — oculomotor

134. For delayed acute subdural hematoma (DASDH) the incidence is _____% in operatively treated acute subdural hematomas.   0.50%   G7 p.899:50mm

135. What are the risk factors for chronic SDH?   G7 p.899:155mm

Hint: catss falls

a. c_____ — coagulopathies

b. a_____ — alcohol abuse

c. t_____ — trauma

d. s_____ — shunts

e. s_____ — seizures

f. f_____ — falls

136. For treatment of chronic subdural hematoma, the following are recommended: G7 p.901:75mm

a. Surgery type is _____. — large craniectomy at least 2.5 cm

b. Membrane treatment is _____. — coagulate outer membrane

c. Drain until _____. — drainage negligible 24 to 48 hours

d. Postoperative position of patient is _____. — flat in bed

e. During treatment if you notice that it has a membrane it is at least _____ days old. — 4

f. During treatment if the CT scan shows it is isodense it is _____ weeks old. — 2

27

137. **Complete the following regarding chronic subdural hematomas:**
G7 p.901:105mm
  a. Repeat surgery is needed in _____%.   19%
  b. Is the use of a drain recommended?   yes
  c. With a drain the need to repeat surgery is reduced to _____%.   10%

138. **Complete the following about chronic subdural hematoma outcomes:**
G7 p.901:167mm
  a. Persistent fluid at 10 days _____%   78%
  b. Persistent fluid at 40 days _____%   15%
  c. How long till full resolution?   may take 6 months
  d. One operation is successful in _____% of patients.   80%
  e. Two operations are successful in _____% of patients.   90%

139. **What are the complications of surgical treatment of chronic SDH?**
G7 p.902:25mm
  Hint: hherps
  a. h _____   hemorrhage
  b. h _____   hyperemia
  c. e _____   empyema
  d. r _____   reexpansion failure
  e. p _____   pneumocephalus
  f. s _____   seizures

140. **Complete the following regarding chronic subdural hematomas:**
G7 p.902:60mm
  a. complication associated with rapid decompression _____   hyperemia
  b. age group _____   elderly (over age 75)
  c. overall mortality of CSDH _____%   4 to 8%

141. **Answer the following about subdural hematoma:**
G7 p.902:80mm
  a. True or false. They are invariably caused by trauma.   false
  b. There is an entity called _____ subdural hematoma.   spontaneous
  c. Possible etiologies are
    i. a_____   aneurysms
    ii. a_____-v_____ malformations   arterio-venous
    iii. c_____   coagulopathies
    iv. i_____ h_____   Intracranial hypotension

27

142. **Complete the following regarding formation of subdural hygromas:**   G7 p.903:68mm
    a. Are they associated with trauma?   yes
    b. Do skull fractures occur? _____%   yes; 39%
    c. Do they have membranes?   no
    d. Fluid on CT is similar to _____.   CSF
    e. They are created by
        i. _____ and   arachnoid tear
        ii. _____.   ball valve flap
    f. Another mechanism is _____   after *Haemophilus influenzae*
        _____.   meningitis effusion

143. **Complete the following regarding traumatic subdural hygromas:**   G7 p.903:115mm
    a. What chemical is found in hygroma fluid that helps in diagnosis?   prealbumin
    b. Is this found in CSF?   yes
    c. Is this found in subdural hematomas?   no
    d. This suggests that hygroma originates from _____ _____.   arachnoid tears
    e. If surgery is needed what may reduce recurrences?   leave a drain

144. **When extraaxial fluid looks dark on CT how can we differentiate CSF/hygroma from chronic subdural hygroma?**   fluid from hygroma and CSF contains prealbumin not found in subdural hematoma   G7 p.903:120mm
    a. Test for _____.   prealbumin
    b. CSF/hygroma will _____ _____.   have prealbumin
    c. Subdural hygroma will _____ _____ _____.   not contain prealbumin

145. **True or False. The following is a common clinical finding in traumatic subdural hygroma:**   G7 p.903:115mm
    a. spontaneous eye opening   true
    b. disorientation or stupor   true
    c. mental status changes without focal signs   true
    d. seizures (usually generalized)   true
    e. hemiparesis   true

146. **Matching. What is the treatment of choice for subdural hygroma? Choose one or more:**   G7 p.903:180mm
    ① subdural to peritoneal shunt; ② no treatment; ③ burr hole drainage; ④ external subdural drain; ⑤ repeat burr hole drainage
    a. asymptomatic   ②
    b. symptomatic   ③ or ④
    c. recurrent   ⑤ or ①

27

147. **List the differential diagnosis of extraaxial fluid collections in children.**

G7 p.904:50mm

a. a_____ s_____

b. b_____ s_____

c. c_____ s_____

d. c_____ a_____

e. c_____ d_____
f. e_____ h_____

acute SDH in a child with low Hct
benign subdural (extraaxial) collections of infancy
chronic symptomatic extraaxial fluid collections
cerebral atrophy external hydrocephalus (EH)
craniocerebral disproportion
external hydrocephalus

148. **What is the mean age of presentation of benign subdural (extraaxial) fluid collections of infancy?**

4 months

G7 p.904:130mm

149. **What is the treatment of benign extraaxial fluid collections of infancy?**

G7 p.904:155mm

a. o_____

b. p_____ e_____

c. h_____ c_____

observation (Most cases resolve spontaneously within 8 to 9 months and require no treatment.)
physical examination periodically (Repeat physical exam to identify development of symptoms.)
head circumference every 3 to 6 months (Orbital-frontal head circumference [OFC] should be done at 3- to 6-month intervals to monitor head growth that should parallel normal growth and approach normal at 1 to 2 years.)

d. Most will _____
e. by _____.

resolve
1 to 2 years

150. **Name seven frequent etiologies of symptomatic chronic extraaxial fluid collections in children.**
Hint: subtact

G7 p.905:35mm

a. s_____
b. u_____
c. b_____
d. t_____
e. a_____
f. c_____

g. t_____

shunt (18%)
unknown (16%)
bacterial meningitis (22%)
trauma (36%)
asphyxia
coagulopathy (vitamin K deficiency)
tumors

27

151. **What are the treatment options for**   G7 p.905:90mm
      symptomatic chronic extra-axial fluid
      collections in children?
      Hint: otb sp

a. o_____   observation with serial orbital
                       frontal head circumferences,
                       ultrasound

b. t_____   at least one percutaneous tap
                       should be done to rule out
                       infection

c. b_____   burr-hole drainage ± external
                       drainage

d. s_____ p_____ s_____   subdural collection to
                       peritoneal shunt (unilateral
                       with extremely low pressure
                       valve)

■ Traumatic Posterior Fossa Mass Lesions

152. **Complete the following about**   G7 p.905 :155mm
      traumatic posterior fossa mass lesions:

a. Head injury that involves the posterior   3%
    fossa is less than _____%.

b. The majority are e_____ h_____.   epidural hematomas

c. Parenchymal hemorrhages can be   3
    managed nonsurgically if they are less
    than _____ cm in diameter.

■ Posttraumatic Hydrocephalus

153. **Complete the following about**   G7 p.906:80mm
      posttraumatic hydrocephalus:

a.
  i.   It can occur in up to _____% of   40%
       patients
  ii. who have GCS below _____.   8

b. It can develop up to _____ weeks   8
    post-trauma.

c. It occurs in _____% of patients with   12%   G7 p.906:150mm
    traumatic subarachnoidal hemorrhage.

d. There is an increased incidence with
  i.   a_____   age
  ii.   i_____ hemorrhage   intraventricular
  iii. blood thickness greater than   5
        _____ mm
  iv.   d_____ distribution of blood   diffuse

■ Aspects of General Care in Severe TBI

154. Complete the following about deep vein thrombosis:

G7 p.907:75mm

a. Risk after severe TBI is _____%.   20%

b. Prophylactic measures advised are

 i. c_____ b_____ and   compression boots

 ii. l_____-d_____ h_____.   low-dose heparin

■ Nutrition in the Head-Injured Patient

155. What is the basal energy expenditure (BEE) of the head-injured patient?

G7 p.907:144mm

a. nonparalyzed _____% of BEE   140%

b. paralyzed _____% of BEE   100%

c. What % of replacement should be in the form of protein?   provide ≥ 15% calories as protein

156. Complete the following regarding head trauma:

G7 p.907:155mm

a. When should nutritional supplementation begin?   within 72 hours

b. When should full caloric replacement be achieved?   by 7 days

c. Rested comatose patients have metabolic expenditure that is _____% of normal   140%

G7 p.907:180mm

157. What is the formula for estimation of the BEE?

G7 p.908:55mm

a. The name of the equation is the _____.   Harris-Benedict equation

b. males _____   BEE = 66.5 + 13.8 × W(kg) + 5 × H(cm) - 6.8 × age

c. females _____   BEE = 65.5 + 9.6 × W(kg) + 1.9 × H(cm) - 4.7 × age

d. infants _____   BEE = 22.1 + 31.1 × W(kg) + 1.2 × H(cm)

e. takes into account _____, _____, and _____   weight in kg, height in cm, and age in years

27

■ Outcomes from Head Trauma

158. A 40-year-old male and his 8-year-old daughter were involved in a head-on collision. You examine them in the emergency room. The child is flaccid with both pupils fixed and dilated. The father's pupils are also fixed and dilated. He has decerebrate posture. True or False. The following parts of the history or physical determine which patient will have the worse prognosis:

G7 p.909:13mm

a. mechanism of trauma — false
b. fixed dilated pupils — false
c. flaccid posture — false
d. decerebrate posture — false
e. age — true (In general, the degree of recovery from closed head injury is better in infants and young children than in adults. In most cases decerebrate/flaccid posture and loss of pupillary reflex are associated with poor outcome in adults, but these findings are not as ominous in the pediatric age group.)

159. Head injury factors to consider for predictors of poor outcome include
Hint: bih macs

G7 p.909:35mm

a. b_____ — blood pressure
b. i_____ — intracranial pressure
c. h_____ — hydrocephalus
d. m_____ — mass lesion
e. a_____ — age
f. c_____ — cisterns
g. s_____ — shift of midline

160. True or False. With head injury outcomes an important predictor for poor outcome is

G7 p.909 :44mm

a. mass lesion requiring surgical removal — true (Mass lesions requiring surgical removal are one of the most important predictors of outcome.)

b. hydrocephalus — true
c. obliteration of basal cisterns — true
d. persistent ICP > 20 — true
e. increased age — true
f. hypotension SBP < 90 — true
g. midline shift greater than 15 mm — true

27

G7 p.909:44mm

161. Complete the following about closed head injury:

a. Predictors of poor outcome are
   Hint: a^2mc-sh^{3}lp
      i.   a_____   age
      ii.   a_____   anemia
      iii. m_____ l_____   mass lesion
      iv. c_____   cisterns
      v.   s_____ of m_____   shift of midline
      vi. h_____ SBP below   hypotension/90
                 _____ mm Hg
      vii. h_____   hypercarbia
      viii. h_____   hypoxemia
      ix. I_____ elevated above _____ ICP; 20
      x.   p_____ responses   pupillary
b. High ICP during the _____ hours is first 24
   especially bad.

G7 p.909:75mm

162. Complete the following about midline shift:

a. Midline is measured at the level of the foramen of Monro
   _____ of _____.
b.
      i.   A shift of _____ mm is well   3
         tolerated.
      ii. A shift of _____ mm correlates 6
         with drowsiness.
      iii. A shift of _____ mm correlates 9
         with stuporousness.
      iv. A shift of _____ mm correlates 12
         with coma.
      v.   A shift of _____ mm correlates 15   G7 p.909:168mm
         with death.

G7 p.909:119mm

163. Complete the following about the status of basal cisterns:

a. It is measured at the _____ level. midbrain
b. Study three limbs.   G7 p.909:142mm
      i.   2 _____ cisterns   ambient
      ii. 1 _____ cisterns   quadrigeminal
c. Obliteration of cistern correlates with   G7 p.910:14mm
   mortality
      i.   All limbs open: mortality is   22%
         _____%.
      ii. One or two limbs closed: mortality is 39%
         _____%.
      iii. All 3 absent: mortality is _____%. 77%

27

164. Complete the following: G7 p.910:15mm

a. You obtain a head CT in both father and
daughter. The child's CT demonstrates
diffuse edema with open cisterns and no
hydrocephalus. The father's CT
demonstrates complete obliteration of
the basal cisterns. True or False. The
most probable Glasgow outcome score
in this adult patient is

i.	GOS1	true (GOS 1 mortality)
ii.	GOS2	false
iii.	GOS3	false
iv.	GOS4	false
v.	GOS5	false

b. An adult with obliterated cisterns has a   77%
mortality of _____%.

165. Complete the following: G7 p.910:18mm

a. What is the genotype associated with   apolipoprotein E4 allele
head injury?

b. It is also a risk factor for _____.   Alzheimer disease

166. True or False. Long-term complications   G7 p.910:70mm
from head injury (HI) include the
following:

a. posttraumatic seizures   true (early: severe HI 30%,
                                   mild HI 1%; Late: LOC > 2 min
                                   10 to 13%)

b. Alzheimer disease   true (HI promotes amyloid
                                   deposits.)

c. hypogonadotropic hypogonadism   true (but rare)
d. visual disturbances   true (5% of head-injured
                                   patients injure visual system.)

e. communicating hydrocephalus   true (severe HI: 3.9%)

167. A 28-year-old male sustained a minor   G7 p.911:70mm
head injury at Macy's with a small
forehead laceration but without loss
of consciousness. He comes to your
office 4 months later after being
offered only supportive treatment by
other clinicians. He presents with
headache, dizziness, anosmia,
difficulty concentrating, and loss of
libido. There are no positive findings
on your physical examination. At this
time do you:

a. tell the patient (and the lawyer) that   no
psychiatric evaluation is warranted?

27

b. implement a neurophysiological battery of tests including magnetic resonance imaging (MRI), EEG, brain stem auditory evoked response (BSAER), and head CT?

yes (The patient has persistent symptoms, > 3 months, that include somatic, cognitive, and psychosocial manifestations. Alves and Jane perform a full battery of testing before proceeding with any plan or venturing any prognosis.)

c. send the patient home with Tylenol?

no

168. Complete the following: G7 p.911:75mm

a. The above patient returns after 1 week. You notice in his records that all the tests are normal. At this time do you

   i. tell the patient (and the lawyer) that psychiatric evaluation is warranted?

yes ("If all studies are negative," the authors, Alves and Jane, tell the patient and the lawyer to seek psychiatric evaluation.)

   ii. schedule more testing?

no

   iii. send the patient home with Tylenol?

no

   iv. reassure the patient that symptoms will resolve?

no

b. and if the tests are abnormal? (Choose: i., ii., iii., or iv. from above)

iv. (Noncorrectable abnormalities prompt reassurance that significant symptoms should subside by 1 year.)

169. Neuropathology in chronic traumatic encephalopathy shows   G7 p.911:170mm

a. n_____ t_____ and

neurofibrillary tangles

b. a_____ a_____.

amyloid angiopathy

c. These changes are similar to A_____ disease.

Alzheimer

170. True or False. Chronic traumatic encephalopathy is more likely in boxers who   G7 p.912:20mm

a. have more than 20 fights

true

b. fight for more than 10 years

true

c. have the apolipoprotein E4 allele

true

d. have cerebral atrophy

true

e. have cavum septum pellucidum

true (13%)

f. also known as d_____ p_____

dementia pugilistica

27

■ Gunshot Wounds to the Head

171. **True or False. Regarding gunshot wounds (GSWs):**   G7 p.912:140mm

a. GSWs represent 35% of all deaths from brain injury in the older population (> 45).

false (GSWs represent 35% of deaths by head injury in the population aged < 45.)

b. GSWs are the most lethal type of head injury; one fourth die at the scene.

false (It is lethal and two thirds of patients die at the scene.)

c. 90% of victims die.

true (Ultimately 90% of patients will die directly or from complications related to GSW regardless of their expression of APO E4 allele.)

d. Poor outcome in GSWs is related to APO E4 allele.

false (APO E4 allele relates well to the poor closed head injury outcome and Alzheimer disease but not to GSW.)

172. **For GSWs to the head the mechanisms of injury include**   G7 p.912:155mm
Hint: Capone gang shootings land in the East River

a. c_____   cavitation, coup-contrecoup
b. g_____   gas
c. s_____   shock waves
d. l_____   low pressure
e. i_____   impact
f. e_____   explosive
g. r_____   ricochet

173. **Complete the following:**   G7 p.913:84mm

a. Higher impact velocity is correlated with ICP that is _____.

higher

b. The size of the entrance wound is _____ compared with the exit wound.

smaller

c. Edges of entrance wound show a beveled _____ table.

inner

d. Edges of exit wound show a beveled _____ table.

outer

174. **Angiography in penetrating injury to the brain should be considered if there is**   G7 p.914:160mm

a. a trajectory near major _____ or   arteries
b. _____ and   sinuses
c. a large _____.   hematoma

175. Complete the following:

G7 p.915:135mm

a. What is the most important prognostic factor after a gunshot wound to the head (GSWH)?

level of consciousness on admission

b. What is the mortality/morbidity in GSWH if the patient is unconscious?

94% of patients comatose on admission die; 3% are severely disabled

c. The prognosis is worse if the path of the bullet
   i. c_____ the m_____
      crosses the midline
   ii. passes through the g_____ c_____
      geographic center of the brain
   iii. t_____ the v_____
      traverses the ventricle
   iv. passes through m_____ l_____
      multiple lobes

■ Non-missile Penetrating Trauma

176. Complete the following:

G7 p.916:45mm

a. Because of low velocity only l_____ d_____ is needed.

local debridement

b. These are more or less contaminated than gunshot wounds?

more

G7 p.916:133mm

c. Prophylactic antibiotics are or are not advised?

are

d.
   i. Would you consider an angiogram?
      yes
   ii. If so why? To rule out a t_____ a_____
      traumatic aneurysm

■ High-Altitude Cerebral Edema

177. In your last trip to Machu Picchu in the high Andes you notice that the passenger sitting beside you in the train starts gasping for air and complains of severe headaches. Within minutes he becomes confused and minutes later becomes paralyzed. You suspect high altitude pulmonary edema (HAPE) with or without cerebral edema (HACE).

G7 p.916:150mm

27

a. You pull out your handy ophthalmoscope and find in the fundus:
   i. p_____
      papilledema
   ii. r_____ h_____
      retinal hemorrhages
   iii. nerve fiber layer i_____
      infarction
   iv. vitreous h_____
      hemorrhage

b. This is compatible with the diagnosis of h_____ a_____ c_____ e_____.

HACE—high altitude cerebral edema (A milder case of acute high altitude sickness [AHAS] that presents without ocular findings is called HAPE.)

c. Prevent fundus deterioration by
  i. g_____ d_____ and
  ii. avoiding _____.

gradual descent
ETOH

d. Treat with
  i. o_____
  ii. s_____

6 to 12 L/min O_2
steroids may be of use

178. Complete the following: G7 p.916:163mm

a. At the upcoming neurosurgical meeting in the Rockies, one of your colleagues presents with acute onset of inappropriate behavior, hallucinations, ataxia, and reduced mental status.
  i. If the breathalyzer is negative, what diagnosis should you consider?
  ii. At 7000 ft you would be correct _____% of the time.
  iii. At 15,000 ft you would be correct _____% of the time.

high altitude cerebral edema (HACE)
25%

50%

b. What else might you see with this condition?
  i. r_____ h_____
  ii. p_____
  iii. v_____ h_____
  iv. s_____ h_____

retinal hemorrhage
papilledema
vitreous hemorrhage
severe headache

c. What treatment should be initiated in a severe case?
  i. location: i_____ d_____
  ii. breathe: o_____

  iii. medication: d_____

immediate descent
oxygen (6 to 12 L/min by NC or FM)
dexamethasone 8 mg/PO/IV followed by 4 mg in 96 hours

■ Pediatric Head Injury

179. Complete the following regarding children hospitalized for trauma: G7 p.917:54mm

a. What percent have head injury?
b. The mortality overall is _____%.
c. If presenting with decerebrate posturing mortality is _____%.

75%
10 to 13%
71%

180. **True or False. A mother brings a 5-day-old baby born via vaginal delivery with a large, right-sided, soft scalp swelling that stops at the suture. You should**

G7 p.918:100mm

a. percutaneously aspirate the lesion

false (Cephalohematoma is most commonly seen associated with parturition. 80% resorb usually within 2 to 3 weeks. Avoid the temptation of puncturing the lesions because the risk of infection exceeds cosmetic benefits.)

b. tell the mother that 50% of these calcify

false—occasionally only

c. tell the mother that the baby may develop jaundice as late as age 10 days

true (Infants may develop hyperbilirubinemia and jaundice as blood is resorbed from this cephalohematoma [subperiosteal hematoma] as late as 10 days after onset.)

d. surgically excise the lesion

false (Surgery is considered only after 6 weeks if a CT demonstrates calcifications.)

e. consider child abuse

true (Child abuse needs to be excluded always.)

f. treat this differently if the soft area crosses sutures

false (called subgaleal hematoma)

181. **If a child is in the ER under age 10 with trauma**

G7 p.918:130mm

a. one must think _____, which will be true in

child abuse

b. _____% of cases.

10%

c. Examine _____ for _____.

retina; hemorrhages

182. **Answer the following regarding child abuse:**

G7 p.918:142mm

a. True or false. There are pathognomonic findings in child abuse.

false

b. Suspicious findings are

i. r_____ h_____

retinal hemorrhage

ii. b_____ c_____ s_____ h_____

bilateral chronic subdural hematomas

iii. s_____ f_____

skull fractures

183. **Retinal hemorrhage in a baby is pathognomonic of**
    s_____/i_____ b_____
    s_____.

shaken/impact baby syndrome

G7 p.919:40mm

27

28

Spine Injuries

■ Spine Injuries

1. Complete the following: G7 p.930:35mm
a. What must you look for in a patient with a major spinal injury?   a second spinal injury
b. It occurs in _____%.   20%

2. Complete the following: G7 p.930:105mm
a. In spinal cord injury, any residual motor or sensory function more than three segments below the level of injury represents an _____ lesion.   incomplete
b. Signs of this being the case include
    i. s_____   sensation (include position sense)
    ii. v_____ m_____   voluntary movement in the lower extremities
    iii. s_____ s_____   sacral sparing (Preserved sacral reflexes alone do not qualify as incomplete injury. Also requires preserved sensation around the anus.)
c. Types of this lesion include these syndromes:
    i. c_____ c_____   central cord
    ii. B_____-S_____   Brown-Séquard
    iii. a_____ c_____   anterior cord
    iv. p_____ c_____   posterior cord

3. A complete spinal cord lesion G7 p.930:144mm
a. is defined as no
    i. m_____ or   motor
    ii. s_____ function   sensory
    iii. t_____ levels below lesion.   three
b. What percent of patients with no function on initial exam will develop some recovery within 24 hours?   3% G7 p.930:147mm
c. A complete spinal cord injury that persists for 72 hours indicates that _____ _____ _____ _____ _____ .   no distal recovery will occur

4. **Complete the following regarding spinal shock:**

G7 p.930:160mm

a. hypotension:
   i. interruption of _____ _____   sympathetic activity
   ii. loss of _____ _____   vascular tone
b. bradycardia: unopposed _____   parasympathetic
   activity
c. relative hypovolemia:
   i. loss of _____   muscle tone due to skeletal
       muscle paralysis below level
       of injury
   ii. resulting in _____ _____   venous pooling
d. true hypovolemia: loss of _____   blood from associated
       wounds

■ Whiplash-Associated Disorders

5. **What is the most common nonfatal automobile injury?**   whiplash

G7 p.931:57mm

6. **Describe the five grades of whiplash-associated disorders and clinical evaluation of each.**

G7 p.931:80mm

a. grade 0
   i. clinical   no complaint
   ii. radiological studies   none required
b. grade 1
   i. clinical   neck pain
   ii. radiological studies   no x-rays needed
c. grade 2
   i. clinical   reduced ROM/point
       tenderness
   ii. radiological studies   CS x-ray flexion/extension
       (F/E) views
d. grade 3
   i. clinical   weakness, sensory deficit,
       deep tendon reflexes (DTR)
       abnormality
   ii. radiological studies   CT, MR, treatment as SCI
e. grade 4
   i. clinical   fracture or dislocation
   ii. radiological studies   CT, MR, treat as spinal cord
       injury

28

■ Pediatric Spine Injuries

7.   Complete the following: G7 p.932:80mm

a.   Due to ligamentous laxity together with   ligamentous
immaturity of paraspinal muscles and
underdeveloped uncinate processes,
pediatric spinal injury tends to involve
_____ types of injury.

b.   In the age group ≤ 9 years, the_____   cervical
spine is the most vulnerable segment.

c.   In cervical spine injuries in the pediatric   upper 3 (occiput-C2)
population, 67% occur in the _____
segments of the cervical spine.

8.   Complete the following about   G7 p.933:50mm
pediatric spine injuries:

a.   "Pseudospread of the atlas" is a   children
phenomenon occurring in _____.

b.   It could be confused with _____   Jefferson fracture
_____.

9.   Answer the following about Jefferson   G7 p.933:70mm
fractures:

a.   True or False. Jefferson fractures are   false
common in pediatric cervical spine
injury.

b.   They are more common during the   teenage
_____ years.

■ Initial Management of Spinal Cord Injuries

10.   Complete the following: G7 p.933:135mm

a.   The major causes of death in spinal cord
injury are
i.   _____ and   aspiration
ii.   _____.   shock

b.   Associated findings suggestive of spinal
cord injury include
i.   _____ _____ and   abdominal breathing
ii.   _____.   priapism (autonomic
dysfunction)

11.   True or False. In caring for an injured   false (Do not remove the   G7 p.934:90mm
athlete, prompt removal of the helmet   helmet in the field—National
is recommended.   Athletic Trainers Association
[NATA] guidelines.)

12.   Complete the following: G7 p.934:125mm

a.   In spinal cord injury with hypotension in   dopamine
the field, the agent of choice is
_____.

b.   Avoid _____.   phenylephrine—noninotropic,
and possible reflex increase in
vagal tone with bradycardia

28

13. **In evaluating spinal cord injury in the field, hypopnea may be related to three conditions:**   G7 p.934:175mm
   a. paralyzed i_____ m_____   intercostal muscles
   b. paralyzed d_____   diaphragm (phrenic nerve = C3, C4, C5)
   c. depressed _____   LOC

14. **Complete the following:**   G7 p.936:26mm
   a. True or False. Spinal cord injury can cause loss of temperature regulation.   true
   b. This is called p_____   poikilothermy
   c. and is caused by v_____ p_____. vasomotor paralysis

15. **Complete the following about initial management of spinal cord injuries:**   G7 p936:32mm
   a. True or False. Spinal cord injury can cause electrolyte disturbances   true
   b. due to
      i. _____ and   hypotension
      ii. _____,   hypovolemia
   c. which cause an increase in _____   plasma aldosterone
      _____,
   d. which leads to _____.   hypokalemia

16. **Complete the following: (Note: Practice parameter caution regarding use of steroids.)**   G7 p.936:165mm
   a. In adhering to the spinal cord injury steroid protocol, methylprednisolone needs to be administered within _____ hours of injury to improve outcome.   8
   b. What may occur if given later?   worse outcome at 1 year

17. **True or False. Methylprednisolone protocol has been shown to be useful for patients with**   G7 p.936:177mm
   a. cauda equina syndrome   false
   b. gunshot wounds to the spine   false
   c. children   false
   d. pregnant women   false

18. **Discuss administration of methylprednisolone protocol in spinal cord injury.**   G7 p.937:35mm
   a. Initial bolus is _____ mg/kg IV.   30
   b. Over how long a period of time?   15 minutes
   c. Followed by a _____.   45-minute pause
   d. Follow with maintenance infusion of _____.   5.4 mg/kg/hr IV
                                               G7 p.937:73mm
   e. Over how long a period of time?
      i. If started within 3 hours of injury, _____ hours.   23
      ii. If started between 3 and 8 hours, _____ hours.   47

28

19. True or False. Regarding deep vein thrombosis (DVT) in spinal cord injury (SCI):
G7 p.937:130mm;

a. Heparin 5000 U subcutaneous (SQ) twice a day is more effective than SQ heparin to titrate partial thromboplastin time (PTT) to 1.5 times normal.   false (Better to titrate SQ heparin to PTT 1.5 times control.)

b. Pneumatic boots should be used initially.   true

20. Complete the following about spinal cord injury and deep vein thrombosis:
G7 p.637:132mm

a. incidence _____%   100%

b. mortality _____%   9%

c. prevent with _____ _____ boots   pneumatic compression

d. and subcutaneous _____   heparin

e. preferably titrated to a partial thromboplastin time (PTT) of _____   1.5 times control

f. What medication can cause thrombocytopenia and osteoporosis?   heparin

21. Matching. In assessing C-spine in these categories of trauma patient, perform the following tests:
G7 p.938:73mm

Test to perform:
① none needed; ② CT from occiput to T1; ③ plain C-spine x-rays; ④ flexion-extension; ⑤ MRI

Category of trauma patient:

a. Alert, denies neck pain   ①

b. Alert, complains of neck pain   ②

c. Obtunded or inebriated   ②

d. Abnormal CT   ⑤

e. Neurological deficit   ② and ⑤

22. When do we do
G7 p.938:148mm

a. Plain C-spine x-ray? If _____ is not available   CT

b. Flexion extension views

   i. in an _____ patient   alert

   ii. who complains of _____ _____   neck pain

   iii. and in whom _____ is normal   CT

   iv. and _____ is not available   MRI

23. Factors associated with increased risk of failing to recognize spinal injuries during radiographic evaluation include
G7 p.939:49mm

a. decreased _____ of _____   level of consciousness

b. multiple _____   injuries

c. inadequate _____   x-rays (technically)

28

24. Radiographic signs of C-spine trauma include

G7 p.939:80mm

a. retropharyngeal space > _____ mm   7 mm
b. retrotracheal space > _____ mm in adult   14 mm
c. or > _____ mm in pediatrics   22 mm
d. atlantodental interval (ADI) > _____ mm in adult   3 mm
e. > _____ mm in pediatrics   4 mm
f. In the neurologically intact patient, subluxation up to _____ mm may be normal.   3.5 mm
g. To prove it is normal do _____.   flexion-extension views

25. When should we order anteroposterior (AP) and lateral views of the thoracic and lumbosacral spine?
Hint: btuf

G7 p.940:90mm

a. b_____   back pain complaints
b. t_____   thrown from a vehicle
c. u_____   unconscious
d. f_____   fell more than 6 feet

26. Complete the following:

G7 p.940:115mm

a. How can we tell an old injury from an acute one?   bone scan
b. We should test between _____ and _____ days.   2 and 21 days
c. Test will remain abnormal for _____ _____.   1 year

27. During evaluation of occult cervical spine trauma, what are the contraindications for flexion-extension cervical spine x-rays?

G7 p.940:58mm

a. patient who is not _____   cooperative
b. patient who has _____ impairment   mental
c. subluxation of _____ or more   3.5 mm
d. neurologic deficit of _____   any degree

28. True or False. A normal flexion-extension study of the cervical spine x-ray may demonstrate slight anterior subluxation distributed over all cervical levels with preservation of the normal contour lines.   true

G7 p.941:35mm

28

29. Complete the following:

G7 p.941:77mm

a. Lumbar puncture is dangerous in complete spinal block and may cause deterioration in _____%.   14%
b. Avoid this with a _____ or _____.   lateral cervical puncture or MRI

30. **Indications for emergent myelogram or magnetic resonance imaging (MRI) in spinal cord injury includes neurologic deficit**
    G7 p.941:98mm
    a. that is not _____   explained
    b. after closed _____   reduction
    c. after _____ surgery   spinal

31. **Complete the following about MRI in spine:**
    G7 p.941:147mm
    a. It is appropriate when
       i.   CT of spine is _____,   inconclusive
       ii. patient has neurological _____.   deficits
    b. It should be done within _____   48 to 72
       hours.
    c. Most useful sequences are
       i.   _____ and   T2W1
       ii. F_____.   FLAIR

32. **Contraindications to traction/reduction of cervical spine injuries include**
    G7 p.942:95mm
    a. atlanto-occipital _____   dislocation
    b. types of axis fractures called _____ or   type II A, or III hangman's
       _____   fracture
    c. a defect in the _____   skull at an anticipated pin site
    d. the patient is less than _____ years of   3
       age

33. **Complete the following:**
    G7 p.943:90mm
    a. After placing the patient in tongs we   lateral cervical spine x-ray
       must obtain a _____
    b. and measure the distance between the
       i.   _____ and the   basion
       ii. _____,   odontoid
    c. which should be less than _____ mm   2 mm
       in adults
    d. and less than _____ mm in children.   10 mm

34. **What is considered proper pin care?**
    G7 p.943:117mm
    a. Clean with _____.   half-strength hydrogen
                                     peroxide
    b. Apply _____.   povidone-iodine
    c. This may reduce the incidence of   osteomyelitis
       _____.

35. **Complete the following:**
    G7 p.943:75mm
    a. Closed reduction of cervical dislocations   retropulsed cervical disc
       may be associated with neurologic
       deterioration, and this may be due to a
       r_____ c_____ d_____.
    b. If neurologic deterioration occurs after
       closed reduction what tests must you do
       immediately?
       i.   l_____ c_____ p_____   lateral cervical puncture
                                                   followed by myelogram/CT
       ii. _____   MRI

28

36. **Complete the following:**   G7 p.944:50mm
   a. True or False. Patient with recent onset of loss of function due to spinal cord injury should have a decompressive laminectomy.

   false (Recent acute injury is not the time for surgery; it may be associated with neurologic deterioration.)

   b. If surgery is done it is usually combined with _____.

   a stabilization procedure

37. **Contraindications to emergent operation for acute spinal cord injury include**   G7 p.944:140mm
   a. complete _____ _____ _____ for more than 24 hours

   spinal cord injury

   b. unstable _____

   medically

   c. central _____ _____

   cord syndrome

■ Neurological Assessment

38. **Complete the following:**   G7 p.944:180mm
   a. Cervical nerves exit _____ their like-numbered vertebra.

   above

   b. Thoracic and lumbar nerves exit _____ their like-numbered vertebra.

   below

   c. For a segment of cord that lies under a given vertebra T2 to T10 add _____ _____ _____.

   two cord levels   G7 p.945:30mm

   d. Under T11, T12, L1 lie the _____.

   lowest 11 spinal segments

   e. The conus lies behind _____.

   L1 or L2

39. **Give the location of the key sensory landmarks.**   G7 p.945:55mm
   a. occipital protuberance   C2
   b. supraclavicular fossa   C3
   c. shoulders   C4
   d. lateral side of antecubital fossa   C5
   e. thumb   C6
   f. middle finger   C7
   g. little finger   C8
   h. medial side of antecubital fossa   T1
   i. nipples   T4
   j. xyphoid   T6
   k. umbilicus   T10
   l. inguinal ligament   T12
   m. medial femoral condyle   L3
   n. medial malleolus   L4
   o. great toe   L5
   p. lateral malleolus   S1
   q. popliteal fossa in midline   S2
   r. ischial tuberosity   S3
   s. perianal area   S4-5

28

40. Write out the American Spinal Injury Association (ASIA) motor scoring system—upper extremity—for the indicated root, muscle, and action to test.

G7 p.945:55mm

   a. root C5

     i.   muscle: d_____ or b_____   deltoid or biceps

     ii. action: s_____ a_____ or   shoulder abduction or elbow

          e_____ f_____   flexion

   b. root C6

     i.   muscle: w_____ e_____   wrist extensors

     ii. action: e_____ w_____   extend wrist

   c. root C7

     i.   muscle: t_____   triceps

     ii. action: e_____ e_____   extend elbow

   d. root C8

     i.   muscle: f_____ d_____   flexor digitorum profundus

          p_____

     ii. action: s_____ h_____   squeeze hand

   e. root T1

     i.   muscle: h_____ i_____   hand intrinsics

     ii. action: a_____ l_____   abduct little finger

          f_____

41. Write out the ASIA motor scoring system—lower extremity—for the indicated root, muscle, and action to test.

G7 p.945:56mm

   a. root L2

     i.   muscle: i_____   iliopsoas

     ii. action: f_____ h_____   flex hip

   b. root L3

     i.   muscle: q_____   quadriceps

     ii. action: s_____ k_____   straight knee

   c. root L4

     i.   muscle: t_____ a_____   tibialis anterior

     ii. action: d_____ f_____   dorsiflex foot

   d. root L5

     i.   muscle: e_____ h_____   extensor hallucis longus (EHL)

          l_____

     ii. action: d_____ g_____   dorsiflex great toe

          t_____

   e. root S1

     i.   muscle: g_____   gastrocnemius

     ii. action: p_____ f_____   plantar flex foot

          f_____

28

42. **Matching. Match the main nerve root responsible for the following motor action:**

G7 p.946:45mm

Nerve root:
① L3; ② L4; ③ L5; ④ S1
Motor action:
a. great toe extension   ③ (+S1)
b. ankle dorsiflexion   ② (+L5)
c. knee extension   ① (+L4)
d. ankle plantar flexion   ④ (+S2)

43. **Complete the following regarding Beevor sign:**

G7 p.946:75mm

a. It tests the level of spinal cord injury at about T_____.   T9
b. It is performed by
   i. flexing the _____.   neck
   ii. Note that the _____ moves cephalad.   umbilicus

44. **Complete the following regarding the abdominal cutaneous reflex:**

G7 p.946:83mm

a. The upper quadrant is served by _____.   T8-9
b. The lower quadrant is served by _____.   T10-11-12
c. Its presence indicates (at least some) function of the _____ _____.   spinal cord
d. There is _____ _____ spinal cord injury   no complete
e. because the reflex _____ to the _____ and then _____to the abdominal muscles.   ascends to the cortex and then descends

45. **Complete the following about priapism:**

G7 p.946:108mm

a. After spinal cord trauma it indicates injury to the _____ tone   sympathetic
b. and a dominance of _____ tone.   parasympathetic
c. Priapism indicates _____ prognosis for spinal cord recovery of function.   poor

28

46. **There is a sensory region that is not represented on the trunk.**

G7 p.946:148mm

a. It jumps from C_____ to T_____.   C4 to T2
b. These levels are distributed exclusively on the u_____ e_____.   upper extremities

47. **Give the motor and sensory**   G7 p.947:120mm
     descriptions for each class in the ASIA
     impairment scale as modified from the
     Frankel neurologic performance scale.
  a. class A
      i.   motor   no motor
      ii. sensory   no sensory, (class
                                        A = complete motor and
                                        sensory paralysis below
                                        lesion)

  b. class B
      i.   motor   no motor
      ii. sensory   some sensory, (class
                                        B = complete motor paralysis,
                                        some residual sensory
                                        perception below lesion)

  c. class C
      i.   motor   useless motor
      ii. sensory   good sensory, (class
                                        C = residual motor function
                                        but no practical use)

  d. class D
      i.   motor   some motor
      ii. sensory   good sensory, (class
                                        D = useful but subnormal
                                        motor function below lesion)

  e. class E
      i.   motor   good motor
      ii. sensory   good sensory (class
                                        E = normal)

■ Spinal Cord Injuries

48. **True or False. Regarding central cord**   G7 p.948:85mm
     injuries:
  a. They usually result from a hyperflexion   false (hyperextension)
      injury.
  b. Motor deficit is greater in the arms than true
      legs.
  c. Hyperpathia is uncommonly seen.   false (Hyperpathia is
                                                 commonly seen.)
  d. It is the most common type of   true   G7 p.948:140mm
      incomplete spinal injury.
  e. The cord's centermost region is a   true
      watershed zone.
  f. Somatotopic organization places fibers   false (more lateral)
      to lower extremities more medial.
  g. BP must be maintained at an MAP of   true   G7 p.949:107mm
      85 to 90 for at least 1 week.
  h. Prompt surgery for decompression is   false
      advised.

28

49. **A 45-year-old alcoholic male trips and falls, briefly losing consciousness. He was unable to move for 15 minutes, but currently complains only of weakness of both hands. He has an abrasion of his forehead. Computed tomographic (CT) scan of his head was negative. X-ray of C-spine reveals only spondylosis. True or False. Regarding this lesion:**

G7 p.949:140mm

a. It has the best prognosis of all incomplete spinal cord injuries.

false (Brown-Séquard has the best prognosis.)

b. There may be sparing of sensation around the anus with an intact voluntary anal sphincter.

true

c. Immediate surgery is recommended even for patients without spinal instability.

false

d. Urinary catheterization is recommended for patients in spinal shock.

true

50. **Complete the following about surgical intervention in patients who have had a central spinal cord injury:**

G7 p.949:140mm

a. Indications for surgical intervention are
    i. spine _____

instability

    ii. continued spinal cord compression in a patient who fails to _____ or _____

improve or deteriorates

b. What surgery should be done?

decompressive laminectomy and lateral mass or pedicle screw fixation and fusion

51. **What is the prognosis in patients with central cord injury?**

G7 p.950:82mm

a. _____% will recover enough to ambulate.

50%

b. Bowel and bladder function _____.

recovers

c. Upper extremities (do/don't) _____ recover well.

don't

d. Elderly patients (do/don't) _____ recover well.

don't

52. **Answer the following about anterior cord syndrome:**

G7 p.950:105mm

a. True or False. Motor findings are of hemiplegia below the lesion.

false (paraplegia)

b. True or False. There is loss of pain sensation, with preservation of deep pressure sensation.

true (deep pressure sensation is via posterior columns)

c. It may result from _____.

occlusion of anterior spinal artery

28

d. Sensory pattern is termed "dissociated" because there is loss of
  i. _____ _____ and preservation of — spinothalamic tract
  ii. _____ _____ _____. — posterior column function

53. **Answer the following about a Brown-Séquard syndrome:**   G7 p.950:116mm
  a. True or False. There is contralateral pain loss beginning 1 to 2 levels above the lesion. — false (Pain loss is 1 to 2 levels below the lesion.)
  b. True or False. Contralateral position sense is preserved. — true
  c. Prognosis compared with all other incomplete cord lesions is _____. — best of all the incomplete cord lesion types
  d. What% will eventually walk? — 90%

■ Cervical Spine Fractures
Atlanto-occipital Dislocation

54. **Complete the following:**   G7 p.951:156mm
  a. Incidence in spinal injury is approximately _____%. — 1%
  b. Are they more common in pediatrics or in adults? — pediatrics (twice as common)
  c. Mortality results from _____ _____ _____ _____. — respiratory arrest causing anoxia

55. **Complete the following about the three types of atlanto-occipital dislocation:**   G7 p.952:17mm
  a. Type I: occiput in relation to atlas is dislocated _____. — anteriorly
  b. Type II: occiput in relation to atlas is dislocated _____. — longitudinally distracted
  c. Type III: occiput in relation to atlas is dislocated _____. — posteriorly

56. **Name the ligaments at the following sites:**   G6 p.718:15mm
  a. atlas to occiput
    i. a_____ a_____-o_____ m_____ — anterior atlanto-occipital membrane (continuation of the ALL)
    ii. p_____ a_____-o_____ m_____ — posterior atlanto-occipital membrane
    iii. a_____ b_____ (of c_____ l_____) — ascending band (of cruciate ligament)
  b. axis to occiput (via dens)
    i. t_____ m_____ — tectorial membrane (continuation of the PLL)
    ii. a_____ l_____ — alar ligaments (occipital-alar portion)
    iii. a_____l_____ — apical ligament

c. atlas to axis
   i.   t_____ l_____   transverse ligament
                                                    (horizontal part of cruciate)
   ii. a_____ l_____   alar ligaments (atlanto-alar
                                                      portion)
   iii. d_____ b_____ (of   descending band (of cruciate
          c_____ l_____)   ligament)

57. Complete the following: G6 p.718:100mm
  a. What structure is the cephalad extension
     of the
     i.   anterior longitudinal ligament?   anterior atlanto-occipital
                                             membrane
     ii. posterior longitudinal ligament? tectorial membrane
  b. Which structures are most important in
     maintaining atlanto-occipital stability?
     i.   t_____ m_____   tectorial membrane
     ii. a_____ l_____   alar ligaments

58. Complete the following: G6 p.719:60mm
  a. Name the horizontal component of the transverse ligament
     cruciate ligament.
  b. What does it hold together?   odontoid and atlas
  c. What is the strongest ligament in the   transverse ligament
     spine?

59. Complete the following: G7 p.952:55mm
  a. The best method by which to measure is BAI-BDI (basion axial interal-
     the _____.   basion dental interval)
  b. It is considered normal if each is less than 12
     _____ mm.
  c. Another method is called the _____ Powers ratio
     _____.
  d. Traction may be used but _____% of 10%
     patients deteriorate.

60. Complete the following: G7 p.952:145mm
  a. A measurement used in evaluating   Powers ratio
     atlanto-occipital dislocation (AOD) is
     called _____ _____.
     i.   divide distance from basion to   post prior arch of atlas
         _____ _____ _____ of
         _____
     ii. by distance from opisthion to   anterior arch of atlas
         _____ _____ of _____
  b. It is considered normal if below _____. 0.9, > 0.9 and < 1 = gray zone
  c. It is definitely abnormal if above   1 = AOD (assumes an intact
     _____.   atlas and foramen magnum)

**61. Powers ratio greater than _____ is 1.0   G7 p.952:145mm
    diagnostic of atlanto-occipital
    dislocation.**

62. AOD is suspected if   G7 p.953:70mm
  a. the atlanto-occipital interval is greater 2
     than _____ mm and/or
  b. there is blood in the _____ _____. basal cisterns   G7 p.954:45mm

28

■ Occipital Condyle Fractures

63. **Complete the following:**   G7 p.954:130mm
  a. Can they involve the hypoglossal nerve?   yes
  b. List the types.
    i.   I is a _____ fracture.   comminuted
    ii. II has a _____ fracture.   linear
    iii. III has an _____ fracture.   avulsion
  c. Treatment is with _____ or   collar or halo
    _____.

  d. Incidence in trauma patients is   0.4%   G7 p.955:35mm
    _____%.

■ Atlanto-axial Dislocation

64. **Answer the following about atlanto-**   G7 p.955:120mm
    axial dislocation:
  a. True or False. It has less morbidity and   true
    mortality than atlanto-occipital
    dislocation.
  b. Name and describe the three types.
    i.   rotatory subluxation
    ii. atlanto-axial dislocation
        type I
        transverse ligament _____   intact
        facet capsule _____   bilateral injury
        treatment _____   soft collar
        type II
        transverse ligament _____   injured
        facet capsule _____   unilateral injury
        treatment _____   Philadelphia collar or SOMI
        type III
        transverse ligament _____   injured
        facet capsule _____   bilateral injury
        treatment _____   halo
    iii. anterior atlanto-axial dislocation
        o_____ f_____   odontoid fracture
        c_____ h_____   congenital hypoplasia
        d_____ of t_____ l_____   disruption of transverse
        ligament

65. **Complete the following regarding**   G7 p.956:40mm
    atlanto-axial rotatory subluxation:
  a. Name four causes.
    Hint: stur
    i.   s_____   spontaneous
    ii. t_____   trauma
    iii. u_____   upper respiratory tract
        infection (Grisel syndrome)
    iv. r_____   rheumatoid arthritis
  b. Competence of the _____ _____   transverse ligament
    must be assessed.

28

c. What is the characteristic head position? — "cock robin" (20 degrees lateral tilt, 20 degrees rotation opposite, slight flexion)

d. Patients are usually _____.   young   G7 p.956:70mm
e. It can occlude the _____ arteries.   vertebral

66. **Complete the following regarding the rule of Spence:**   G7 p.957:120mm
a. It is designed to determine if the _____ _____ is disrupted.   transverse ligament
b. If disrupted what effect does it have on treatment?   halo versus collar
c. It is performed by studying what view on x-ray?   open-mouthed AP odontoid view
d. To assess what structures?   lateral masses of C1-C2 overhang
e. The critical reference number is _____.   7 mm—sum of both sides

◼ Atlas (C1) Fractures

67. **Complete the following:**   G7 p.957:165mm
a. isolated fracture _____%   56%
b. combined with C2 fracture _____%   44%
c. additional spine fracture _____%   9%
d. combined with head injury _____%   21%

68. **True or False. Regarding a Jefferson fracture:**   G7 p. 958:35mm
a. It involves a single fracture through the arch of C1.   false (At least 2 fracture sites—it's a ring!)
b. It is generally a stable fracture.   false (But without neurologic deficit.)
c. "Rule of Spence" assesses displacement of the dens on a lateral C-spine x-ray.   false (Rule of Spence assesses the lateral movement of the C1 lateral masses; if sum of overhang of both sides > 7 mm, halo will be necessary for treatment; assessed on AP C-spine x-ray.)
d. Treatment is generally surgical (fusion).   false (Treatment is generally with external immobilization—soft collar or rigid external device.)

28

◼ Atlas (C2) Fractures

69. **Complete the following about acute fractures of the axis:**   G7 p.959:35mm
a. Represent _____% of cervical fractures   20%
b. Neurologic deficit occurs in _____%.   10%

70. Complete the following: G7 p.960:13mm

a. True or False. Regarding hangman's fracture:

    i.   In contrast to judicial hanging, modern-day hangman's fractures result from hyperextension and distraction.   false (hyperextension and axial loading)

    ii. This is usually a stable fracture.   true

    iii. There is a common occurrence of nonunion, hence the need for surgery.   false (usually heal with external immobilization)

b. Hangman's fracture results in a fracture through the _____.   pars interarticularis bilaterally

c. It is also known as _____.   traumatic spondylolisthesis of the axis

71. Complete the following regarding hangman's fracture: G7 p.960:58mm

a.

    i.   Subluxation of C2 and C3 by more than _____ mm   3

    ii. indicates _____ disruption.   disc

b.   G7 p.961:106mm

    i.   This is a marker for _____   instability

    ii. and usually requires _____.   stabilization

72. Classify hangman's fractures and give the subluxation, angulation, and neurologic deficit.   G7 p.960:70mm

a. Type I

    i.   subluxation: _____   < 3 mm

    ii. angulation: _____   0

    iii. neurologic deficit: _____   0

b. Type IA

    i.   subluxation: _____   2 to 3 mm

    ii. angulation: _____   0

    iii. neurologic deficit: _____ %   33%

c. Type II

    i.   subluxation: _____   > 3 mm

    ii. angulation: _____   not specified   G7 p.960:150mm

    iii. neurologic deficit: _____   rare

d. Type IIA

    i.   subluxation: _____   < 3 mm

    ii. angulation: _____   > 15 degrees

    iii. neurologic deficit: _____ %   10%

e. Type III

    i.   subluxation: _____   yes

    ii. angulation: _____   facets locked

    iii. neurologic deficit: _____   deficit: ± fatal: occasionally

f. A special caution for fractures IIA and III it is best to avoid the use of _____.   traction

g. Whose classification is this?   Effendi

28

73. Describe radiologic abnormalities of hangman's fractures.

G7 p.960:82mm

a. Type I
   i.   vertical pars fracture   yes
   ii. disruption   none
b. Type IA
   i.   vertical pars fracture   yes, nonparallel
   ii. disruption   none
c. Type II
   i.   vertical pars fracture   yes
   ii. disruption   C2-3 disc
d. Type IIA
   i.   vertical pars fracture   yes, oblique
   ii. disruption   none
e. Type III
   i.   vertical pars fracture   yes
   ii. disruption   facets of C2/C3 subluxed or locked

74. Classify hangman's fractures.

G7 p.960::90mm

a. Type I
   i.   subluxation less than _____ mm   3 mm
   ii. angulation _____   none
b. Type IA
   i.   C2 appearance   elongated
   ii. canal   narrowed
   iii. typical?   atypical
   iv. paralysis?   33%
c. Type II
   i.   subluxation more than _____ mm   3 mm
   ii. angulation more than _____   11 degrees (indicates disruption of C2-3 disc and PLL)
d. Type IIA
   i.   subluxation is _____   < 3 mm
   ii. angulation _____   more angulation than type II
e. Type III
   i.   facets are _____ and   C2-3 facets disrupted (conceptually similar to bilateral jumped facets)
   ii. _____ with traction   nonreducible

75. Most hangman's fracture patients

G7 p.961:60mm

a. present neurologically _____ and   intact
b. need MRI to assess _____ disc.   C2-C3

G7 p.962:26mm

c.
   i.   It can be treated with _____   immobilization
   ii. for _____ weeks.   12
d. Average time to heal is _____ weeks,   11.5

28

76. **Describe treatment of Effendi**   G7 p.963:110mm
       classification fractures
   a. Type I: c_____   collar
   b. Type IA: c_____   collar
   c. Type II: Less than 5 mm sublux and less
      than 10 degrees angulation
      i.   t_____   traction
      ii. h_____   halo
   d. Type IIA: More than 5 mm sublux or   surgical fusion
      more than 10 degrees angulation

      _____
      i.   no t_____   traction
      ii. h_____   halo
   e. Type III:
      i.   M_____   MRI
      ii. s_____   surgery (ORIF)

77. **Describe the radiologic criteria of**   G7 p.963:110mm
       good fusion.
   a. Across the fracture site we should see   trabeculations
      _____.
   b. Flexion-extension radiographs should   movement
      show no _____.

■ Odontoid Fractures

78. **Complete the following about**   G7 p.963:160mm
       odontoid fractures:
   a. Odontoid fractures represent   10 to 15%
      approximately _____% of all cervical
      spine fractures.
   b. Mechanism of injury is usually _____. flexion
   c. They are fatal in about _____%.   25 to 40%
   d. Major deficits in type II is _____%.   10%
   e. In Type III it is _____ to have   rare
      neurologic deficit.
   f. A displacement
      i.   of _____ mm   6 mm
      ii. results in a nonunion rate of   70%
           _____%
      iii. therefore the treatment advised is   surgical
           _____

79. **True or False. Regarding odontoid**   G7 p.963:170mm
       fractures:
   a. They are a hyperflexion injury in most   true
      instances.
   b. Most patients have presenting   false
      neurological deficit.
   c. Neck pain is infrequent.   false

28

80. **Complete the following:**   G7 p.964:50mm
   a. Regarding odontoid fractures:
      i.   Type I is fracture through the   apical dens (rare)
           _____.
      ii. Type II is fracture through the   base of the dens
           _____.
      iii. Type III is fracture through the   body of C2
           _____.
   b. True or False. The spinal cord occupies   false (Steele's rule of thirds:
      50% of the canal at C1.   dens, space, spinal cord.)
   c. True or False. The ossiculum terminale   false (Os
      results from posttraumatic fracture of   odontoideum = fracture of
      the apical dens.   apical dens or avulsion of alar
                                                   ligament. Ossiculum
                                                   terminale = nonunion of
                                                   secondary ossification
                                                   center.)

81. **Complete the following:**   G7 p.965:75mm
   a. List indications for surgical treatment of
      Type II odontoid fractures.
      i.   displacement of dens more than   5 mm (4 to 5 or 6 mm used
           _____ mm   by some)
      ii. despite halo there is _____   instability
      iii. despite immobilization there is   nonunion
           _____
      iv. patient is older than _____   50
      v.   disruption of the _____   transverse ligament
           _____
   b. True or False. Most odontoid type III   false (Most [90%] heal with
      fractures should be treated surgically   external immobilization.)
      due to low union rate by rigid external
      immobilization (halo).

■ Os Odontoideum

82. **The appearance of os odontoideum is**   G7 p.966:135mm
   a. a _____ bone   separate
   b. with _____ borders   smooth
   c. near a _____ odontoid peg.   short
   d. It may fuse with the _____.   clivus
   e. It may mimic an _____ fracture.   odontoid

83. **Complete the following about os**   G7 p.966:142mm
    odontoideum:
   a. Postulated etiologies
      i.   c_____   congenital
      ii. a_____   acquired—avulsion of alar
                                                   ligament
   b. Does treatment depend on the etiology?   no
   c. Myelopathy correlates with an AP canal   13 mm
      diameter of less than _____.
   d. Will immobilization result in fusion?   no

28

e. Treatment
   i.   p_____ w_____   posterior wiring C1-C2
   ii.   t_____ s_____   transarticular screw
f. Do we need a halo with each of these   not with transarticular screws
   procedures?

■ Combined C1 and C2 Fractures

84. Complete the following about   G7 p.967:123mm
combined C1 and C2 fractures:
a. Treatment is decided based on type of   C2
   _____ fracture.
b. An odontoid fracture type II that is
   displaced more than
   i.   _____ mm is considered   5 mm
   ii.   _____.   unstable
c. Treatment is with _____ _____   posterior surgical fusion
   _____.

■ Subaxial (C3 through C7) Injuries/Fractures

85. Answer the following about SCIWORA: G7 p.975:20mm
a. True or False.
   i.   There is a higher incidence in age   true
       ≤ 9 years.
   ii.   There is a risk of SCIWORA among   true
       young children with asymptomatic
       Chiari I.
   iii.   Dynamic flexion/extension (F/E)   true
       films are normal.
   iv.   54% of children have a delay   true
       between injury and the onset of
       objective sensorimotor dysfunction.
b. SCIWORA stands for _____.   spinal cord injury without
                                       radiological abnormality

86. Matching. For the following   G7 p.968:100mm
conditions, choose the most
appropriate mechanism producing the
cervical fracture.
Mechanism:
① hyperextension; ② vertical
compression; ③ hyperflexion; ④ flexion
plus rotation
Condition:
a. burst fracture   ②
b. unilateral locked facet   ④
c. bilateral locked facet   ③
d. laminar fracture   ①

87. Clay shoveler's fracture usually   C7   G7 p.969:160mm
involves the spinous process of
_____.

28

88. Guidelines for determining clinical instability include   G7 p.970:20mm

a. compromise of the anterior elements produces more instability in _____.   extension

b. compromise of the posterior elements produces more instability in _____.   flexion

c. extension will demonstrate more instability if the _____ elements are injured.   anterior

d. flexion will demonstrate more instability if the _____ elements are injured.   posterior

89. Give radiographic criteria for clinical instability.   G7 p.970:60mm

a. A sagittal plane displacement of _____ mm and   > 3.5 mm

b. relative sagittal plane angulation of _____ degrees (on neutral position lateral C-spine films) are associated with instability.   > 11 degrees

90. True or False. The following is true of teardrop fractures: G7 p.970:135mm

a. They usually result from
   i. hyperflexion injuries   true
   ii. compression flexion injury   true
   iii. hyperextension injury   false

b. They are stable fractures.   false (Teardrop fractures are unstable due to complete disruption of the ALL, PLL, and facet joints.)

c. The fractured vertebra is usually displaced posteriorly into the spinal canal.   true

d. They are often associated with a fracture through the sagittal plane of the vertebral body.   true

e. The patient is often quadriplegic.   true

f. A "teardrop" chip of bone is at the anterior-superior edge of the vertebral body.   false (Teardrop is at the anterior-inferior edge of the vertebral body.)

91. Complete the following: G7 p.971:37mm

a. A teardrop fracture must be distinguished from an _____ _____.   avulsion fracture

   i. _____ is unstable and requires _____, and   Teardrop; surgery

   ii. _____ is stable.   avulsion

28

b. How can we distinguish them? Serious teardrop will have:
Hint: sansfhh

    i. size of fracture _____   small chip
    ii. alignment _____   displaced
    iii. neurological _____   injured
    iv. soft tissue _____   swelling
    v. fracture _____   through vertebra
    vi. height of disc _____   reduced
    vii. height of vertebral body _____   reduced or wedged

c. If in doubt perform _____ views.   flexion-extension views
d. If negative repeat _____ _____ in   flexion-extension views in 4 to
_____ to _____ days.   7 days
e. The fractured vertebra is displaced _____.   posteriorly

f. True teardrop fractures should be   combined anterior and
treated with c_____ a_____ and   posterior fusions
p_____ f_____.

92. Quadrangular fractures have four features.   G7 p.971:140mm

a. feature 1: an _____ fracture   oblique
    i. from _____-_____   anterior-superior
    ii. to _____ _____ _____   inferior end plate
b. feature 2: subluxation of superior   posteriorly
vertebral body (VB) on the inferior VB _____

c. feature 3: with angular _____   kyphosis
d. feature 4: disruption of
    i. _____   disc
    ii. _____   ALL
    iii. _____   PLL
e. Treat with _____ _____   combined anterior and
_____ _____ _____.   posterior fusion

93. Describe distraction flexion injuries.   G7 p.971:165mm

a. Flexion injuries include _____.   strain, subluxation, locked facets
b. Which ligament is injured early?   posterior ligamentous complex
c. X-rays demonstrate this by showing _____.   widening of the interspinous distance
d. We may need to test by performing _____.   flexion-extension views (or MRI)
e. If symptoms persist 1 to 2 weeks we should _____.   repeat the flexion-extension views
f. Ligamentous instability is confirmed if there is a
    i. subluxation of _____ mm or angulation of   3.5 mm
    ii. _____ degrees.   11

94. Describe locked facets.   G7 p.972:85mm

a. Normally the inferior facet of the level   posterior
   above is _____ to the superior facet
   of the level below.

b. In locked facets there is _____   disruption

c. of the facet _____.   capsule

d. Flexion and rotation produces _____   unilateral locked facet

   _____ _____.

e. Hyperflexion produces _____   bilateral locked facets

   _____ _____.

f. Neurological injury is _____ for cord   frequent
   and/or root injury.

g. In patients with locked facets the inferior   anterior
   facet of the level above is _____ to
   the superior facet of the level below.

95. Describe evidence of locked facets on   G7 p.973:25mm
x-ray.

a. In unilateral locked facets the spinous   unilateral locked facet
   process is rotated to the side of the

   _____ _____ _____.

b. Facets look like a _____ _____.   bow tie

c. Interspinous space is _____.   widened

d. Neural foramen is _____.   blocked

e. Articular surfaces of the facets are   on the wrong side

   _____ _____ _____

   _____.

96. Complete the following regarding   G7 p.973:60mm
locked facets:

a. When the articulating surfaces of the   naked facet
   facets are on the wrong side, this is
   called the "_____ _____ sign."

b. In bilateral locked facets traumatic disc   80%
   herniation is found in _____%.

c. Attempt at closed reduction of locked   10
   facets by traction must not exceed
   _____ lb per vertebral level.

d. Disc space height must not exceed   10
   _____ mm.

e. If neurologic worsening occurs you   disc herniation
   should suspect _____ _____

f. and plan for _____ _____.   prompt surgery

g.   G7 p.973:120mm

   i.   Closed reduction is c_____   contraindicated
   ii. until MRI assesses for t_____   traumatic herniated disc
        h_____ d_____.

28

97. **Answer the following about locked facets:**

G7 p.974:60mm

a. True or False. Stabilization is more likely to be successful in halo if there are
 i. multiple fractures of the facets　true
 ii. no fractures of the facets　false
b. Halo alone is successful for good anatomical result in _____%.　23%
c. Failure of good anatomical result occurs in _____%.　77%
d. True or False: Surgical fusion is therefore more or less clearly indicated in cases without facet fracture fragments.　true

98. **Complete the following about subaxial (C3 through C7) injuries/fractures:**

G7 p.974:155mm

a. Extension injuries can produce
 i. _____ in adults and　central cord syndrome
 ii. _____ in children.　SCIWORA
b. The ligament that is most often injured in extension injuries is the _____.　ALL
c. Is disc injury possible?　yes
d. What vascular injury can occur?　carotid artery dissection

99. **Complete the following:**

G7 p.978:25mm

a. When combined anterior and posterior cervical fusion is needed which should be done first?　anterior
b. When the mechanism of injury is flexion what is the procedure of choice?　posterior fusion
c. When the mechanism of injury is extension what is the procedure of choice for
 i. teardrop fracture is c_____ a_____ and p_____ fusion　combined anterior and posterior
 ii. burst fracture is c_____ a_____ and p_____ fusion　combined anterior and posterior

100. **Complete the following about cervical corpectomy:**

G7 p.978:110mm

a. Decompression of the cord usually requires corpectomy that is at least _____ mm wide.　16 mm
b. It is advised to note position of _____ _____.　vertebral arteries

101. **Complete the following about football-related cervical spine injuries:**

G7 p.980:85mm

a. stinger
 i. involves _____　one extremity
 ii. represents _____　compression of a root
b. burning hands
 i. involves _____　both arms
 ii. represents _____　mild central cord syndrome

28

   c. neuropraxia
     i. involves _____   four extremities
     ii. represents _____   cervical cord injury
   d. must rule out _____   cervical stenosis
   e. by performing an _____   MRI

102. Complete the following: G7 p.980:140mm
   a. A football player who uses his helmet as   spear tackler
       a battering ram is called a _____.
   b. What evidence may be present on his
       spine x-rays?
     i. loss of _____   lordosis
     ii. evidence of _____ _____   prior trauma
     iii. presence of _____ _____   cervical spinal stenosis
        _____
   c. When may the athlete resume play?   when lordosis returns

103. True or False. Contact sports are   G7 p.981:45mm
**   permitted in**
   a. Klippel-Feil with symptoms   false
   b. Klippel-Feil without symptoms   true
   c. spina bifida   true
   d. status post-anterior cervical discectomy   true
       and fusion (ACDF) 1 level
   e. status post-ACDF 2 levels   false
   f. status post-ACDF 3 levels   false

104. Delayed cervical instability is defined   20   G7 p.982:35mm
**   as instability identified after _____**
**   days.**

105. Complete the following about blunt   G7 p.982:115mm
**   cerebrovascular injuries (BCVI):**
   a. The usual injury is _____.   dissection
   b. It occurs in _____% of BCVI patients.   1 to 2%
   c. Mortality occurs in _____%.   13
   d. Which is a better test: MRI or CTA?   CTA
   e.   G7 p.984:52mm
     i. Treatment is with h_____   heparin
     ii. or occasionally with e_____   endovascular
        techniques.

106. Complete the following regarding   G7 p.985:55mm
**   blunt vertebral artery injury:**
   a. most common etiology _____   motor vehicular accidents
   b. treatment to strongly consider is   IV heparin
       _____ _____
   c. because strokes were _____   more frequent
       _____ in those patients not treated
   d. incidence is _____% but   0.5 to 0.7%   G7 p.985:85mm
   e. increases to _____% if cervical   6%
       fracture or ligament injury
   f. Is there a warning "TIA"?   no   G7 p.985:130mm
   g. Can occur from _____ hours to   8; 12
       _____ days

28

h. Is any cervical fracture pattern a   no   G7 p.985:145mm
    predictor of blunt vertebral injury?
i. Overall mortality was _____%   16%   G7 p.986:17mm
j. Bilateral VA dissection is highly   fatal
    _____.

■ Thoracolumbar Spine Fractures

107. Complete the following about thoracic   G7 p.986:48mm
and lumbar spine fractures:
a. Percent of spinal fractures that occur at   64%
    T11, T12, L1 is _____%.
b. Percent that have neurological deficits is 30%
    _____%.

108. Matching. Match the following   G7 p.986:100mm
structures with the appropriate Denis
column:
① anterior; ② middle; ③ posterior
a. anterior half of disc   ①
b. posterior half of disc   ②
c. posterior arch   ③
d. anterior half of vertebral body   ①
e. posterior half of vertebral body   ②
f. facet joints and capsule   ③
g. anterior anulus fibrosus   ①
h. posterior anulus fibrosus   ②
i. interspinous ligament   ③
j. supraspinous ligament   ③
k. anterior longitudinal ligament   ①
l. posterior longitudinal ligament   ②
m. ligamentum flavum   ③

109. True or False. The following are   G7 p.986:165mm
considered minor fractures of the
lumbar spine:
a. fracture of transverse process   true
b. fracture of spinous process   true
c. fracture of superior articular process   true
d. fracture of inferior articular process   true
e. fracture of superior end plate of   false (Fracture of the superior
    vertebral body   end plate of the vertebral
                                               body is not considered a
                                               minor fracture.)

110. True or False. Major injuries of the   G7 p.987:110mm
spine include:
a. compression fracture   true
b. burst fracture   true
c. seat belt fracture   true
d. fracture of articular process   false (Fracture of the articular
                                               process is a minor fracture.)
e. fracture dislocation   true

111. **True or False. Subtypes of burst fracture include the following:**

G7 p.987:75mm

a. fracture of both end plates — true
b. fracture of superior end plate — true
c. fracture of inferior end plate — true
d. fracture of pars interarticularis — false (Fracture of the pars interarticularis is not a burst fracture.)
e. burst rotation — true

112. **True or False. Regarding burst fracture:**

G7 p.987:78mm

a. It occurs mainly at thoracolumbar junction — true
b. Mechanism—axial load — true
c. Mechanism—flexion and compression — false (Mechanism is not flexion and compression but pure axial loading and in some subtypes added flexion.)
d. It is a consequence of fracture of the anterior and middle column. — true
e. The most common subtype is fracture of the superior end plate. — true

113. **True or False. Radiographic evaluation of burst fracture might show the following on**

G7 p.987:100mm

a. lateral x-ray—cortical fracture of posterior vertebral wall — true
b. AP x-ray—increase in interpedicular distance — true
c. lateral x-ray—loss of posterior vertebral height — true
d. CT—fracture posterior wall with retropulsed bone — true
e. myelogram—large central defect — true

114. **True or False. Seat belt fracture has all of the following subtypes:**

G7 p.987:145mm

a. chance fracture, one-level through bone — true
b. one-level through ligaments — true
c. two-level, bone in middle column ligaments in anterior and posterior columns — true
d. pedicle fracture — false (A pedicle fracture is not one of the subtypes of seat belt fracture.)
e. two-level through ligaments in all three columns — true

28

115. State which of the following are stable or unstable fractures of the spine: G7 p.988:160mm

a. three or more consecutive compression fractures — unstable

b. a single compression fracture with loss of > 50% of height with angulation — unstable

c. kyphotic angulation > 40 degrees at one level or > 25% — unstable

d. Chance fracture — stable

e. progressive kyphosis — unstable

116. State whether the following are stable or unstable fractures of the spine: G7 p.989:60mm

a. middle column fracture above T8 below T1 if ribs and sternum intact is _____ — stable

b. middle column fracture below l4 if posterior column is intact is _____ — stable

c. posterior column fracture is _____ — stable

d. compression fracture in three consecutive segments is _____ — unstable

117. True or False. Regarding burst fractures: G7 p.989:153mm

a. Surgical treatment is recommended if angular deformity > 20 degrees. — true

b. Surgical treatment is recommended for patients with neurologic deficit. — true

c. Surgical treatment is recommended for anterior body height reduction ≥ 50% compared with the posterior body height. — true

d. Surgery is recommended for canal reduction ≥ 50%. — true

e. The anterior approach is recommended if a dural tear is present. — false (A posterior approach is recommended if there is a dural tear.)

118. Burst fractures are unstable if   G7 p.989:154mm
Hint: KIPHD

a. K—Kyphosis is more than _____ — 20

b. I—Interpendicular distance is _____ — Increased

c. P—Progressive _____ occurs — Kyphosis

d. H—Height of anterior body is less than _____% _____ — 50; posterior

e. D—Deficit in n_____ status — neurological

119. True or False. Regarding L5 burst fractures: G7 p.990:40mm

a. They are very common. — false

b. It is difficult for instrumentation to maintain alignment at this level. — true

c. Patients will lose ~15 degrees of lordosis between L4 and S1 even with instrumentation. — true

28

d. If treatment is nonsurgical a thoracolumbar-sacral orthosis (TLSO) brace is recommended for 4 to 6 months.

true

e. If treatment is surgical a posterior approach with fusion and fixation L5-S1 is recommended.

true

f. If "ligamentotaxis" is expected, distraction should be done within _____ hours.

48

G7 p.990:165mm

120. Complete the following about post-spinal fusion wound infections:

G7 p.991:155mm

a. They are usually due to _____ _____.

Staph aureus

b. They may respond to _____ alone.

antibiotics

c. Rarely _____ may be necessary.

debridement

d. Only occasionally must instruments be _____.

removed

121. Complete the following regarding demographics of osteoporotic spine fractures:

G7 p.992:28mm

a. True or False. There are ~700,000 osteoporotic fractures per year in the United States.

true

b. True or False. Risk factors include weight > 58 kg (127 lb).

false (Risk factors include weight below 58 kg [127 lb].)

c. There is a risk with the use of which anticonvulsant?

phenytoin

d. There is a risk with the use of which anticoagulant?

warfarin

e. There is a risk with consumption of which beverage?

ETOH

f. There is a risk with the use of c_____.

cigarettes

g. There is a risk with the use of which anti-inflammatory drug?

steroids

122. Complete the following regarding osteoporotic spine fractures:

G7 p.992:35mm

a. The most likely population is _____ _____ _____.

elderly white females

b. Can these fractures occur in premenopausal women?

yes

c. The lifetime risk for women is _____%.

16%

d. The lifetime risk for men is _____%.

5%

e. The best predictor of fractures is

i.   the _____ _____ _____ test

bone mineral density

ii. measured at the _____ _____.

proximal femur

28

123. **True or False. Regarding bone mineral density (BMD):**

G7 p.992:110mm

a. It is not the correct predictor of bone fragility. false

b. It is measured by Dexa Scan at the proximal femur. true

c. The AP view of the lumbosacral spine underestimates BMD. false (It overestimates BMD.)

d. The *T*-score of BMD compares to normal subjects. true

e. The *Z*-score defines osteoporosis compared with subjects of the same age and sex. true

124. **True or False. Regarding sodium fluoride:**

G7 p.993:59mm

a. 75 mg/d increases bone mass. true

b. 75 mg/d decreases fracture rate. false (It increases bone mass but did not reduce the fracture rate.)

c. 25 mg by mouth twice a day (slow fluoride) decreases the fracture rate. true

d. 25 mg PO BID (slow fluoride) increases the fragility of the bone. true

e. Fluoride increases the demand for Ca. true

f. If you use fluoride also use Ca and vitamin D. true

125. **True or False. The following drugs reduce bone resorption:**

G7 p.993:80mm

a. estrogen true

b. calcium true

c. vitamin D true

d. calcitonin true

126. **Calcitonin is derived from s_____.** salmon

G7 p.993:150mm

127. **How do the bisphosphonates work?**

G7 p.993:170mm

a. They inhibit _____ _____ bone resorption

b. by destroying _____. osteoclasts (They are carbon-substituted analogues of pyrophosphate.)

128. **True or False. The following are bisphosphonates that inhibit bone resorption:**

G7 p.993:183mm

a. etidronate (Didronel) true

b. alendronate (Fosamax) true

c. risedronate (Actonel) true

28

G7 p.994:92mm

129. **True or False. Recommended treatment for osteoporotic vertebral body fracture includes**
    a. sufficient pain medications   true
    b. bed rest for 3 to 4 weeks   false (7 to 10 days)
    c. DVT prophylaxis is contraindicated.   false
    d. Start physical therapy in 7 to 10 days.   true
    e. lumbar brace for pain control and comfort   true

G7 p.994:140mm

130. **True or False. Regarding PVP:**
    a. PVP stands for percutaneous vertebroplasty.   true
    b. It involves injection of polymethylmethacrylate (PMMA) into compressed bone.   true
    c. Goals include prevention of progression of kyphosis.   true
    d. Goals include correction of kyphosis.   false
    e. Goals include shortened duration of pain.   true

G7 p.995:45mm

131. **True or False. Indications for PVP include the following:**
    a. severe pain that interferes with activity   true
    b. painful osteoporotic compression fracture with < 10% of height reduction   false (We do not treat for less than 10% reduction in height.)
    c. failure to control pain with pain medications   true
    d. progressive vertebral hemangioma   true
    e. pedicle screw salvage   true

G7 p.995:100mm

132. **True or False. Vertebroplasty contraindications include**
    a. international normalized ratio (INR) of 3.4   true
        i.   because patient has _____   coagulopathy
    b. injury occurred > 8 months ago   true
        i.   because patient has _____   completely healed
        _____
    c. fever, chills, elevated WBCs   true
        i.   because patient has _____   active infection
        _____
    d. burst fracture   true
        i.   because of concern for _____   leakage of PMMA
        _____

28

133. **Matching. Match the complications of PVP with the order in which they are more likely to occur with.** G7 p.995:140mm
     Occurrence:
     ① highest; ② second highest; ③ least complications
     Complications:
     a. vertebral hemangiomas   ②
     b. pathologic fractures   ①
     c. osteoporotic compression fractures   ③

134. **True or False. Complications of PVP include** G7 p.995:145mm
     a. PMMA leak   true
     b. pedicle fracture   true
     c. transverse process fracture   true
     d. spinous process fracture   false
     e. rib fracture   true

135. **True or False. Post-PVP recommendations include the following:** G7 p.997:25mm
     a. discharge home the same day   false (Patients are usually admitted overnight.)
     b. watch for chest pain   true
     c. watch for fever   true
     d. watch for neurologic deficit   true
     e. gradual mobilization after 2 hours   true

■ Sacral Fractures

136. **Complete the following:** G7 p.997:65mm
     a. Look for in patients who have _____ fractures   pelvic
        i. because _____% will also have sacral fractures   17%
     b. accompanied in _____% by neurologic deficits.   20 to 60%
     c. Sacral fractures are divided into _____ zones.   three
        i. I involves _____ _____.   ala only
        ii. II involves _____ _____.   sacral foramina
        iii. III involves _____ _____. sacral canal
     d. The fractures that involve neurologic deficits are those involving zone _____ and zone _____.   II and III
     e. Which fracture can cause bowel and bladder incontinence?   zone III (bilateral nerve injury)
     f. Which fracture can cause L5 root injury?   zone I   G7 p.997:132mm

28

■ Gunshot Wounds to the Spine

137. **Name the surgical indications for gunshot wounds (GSW) to the spine.**
G7 p.998:60mm
Hint: rinds

a. remove _____-jacketed bullet   copper (local reaction)

b. _____ is more of a concern in _____ than _____ GSW   infection; military; civilian

c. neurologic
  i. cauda e_____ i_____   equina injury
  ii. root _____ c_____   nerve root compression
  iii. leak _____   CSF leak
  iv. hema _____   spinal hematoma/vascular injury

d. delayed complications
  i. migrating _____   bullet
  ii. plumbism means _____ _____   lead toxicity

e. sp_____ inst_____   spinal instability (rare)

138. **True or False. Indications for surgery in gunshot wounds to the spine include the following:**
G7 p.998:60mm

a. injury to cauda equina if root compression is demonstrated   true

b. to remove copper-jacketed bullets from the spine   true

c. CSF leak   true

d. compression of nerve root   true

e. vascular injury   true

f. to improve spinal cord function   false (Surgery will not improve spinal cord function.)

■ Penetrating Trauma to the Neck

139. **Matching. Penetrating wounds of the neck are divided into three zones by anatomical boundaries.**
G7 p.998:145mm
Zone:
① zone I; ② zone II; ③ zone III
Anatomical boundaries:

a. clavicle   ②

b. angle of mandible   ②–③

c. head of clavicle   ①

d. thoracic outlet   ①

e. base of skull   ③

28

140. **True or False. Regarding vascular injuries of the neck:**   G7 p.998:168mm

   a. Venous injuries occur in ≈ 30% of penetrating neck trauma.   false (Venous injury represents 18%.)

   b. Arterial injuries occur in ≈ 12% of penetrating neck trauma.   true

   c. 72% of vertebral artery injuries had no neurological deficits on exam.   true

   d. Common carotid artery injury is the most common vascular injury.   true

141. **True or False. Treatment of penetrating trauma to the neck includes all of the following:**   G7 p.999:89mm

   a. Immediate prophylactic intubation to protect airway   false (Intubation is not needed in stable patients.)

   b. Cricothyroidotomy if apparent mechanical instability of the neck   true

   c. Surgical exploration is recommended for all wounds piercing the platysma and entering the anterior triangle of the neck.   true

   d. Patients in coma are poor candidates for surgical vascular reconstruction.   true

142. **Complete the following regarding vertebral artery (VA) trauma:**   G7 p.999:148mm

   a. It is more common to treat by _____ than by direct repair.   ligation

      i. What must you know about other vessels before you decide on treatment of VA injury?   their patency

      ii. Which vessels?   contralateral VA and posterior inferior cerebellar artery (PICA)

   b. What minimally invasive treatment is available?   endovascular occlusion

   c. Is arterial bypass ever indicated?   yes

28

■ Chronic Management of Spinal Cord Injuries

143. **True or False. Syndromes associated with spinal cord injuries include all of the following:**   G7 p.1000:98mm

   a. autonomic hyporeflexia   false (Autonomic hyperreflexia is associated with spinal cord injury.)

   b. DVT   true

   c. syringomyelia   true

   d. spasticity   true

   e. osteoporosis   true

   f. shoulder-hand syndrome   true

144. **True or False. In autonomic hyperreflexia the following is found:**   G7 p.1000:145mm
   a. exaggerated autonomic response to stimuli — true
   b. only in patients with lesion above T6 — true
   c. complaints of headache, flushing, and diaphoresis — true
   d. extreme hypertension — true
   e. epinephrine is released causing this syndrome — false (Norepinephrine is released but not epinephrine.)

145. **True or False. Regarding autonomic hyperreflexia in SCI:**   G7 p.1000:170mm
   a. It occurs only in patients with SCI below T6. — false (It occurs only in patients with SCI above T6.)
   b. Patients complain of pounding headache. — true
   c. It can be life threatening. — true
   d. It occurs in ≈ 30% of quadriplegic patients. — true
   e. There is a lag time of 3 to 4 months. — true

146. **True or False. Regarding autonomic dysreflexia in SCI:**   G7 p.1001:22mm
   a. It often occurs in the first 3 to 4 months after SCI. — false (It occurs after the first 12 to 16 weeks.)
   b. Bladder distension may cause onset. — true
   c. Colorectal distension may cause onset. — true
   d. DVT may cause onset. — true

147. **True or False. Presentation of autonomic hyperreflexia in SCI includes**   G7 p.1001:45mm
   a. paroxysmal hypertension — true
   b. anxiety — true
   c. miosis — false (Mydriasis occurs [dilated pupil].)
   d. penile erection — true
   e. Horner syndrome — true

148. **Complete the following about autonomic hyperreflexia:**   G7 p.1001:46mm
   a. What is the triad of presenting symptoms?
      i. h_____ — headache—cephalgia
      ii. s_____ — sweating—hyperhydrosis
      iii. f_____ f_____ — facial flushing—cutaneous vasodilation
   b. It could be confused with _____. — pheochromocytoma

28

c. Differentiate the two by noting the following:
   i.   flushing limited to face in _____   autonomic hyperreflexia—rest of body is pale
   ii. flushing all over body in _____   pheochromocytoma
d. It occurs in quadriplegia patient with an acutely d_____ b_____.   distended bladder   G7 p.1001:100mm

149. True or False. Prophylaxis in patients with recurrent episodes of autonomic hyperreflexia include the following: G7 p.1001:183mm
  a. phenoxybenzamine   true
  b. beta blockers   true
  c. hydralazine   false
  d. pyridium   true
  e. sympathectomy   true (but radical and may jeopardize reflex voiding)

29

Stroke

■ Cerebrovascular Hemodynamics

1. Complete the following:

a. Cerebral blood flow (CBF) less than _____ mL per 100 g of tissue per minute is associated with ischemia.

20 mL

G7 p.1010:100mm

b. If prolonged, it will result in _____.

cell death

2. Electroencephalography (EEG) becomes flat line at CBF of _____ mL/100 g/min.

16 to 18

G7 p.1010:150mm

3. Complete the following about strokes in general:

a. What is the range of cerebral perfusion pressure in which cerebral blood flow is maintained constant despite changes in cerebrovascular resistance?

50 to 150 mm Hg

G7 p.1010:163mm

b. This is called _____.

autoregulation

4. Complete the following about strokes in general:

a. $CMRO_2$ stands for _____ and

cerebral metabolic rate of oxygen consumption

G7 p.1010:175mm

b. averages _____.

3.0 to 3.8 mL/100 g of tissue per minute

5. Complete the following regarding abrupt onset of new focal deficit caused by:

G7 p.1011:60mm

a. tumor/seizure _____%   5%

b. ischemic infarct _____%   85%

c. hemorrhagic infarct _____%   15%

d. mortality _____%   25%

e. nursing home _____%   25%

f. home _____%   50%

29

6. **True or False. The following is a cause of ischemic infarcts:**   G7 p.1011:75mm

a. lacune   true
b. large artery embolism   true
c. cardiogenic embolism   true
d. aortic arch plaques   true

7. **Modifiable risk factors for stroke include**   G7 p.1011:120mm

a. c_____   cigarettes
b. a_____   alcohol
c. h_____   hypertension
d. l_____   lipids
e. a_____   antiplatelets

8. **Computed tomographic (CT) scan signs of early ischemia include**   G7 p.1012:110mm

a. i_____   insular ribbon lost
b. s_____   shift of midline day 1 to 25
c. c_____   calcification almost never 1 to 2%
d. h_____   hyperdense artery sign
e. e_____   effacement of cerebral sulci
f. m_____   mass effect
g. i_____   interface of gray-white lost
h. c_____   contrast CT should be included on at least one occasion

9. **True or False. The following can be early CT findings of ischemic strokes:**   G7 p.1012:125mm

a. midline shift   true
b. loss of gray-white interface   true
c. hyperdensity of lentiform nucleus   false (Attenuation of the lentiform nucleus may be seen.)
d. enhancement of ischemic area   true (One third of ischemic strokes may enhance early.)
e. normal CT   true
f. hyperdense artery sign   true (usually MCA)   G7 p.1013:40mm

10. **Is there CT enhancement with intravenous (IV) contrast in cerebrovascular accidents (CVAs) in the presence of mass effect?**   no (As a rule of thumb there should not be.)   G7 p.1013:55mm

11. **MRI sequences in stroke are**   G7 p.1013:160mm

a. _____ represents dead tissue.   DWI
b. _____ represents penumbra.   PWI
c. Penumbra is potentially s_____ tissue.   salvageable

29

12. **Components of luxury perfusion are**
Hint: ischemia

G7 p.1014:35mm

a. i_____   ischemia
b. "s"_____   "s" idosis (acidosis)
c. c_____ CO_2 rises
d. h_____   hyperemia
e. e_____   enlargement (dilation) of
                      vessels
f. m_____   mechanism of luxury
                      perfusion
g. i_____   increase blood flow
h. a_____   accelerated circulation
                      adjacent to an infarct

13. **Explain the mechanism of luxury perfusion.**

G7 p.1014:40mm

a. Ischemia produces _____,   acidosis
b. which causes an _____ in PCO_2. increase
c. What does this do to regulation?   loss of autoregulation
d. It results in _____ vessels   dilated
e. and blood flow _____ called   excess; hyperemia
   _____.
f. What happens to blood flow adjacent to   it becomes accelerated
   an infarct?

14. **t-PA works by**

G7 p.1016:145mm

a. converting p_____   plasminogen
b. to the fibrinolytic compound _____.   plasmin
c. The primary agent is a _____.   alteplase

15. **Complete the following regarding the use of recombinant tissue plasminogen activator (rt-PA) compared with control groups:**

G7 p.1016:175mm

a. reduction in stroke _____%   30%
b. recurrent stroke rate _____%   5%—same in both groups
c. mortality _____ vs _____%   17 vs 21%
d. hemorrhage (NINDS study) _____ vs   6.4 vs 0.6%
   _____%
e. hemorrhage ECASSII study _____ vs   8.8 vs 3.4%
   _____%
f. benefit at 90 days in mortality _____   no difference
   _____

29

16. **Facts learned from the ECASS-3 study of t-PA include**   G7 p.1017:16mm
   a. Extended the window of IV treatment to _____ hours   4.5
   b. Improved outcome at 90 days by _____%   7.2%
   c.
      i. Incidence of hemorrhage _____%   7.9%
      ii. And _____% for placebo   3.5%
   d.
      i. Yet no increase in death rate t-PA _____%   7.7%
      ii. Placebo _____%   8.4%
   e. For every 100 patients treated with t-PA
      i. _____ will benefit   32
      ii. _____ will be harmed   3

17. **True or False. The following would exclude a patient with ischemic stroke from treatment with tissue plasminogen activator (t-PA):**   G7 p.1017:70mm
   a. systolic blood pressure (SBP) 180 mm Hg   false (SBP above 185 disqualifies.)
   b. gastrointestinal (GI) bleed 6 months ago requiring transfusion   false (GI bleed within 21 days disqualifies.)
   c. platelet count 120,000/mm^3 false (Below 100,000 disqualifies.)
   d. hip arthroplasty 10 days ago   true (Major surgery within 14 days of an ischemic stroke is a contraindication for t-PA treatment.)
   e. blood glucose 250 mg%   false (Above 400 mg% disqualifies.)

18. **Complete the following about the management of post-t-PA intracerebral hemorrhage:**   G7 p.1018:15mm
   a. Stop _____.   t-PA
   b. Obtain stat _____.   CT
   c. Send labs for PT, PTT, platelet and _____.   fibrinogen
   d. Prepare to administer
      i. 6 to 8 units of c_____   cryoprecipitate
      ii. 6 to 8 units of p_____   platelets
   e. Consider use of _____ _____.   factor VII

19. **Intra-arterial t-PA may be used up to _____ hours after stroke onset.**   6   G7 p.1018:48mm

20. **Merci retriever**   G7 p.1018:48mm
   a. stands for mechanical embolus removal in _____.   cerebral ischemia
   b. It can be used for up to _____ hours.   8
   c. It has a recanalization rate of _____%.   48%

29

21. **Complete the following about strokes in general:**   G7 p.1018:165mm
   a. After a stroke you must monitor electrocardiography (EKG) because
      i. _____% have EKG changes   5 to 10%
      ii. _____% have myocardial   2 to 3%
         infarction (MI)
   b. You must avoid hyperglycemia because hyperglycemia
      i. _____ the ischemia zone, also   extends
         known as the
      ii. _____.   penumbra

22. **Complete the following regarding hypertension treatment:**   G7 p.1019:120mm
   a. If diastolic blood pressure (DBP) is above   140 mm Hg
      _____ it is called malignant
      hypertension.
   b. Decreasing by _____% to DBP of   20 to 30% (112 to 98 mm Hg)
      _____ is desirable.
   c. If SBP is above 230 or DBP is above 120   180; 110
      decrease to SBP of _____ or DBP of
      _____.
   d. For SBP of 180 to 230 or DBP of 105 to   not needed emergently
      120 decrease n_____ n_____
      e_____.
   e. For SBP of less than _____or DBP of   180; 105
      less than _____ antihypertensive
      treatment is not needed.
   f. Approximately _____ / _____ is   180/100
      acceptable.
   g. Add _____ if there is a history of   5
      hypertension.

23. **Complete the following:**   G7 p.1020:40mm
   a. Incidence of recurrent ischemic strokes   2.2%
      in the week following a CVA is
      _____%.
   b. Is it any less if you use heparin?   no
      i. except in _____   cardiogenic emboli
   c. Complication rate of heparin
      i. symptomatic intracerebral   1 to 8%
         hemorrhage (ICH) occurs in
         _____%
      ii. conversion of pale to hemorrhagic   2 to 5%
         CVA _____%
      iii. other bleeding complications   3 to 12%
         _____%
   d. On balance is it justified to use heparin   no
      after an ischemic CVA?
      i. The American Heart Association   doctor
         states that the _____ decides.

29

24. **Complete the following regarding the use of anticoagulants (heparin or warfarin):** `G7 p.1020:40mm`
   a. True or False. They are effective in the prevention of embolic strokes caused by cardiogenic embolism. — true
   b. True or False. They are effective in ischemic strokes. — false
   c. They have a risk of hemorrhage of _____% per year. — 1 to 8%
   d. They will convert pale to hemorrhagic CVA in _____%. — 2 to 5%

25. **CVA and anticoagulation are generally used for** `G7 p.1020:115mm`
   a. c_____ e_____. — cardiogenic emboli
   b. c_____ d_____. — carotid dissection
   c. Complications are worse if the patient has _____. — hypertension
   d. How do you start the drugs? (heparin/warfarin) — simultaneously
      i. Why? Because of initial _____. — hypercoagulability
   e. Stop warfarin after _____. — 6 months
   f. Why? — reduced benefits, increased risks

26. **True or False. Regarding cerebellar infarction:** `G7 p.1021:30mm`
   a. Hydrocephalus may occur. — true
   b. Surgery is appropriate even if patient is in coma. — true (Patient may respond even if in deep coma.)
   c. Steroids should be used. — true (Steroids are suggested for cerebellar stroke.) `G7 p.1020:145mm`
   d. Ventricular drainage should be used. — false (Is to be avoided; it might cause upward herniation.)
   e. Incidence of cerebellar infarction is less than 1%. — true (It is seen on 0.6% of all CT scans.)

27. **Cerebellar infarction of the** `G7 p1021 :30mm`
   a. tonsil implicates the _____ — PICA
   b. inferior vermis implicates the _____ — PICA
   c. superior hemisphere implicates the _____ — SCA
   d. superior vermis implicates the _____ — SCA

28. **True or False. The following may be a late finding in patients with cerebellar infarctions that may prompt surgical decompression:** `G7 p.1021:105mm`
   a. sixth nerve palsy — true
   b. seventh nerve palsy — true
   c. worsening headache — true

29

d. Horner syndrome

false (The late findings in a cerebellar infarction are from hydrocephalus or brain stem compression. Horner syndrome is typically seen with lateral medullary syndrome and is due to an intrinsic brain stem lesion and is not an indication for surgery.)

e. decreased level of consciousness

true

29. **Surgical decompression is appropriate if patient develops:**

G7 p.1021:105mm

a. True or False. Coma — true
b. True or False. Ataxic respiration — true
c. Loss of lateral gaze implicates _____ nerve. — sixth
d. Paresis of face implicates _____ _____. — facial colliculus
e. Confusion and somnolence implicates _____ _____. — hydrocephalus

30. **With MCA infarction, consider hemicraniectomy if**

G7 p.1022:85mm

a. distribution of infarct is in the _____ territory — middle cerebral artery (MCA)
b. age of the patient is _____ — under age 70
c. if CVA is on the _____ side — right (nondominant)
d. it may reduce mortality from _____ to _____% — 80 to 30%

31. **Demographics of cardiogenic stroke include**

G7 p.1022:140mm

a. incidence of _____ — 1 in every 6 strokes (i.e., ~17%)
b. after MI _____% in 2 weeks — 2.5%
c. anterior wall _____% — 6%
d. inferior wall _____% — 1%
e. atrial fibrillation _____% per year without treatment — 4.5%
f. especially if patient has _____ ventriculomegaly — left
g. due to _____ _____ — atrial thrombosis
h. heart valve prostheses with anticoagulation
   i. mitral _____% per year — 3%
   ii. aortic _____% — 1.5%
   iii. without anticoagulation _____% per year — 2 to 4%

G7 p.1022:165mm

29

32. **Complete the following about paradoxical embolus:**   G7 p.1023:55mm
   a. Population incidence of patent foramen ovale is _____%.   10 to 18%
   b. In patients with unexplained CVA, the incidence is _____%.   56%

33. **Complete the following about a cardiogenic brain embolism:**   G7 p.1023:100mm
   a. Transformation from bland to hemorrhagic infarct may occur within _____.   2 days (48 hours)
   b. Based on what three-step mechanism?
      i. i_____   ischemia
      ii. c_____ l_____   clot lysis
      iii. r_____   reperfusion of the infarcted brain
   c. If transformation occurs you can surmise that indeed this large infarction can be attributed to a _____ _____.   cardiac cause

34. **Complete the following:**   G7 p.1023:145mm
   a. What is the only stroke for which anticoagulation is beneficial?   cardiogenic brain embolism
   b. What does anticoagulation accomplish regarding further CVAs?   reduces the incidence
   c. The natural risk without treatment is _____%.   12%
   d. If used, when should anticoagulation be instituted?   not before 48 hours
   e. The size of the infarct should be _____.   not a large one
   f. Aim for an international normalized ratio (INR) of _____.   2 to 3
   g. Coumadin reduces stroke risk in atrial fibrillation by _____%.   66 to 86%

35. **True or False. Anticoagulation should be initiated immediately after detection of stroke caused by cardiogenic embolism.**   false (After 48 hours is the proper time. Hemorrhagic conversion is more likely to occur with cardiogenic embolic strokes and is most likely to occur within 48 hours of the stroke. A CT scan should be obtained 48 hours after the stroke and before the initiation of anticoagulation.)   G7 p.1023:165mm

■ Strokes in Young Adults

36. Complete the following about strokes in young adults:

G7 p.1024:45mm

a. Incidence of all strokes
   i.   Under age 40: _____%   3
   ii. Under age 55: _____%   10

b. Etiologies
   Hint: $mA^3pc^3le^2hv$
   i.   m_____   migraine
   ii.   al_____   alcohol
   iii.   AP_____   APLAS
   iv.   ar_____   arteriosclerosis
   v.   p_____   peripartum
   vi.   coa_____   coagulopathy
   vii.   coc_____   cocaine
   viii. con_____   contraceptives
   ix.   l_____   lupus
   x.   ec_____   ecstasy
   xi.   em_____   embolism
   xii.   h_____   homocystinuria
   xiii. v_____   vasculitis

c. Incidence of main etiologies
   i.   arterio-sclerosis _____%   20%
   ii.   embolism _____%   20%
   iii. vasculitis _____%   10%
   iv. coagulopathy _____%   5%

■ Lacunar Strokes

37. Complete the following about lacunar infarcts:

G7 p.1026:50mm

a. size of infarct _____   3 to 20 mm
b. size of artery involved _____   less than 200 µm in diameter
c. due to _____   lipohyalinosis
d. related to _____   hypertension
e. L'etat Lacunaire is _____ _____.   multiple lacunae
f. Small-step gait is called _____
   _____ _____ _____.   marche á petits pas

38. What is Dejerine-Roussy syndrome?

G7 p.1026:105mm

a. The patient complains of _____.   pain
b. The area of the brain involved is
   _____,   thalamus
c. specifically the _____ _____   posteroventral nucleus
d. due to a _____ infarct.   lacunar (Rare thalamic pain syndrome develops long after a lacunar infarct in the posteroventral [sensory] thalamus.)

29

39. **Name the lacunar syndrome sites.**   G7 p.1026:115mm
  a. pure sensory _____   posterior ventral thalamus
  b. pure motor _____   posterior limb of internal
                                     capsule
  c. ataxia hemiparesis _____   basis pontis
  d. top of the basilar _____   mesencephalothalamic
  e. Weber _____   third-nerve palsy and
                                     contralateral hemiparesis
                                     (cerebral peduncle and
                                     issuing fibers of third nerve)
  f. hemiballismus _____   subthalamic nucleus of Luys
  g. Wallenberg _____   posterior inferior cerebellar
                                     artery (PICA)—vertebral artery

40. **Concerning lacunar infarcts, give the**   G7 p.1026:120mm
    symptoms, anatomic site, and
    distinguishing comment for the listed
    syndromes.
  a. pure sensory
     i. symptom: f_____, a_____,   face, arm, leg numbness
        l_____ n_____
     ii. anatomic site: PVT   PV thalamus
     iii. comment: (first)   most common lacuna
  b. pure motor
     i. symptom: f_____, a_____,   face, arm, leg
        l_____
     ii. anatomic site: PL-IC   posterior limb of IC
     iii. comment: (second)   second most common
  c. ataxia hemiparesis
     i. symptom: a_____   ataxia
     ii. anatomic site: PL-IC   basis pontis (midbrain)
     iii. comment: (lips)   numb lips
  d. top of the basilar
     (mesencephalothalamic)
     i. symptoms: t_____ n_____   third nerve palsy, Parinaud,
        p_____, P_____, a_____   abulia
     ii. anatomic site: b_____   basis pontis (midbrain)
        p_____
     iii. comment: b_____ s_____   butterfly shape
  e. Weber
     i. symptoms: t_____ n_____   third nerve palsy, motor
        p_____, m_____ w_____   weakness
     ii. anatomic site: i_____ a_____ interpeduncular arteries to
        to the m_____   the midbrain
     iii. comment: b_____ a_____   basilar aneurysm

41. **True or False. The following is part of the "top of the basilar" syndrome:**

G7 p.1026:160mm

a. third nerve palsy   true
b. amnesia   true
c. light-near dissociation   true
d. vertical gaze impairment   true
e. dysarthria, clumsy hand   false (Dysarthria—clumsy
                                                hand syndrome—occurs with
                                                lacunar infarction of the basis
                                                pontis or genu of the internal
                                                capsule.)

42. **Matchin. Match the following regarding MCA occlusion and symptoms.**
     Area of MCA occlusion:
     ① complete MI; ② superior division;
     ③ inferior division
     Symptoms:

G7 p.1028:25mm

a. homonymous hemianopsia   ①, ③
b. aphasia   ①, ③
c. paresis   ①, ②
d. hemi-sensory loss   ①, ②

43. **True or False. Complete the following regarding inferior division MCA occlusion:**

G7 p.1028:25mm

a. Patient's visual fields will be normal.   false
b. Patient's speech will be normal.   false
c. Patient will have hemiparesis.   false
d. Patient will have sensory deficit.   false

■ Miscellaneous CVA

44. **Complete the following about the Huebner artery:**

G7 p.1028:121mm

a. also known as the r_____ a_____   recurrent artery
b. also known as m_____ s_____   medial striate artery
    a_____
    i.   arises from A2 in _____% of   78%
         patients
    ii. arises from A1 in _____% of   14%
         patients
    iii. arises from anterior communicating   8%
         artery (A-comm) in _____% of
         patients
    iv. arises within _____ mm of the   5 mm
         A-comm junction
c. diameter is _____ mm: mean range   1 mm: mean range 0.2 to
    _____ to _____   2.9 mm
d. diameter compared with diameter of A1   one third
    is _____

29

e. may be confused at surgery with the
    _____ artery

orbitofrontal artery (second
branch of A2—arises 5 mm or
more from A-comm junction)

f. supplies:
    Hint: capghal
    i.   ca_____   caudate
    ii.   p_____   putamen
    iii. g_____ p_____   globus pallidus
    iv.   h_____   hypothalamus
    v.   a_____ l_____   anterior limb of internal
                                               capsule

**45. Describe the syndrome of occlusion of
      the recurrent artery of Huebner.**
      Hint: Huepb

G7 p.1028:123mm

a. h_____   hemiparesis (mild)
b. u_____   upper extremity—weaker
                                      than lower
c. e_____   expressive aphasia
d. p_____   proximal muscles—weaker
                                      than distal
e. b_____   A2 segment of origin 78%

46. Complete the following:

G7 p.1028:125mm

a. Occlusion of the anterior choroidal artery   posterior
    produces infarct in the _____ limb of
    the internal capsule.
b. The Huebner artery produces infarct in   anterior
    the _____ limb of the internal
    capsule.

**47. Occlusion of the anterior choroidal
      artery causes**

G7 p.1028:125mm

a. c_____ h_____   contralateral hemiplegia
b. c_____ h_____   contralateral hypesthesia
c. c_____ h_____ h_____   contralateral homonymous
                                      hemianopsia

**48. Complete the following about
      Wallenberg syndrome:**

G7 p.1028:155mm

a. also known as l_____ m_____   lateral medullary syndrome
    s_____
b. also known as P _____ s_____   PICA syndrome
c. but most related to _____ artery   vertebral

29

d. Give the structure involved and the symptoms:

i.   structure: v_____ n_____
     symptoms: v_____, n_____
     and v_____, n_____
     structure: vestibular nucleus;
     symptoms: vertigo, nausea and vomiting, nystagmus

ii. structure: v_____ and g_____ n_____
     symptoms: d_____, h_____
     structure: vagus and glossopharyngeal nerve;
     symptoms: dysphagia, hoarseness

iii. structure: n_____ of _____
     symptoms: f_____ p_____, p_____
     structure: nucleus of V;
     symptoms: facial pain and paresthesias

iv. structure: r_____ b_____
     symptom: l_____ a_____
     structure: restiform body;
     symptom: limb ataxia

v.   structure: s_____ t_____
     symptom: H_____
     structure: sympathetic tract;
     symptoms: Horner

vi. structure: s_____ t_____
     symptoms: c_____ p_____ and t_____ l_____
     structure: spinothalamic tract;
     contralateral pain and temperature loss

29

30

SAH and Aneurysms

■ Introduction to SAH

1. True or False. Etiologies of subarachnoid hemorrhage (SAH) include the following:

G7 p.1034:50mm

a. arteriovenous malformation (AVM) rupture — true

b. vasculitis — true

c. encephalitis — false

d. drug use — true

e. coagulopathy — true

2. Complete the following about aneurysms:

G7 p.1034:125mm

a. What is the incidence of aneurysmal SAH per 100,000? — 6 to 8

b. How many are there per year in the United States? — 18,000 to 24,000

c. What% die before reaching the hospital? — 10%

d. What is the risk of rebleeding in 2 weeks? — 15 to 20%

e. What is the risk of death from vasospasm? — 7%

f. What is the risk of severe deficit from vasospasm? — another 7%

g. What% die within the first month? — ~50%

h. What is the number of good results in survivors? — one third of survivors

3. True or False. One month mortality from aneurysmal SAH is closest to

G7 p.1034:143mm

a. 10% — false

b. 25% — false

c. 50% — true

d. 75% — false

4. True or False. Risk factors for SAH include the following:

G7 p. 1035:70mm

a. hypertension — true

b. oral contraceptives — true

c. cigarette smoking — true

d. parturition — true

5. **True or False. SAH may present as any of the following:** G7 p.1035:120mm
   a. meningismus — true
   b. photophobia — true
   c. hearing loss — false
   d. low back pain — true
   e. ptosis — true

6. **True or False. Formal angiography is indicated in** G7 p.1035:145mm
   a. sentinel hemorrhage — true
   b. crash migraine (thunderclap headache) — false
   c. benign orgasmic cephalgia — false

7. **The incidence of sentinel hemorrhage is _____%.** — 30 to 60% G7 p.1035:146mm

8. **True or False. Regarding benign thunderclap headache:** G7 p.1035:160mm
   a. Can be distinguished from SAH — false
   b. Reaches maximal intensity in one minute — true
   c. Is accompanied by vomiting — true
   d. Never recurs — false
   e. Is related to vascular cause — true
   f. CT and LP show no blood — true
   g. Require angiography — false

9. **Complete the following about reversible cerebral vasoconstrictive syndrome:** G7 p.1035:180mm
   a. Has a s_____ onset — sudden
   b. Associated with n_____ deficit — neurological
   c. Angiography shows a _____ of _____ — string of beads
   d. Which clears within _____ months — 3
   e.
      i. Associated with v_____ drugs — vasoconstrictive
      ii. B_____ drinking — binge
      iii. May occur p_____ — postpartum

10. **Complete the following about benign orgasmic headache:** G7 p.1036:35mm
    a. Occurs just before or at time of o_____ — orgasm
    b. Workup is the same as for t_____ headache — thunderclap

11. **Complete the following about meningismus:** G7 p.1036:65mm
    a. aka n_____ r_____ — nuchal rigidity
    b. Signs — Hint:
       bend neck = Brudzinski
       knee bent = Kernig
       i. Bend neck and hip flexes called _____ sign — Brudzinski
       ii. Knee bent then straightened causes _____ pain — hamstring
       iii. Called _____ sign — Kernig

30

12. **True or False. Coma in SAH may be due to the following:**   G7 p.1036:80mm

a.	seizure	true
b.	increased intracranial pressure (ICP)	true
c.	intraparenchymal hemorrhage	true
d.	hydrocephalus	true
e.	low blood flow	true

13. **True or False. The following CSF findings are expected with SAH:**   G6 p.783:50mm

a.	elevated opening pressure	true
b.	nonclotting bloody fluid	true
c.	xanthrochromia	true
d.	red blood cells (RBCs) > 100,000	true
e.	elevated glucose	false

14. **What percentage of patients with subarachnoid hemorrhage have funduscopic abnormalities?**   20 to 40%   G7 p.1036:110mm

15. **Matching. Match the type of ocular hemorrhage with the associated characteristic(s).**   G7 p.1036:120mm

Ocularhemorrhage:
① subhyaloid; ② retinal; ③ vitreous
Characteristic:

a.	bright red blood near optic disc	①
b.	vitreous opacity	③
c.	blood obscures the retinal vessels	①
d.	surrounds the fovea	②
e.	may result in retinal detachment	③

16. **True or False. The following are characteristics of SAH:**   G7 p.1036:23mm

a.	Subhyaloid hemorrhage from SAH occurs near the optic disc.	true
b.	Retinal hemorrhage occurs near the fovea.	true
c.	The prognosis for vision recovery in Terson syndrome is poor.	false (Prognosis in Terson syndrome [hemorrhage in the vitreous] is good in 80%.)
d.	Vitreous hemorrhage may occur with nonaneurysmal causes for increased ICP.	true
e.	Ocular hemorrhage from SAH may be associated with retinal detachment.	true

17. **Complete the following:**   G7 p.1037:80mm

a.	A good-quality computed tomographic (CT) scan will detect SAH in what percentage of patients?	95%
b.	If scanned within how many hours?	48 hours
c.	Ventriculomegaly (hydrocephalus) occurs acutely in _____%.	21%

30

18. **True or False. Regarding head CT for SAH:**

G7 p.1037:81mm

a. Ventricular size needs to be assessed because hydrocephalus can occur acutely.

true

b. There may be intracranial hemorrhage requiring urgent craniotomy.

true

c. The amount of SAH correlates with vasospasm risk.

true

d. If there are multiple aneurysms, the distribution of SAH may reveal which aneurysm ruptured.

true

e. Head CT is a poor predictor of aneurysm location.

false (The head CT scan can predict the aneurysm location in 70% of cases.)

19. **To predict aneurysm location, blood in the**

G7 p.1037:134mm

a. ventricles suggests _____ _____ aneurysm.

posterior fossa

b. Anterior interhemispheric fissure suggests an _____ aneurysm.

A-comm

c. Sylvian fissure is compatible with a
   i. _____ or a
   ii. _____ aneurysm

P-comm
MCA

20. **Complete the following:**

G7 p.1037:140mm

a. The most sensitive test for SAH is _____ _____.

lumbar puncture

b. Lowering the cerebrospinal fluid (CSF) pressure might precipitate rebleeding because it causes an _____ _____ _____ _____.

increase in transmural pressure

c. Therefore, as a precaution
   i. use only a _____-_____ _____.

small-gauge needle

   ii. remove only a _____ _____ of _____.

small amount of fluid

21. **Complete the following about xanthochromia:**

G7 p.1038:20mm

a. Used to differentiate SAH from _____

traumatic tap

b. Does not show up until _____ hours after bleeding

2

c. Is present in 100% of patients by _____ hours

12

d. Lingers for up to _____ weeks

4

30

22. Complete the following about MRI: G7 p.1038:75mm

a. Most sensitive imaging study for detecting blood in the subarachnoid space is the _____ sequence.   FLAIR

b. The sequence that may help you learn which of several aneurysms bleed is the _____ sequence.   FLAIR

c. It is most reliable after _____ to _____ days.   4 to 7

23. Complete the following about MRA: G7 p.1038:85mm

a. Can defect aneurysm larger than _____ mm   3

b. With approximately _____% accuracy   87%

c.   G7 p.1038:11mm

   i. CTA has an accuracy of _____%   97%

   ii. and shows a _____-dimensional image.   three-

24. Complete the following: G7 p.1038:135mm

a. Angiography demonstrates the source of SAH in _____%.   80 to 85%

b. To call an angiogram negative for aneurysm you must see what two areas?

   i. Take off both _____ and   PICAs

   ii. _____   A-commA

c. What percent of aneurysms occur at the posterior inferior cerebellar artery (PICA) origin?   1 to 2%

25. Clinical vasospasm almost never occurs less than _____ days following SAH.   3   G7 p.1038:145mm

26. If infundibulum is located near SAH _____ is advisable.   exporation   G7 p.1039:27mm

27. Complete the following about the infundibulum: G7 p.1039:35mm

a. The three criteria are

   i. shape _____   triangular

   ii. size of mouth less than _____ mm   3 mm

   iii. at apex a _____ _____   vessel is found

b. The most common site is at the _____.   P-comm

28. Infundibula are found in approximately what percentage of normal arteriograms?   10%   G7 p.1039:35mm

29. True or False. Infundibula are most commonly found at   G7 p.1039:52mm

a. carotid bifurcation   false

b. middle cerebral artery (MCA) origin   false

30

c.	supraclinoid segment of carotid	false
d.	origin of posterior communicating artery (P-comm)	true
e.	MCA trifurcation	false

G7 p.1039:95mm

30. **True or False. Regarding coiling the shape of aneurysms. Coiling is more successful if the aneurysm**

a.	is large and above 15 mm in diameter	false
b.	has a narrow neck less than 5mm	true
c.	has a broad neck greater than 5mm	false
d.	has a dome neck ratio greater than 2	true

■ Grading SAH

G7 p.1039:150mm

31. **Matching. Match the hemorrhage grade with when to operate.**
① manage till patient improves;
② immediately; ③ promptly within 24 hours

a.	Hunt and Hess grade 1	③
b.	Hunt and Hess grade 2	③
c.	Hunt and Hess grade 3, 4, or 5	①
d.	Patient with large hematoma	②
e.	Patient with multiple bleeds	②

G7 p.1040:15mm

32. **Complete the World Federation of Neurologic Surgeons (WFNS) grading scale for SAH grade.**

a.	grade 0 _____	unruptured
b.	grade 1 Glasgow Coma Scale (GCS) _____	GCS 15
c.	grade 2 GCS _____	GCS 13 to 14
d.	grade 3 GCS _____	GCS 13 to 14 and major focal deficit (aphasia, hemiparesis)
e.	grade 4 GCS _____	GCS 7 to 12
f.	grade 5 GCS _____	GCS 3 to 6

G7 p.1040:30mm

33. **What is the Hunt and Hess grade in a patient who has a headache and SAH seen on CT scan?**

a.	and a third nerve palsy	Hunt and Hess grade 2
b.	and mild one-sided weakness and confusion	Hunt and Hess grade 3
c.	deep coma and decerebration	Hunt and Hess grade 5
d.	a patient with an incidental aneurysm	Hunt and Hess grade 0

30

■ Initial Management of SAH

34. **List nine potential complications of SAH.**
Hint: veraNdsah   G7 p.1040:95mm

a. v_____	vasospasm
b. e_____	embolus—pulmonary
c. r_____	rebleed
d. a_____	arachnoid granulation blockage
e. N_____	Na metabolism
f. d_____	deep vein thrombosis
g. s_____	seizures
h. a_____	acute hydrocephalus
i. h_____	hyponatremia

35. **Complete the orders for SAH patient.**   G7 p.1041:135mm

a. intravenous (IV) fluids	normal saline (NS) and 20 milliequivalents (mEq) KCl
b. rate	2 cc/kg/hour
c. anticonvulsants?	yes—Dilantin-fosphenytoin
d. amount	17 mg/kg load and 100 mg three times a day (or Keppra 500 mg every 12 hours)

36. **For the listed SAH conditions, give the frequency of seizure incidence.**   G7 p.1041:145mm

a. during acute illness	3%
b. immediate postop	5%
c. during 5-year follow-up	10%
d. middle cerebral artery (MCA)	20%
e. posterior cerebral artery (PCA)	9%
f. anterior cerebral artery (ACA)	2.5%

37. **The dosage of Keppra should be**   G7 p.1041:182mm

a. _____ mg IV	500
b. every _____ hours.	12

38. **During the postsubarachnoid hemorrhage period, with the aneurysm unclipped, phenothiazines should be avoided because**   G7 p.1042:35mm

a. True or False. They may be overly sedating and obscure neurological assessment.	false
b. True or False. They may lower seizure threshold.	true
c. True or False. They cause elevation of systolic blood pressure.	false
d. True or False. Their metabolites may hasten vasospasm.	false
e. Instead use _____.	Zofran (ondansetron)

39. **Ideal systolic blood pressure should be in the range of _____ to _____.**   120 to 150   G7 p.1042:145mm

40. True or False. The following is the most reliable parameter to differentiate syndrome of inappropriate diuretic hormone (SIADH) from cerebral salt wasting syndrome:

G7 p.1043:55mm

a. serum atrial natriuretic factor (ANF) and brain natriuretic factor (BNF)

false

b. urine Na^+ and osmolarity

false

c. serum Na^+ and osmolarity

false

d. extracellular fluid volume

true (Extracellular fluid volume is low in CSW and normal or elevated in SIADH.)

e. 24-hour urine output

false (ANF = atrial natriuretic factor, BNP = brain natriuretic peptide. If they rise after SAH, it is more likely that the patient will develop negative fluid balance.)

41. Complete the following:

G7 p.1043:56mm

a. True or False. Cerebral salt wasting (CSW) is best differentiated from SIADH by measuring the:
   i. serum sodium

   false

   ii. intravascular volume

   false

   iii. urine osmolarity

   false

   iv. fluid restriction

   false

   v. fluorocortisone trial

   false

   vi. extracellular fluid volume

   true (Measurement [i.e., clinical estimation] of extracellular fluid volume is decreased in CSW.)

b. Keeping serum Na levels normal is important because hyponatremic patients have three times the rate of d_____ c_____ i_____ as do normal natremic patients.

delayed cerebral infarction

42. Cerebral salt wasting is

G7 p.1043:90mm

a. more common after SAH than _____.

SIADH

b. Treat with _____ _____.

normal saline

c. Use caution regarding the rate of treatment because you risk producing _____ _____ _____.

central pontine myelinolysis

43. True or False. Regarding SAH:

G7 p.1043:115mm

a. The maximum frequency of rebleeding from SAH is on day 7.

false (4% on day 1, maximum)

b. SAH is associated with stunned myocardium.

true

c. Approximately 50% of ruptured aneurysms will rebleed within 6 months.

true

d. Epsilon-aminocaproic acid may decrease the risk of rebleeding.

true

G7 p.1044:20mm

30

44. **Complete the following:**   G7 p.1043:116mm
a. Maximum frequency of rebleeding is on   first
   the _____ day
b. at a rate of _____%   4%
c. then at _____%   1.5%
d. for _____ days.   13
e. Total of rebleed in 2 weeks = _____%   15 to 20%
f. _____% in 6 months   50%
g. Thereafter rebleed rate is _____% per   3%
   year.
h. Time period of the highest risk of   first 6 hours
   rebleeding is the _____.

45. **Complete the following about acute**   G7 p.1043:130mm
post-SAH hydrocephalus:
a. The proper treatment is placement of a   ventriculostomy drain
   _____ _____.
b. Drain fluid _____.   slowly
c. It is recommended to keep the ICP in the   15 to 25
   range of _____ mm Hg.
d. This reduces the tendency to _____.   rebleed
e. A similar concern is present in use of   lumbar spinal drainage
   _____ _____ _____.
f. Risk of aneurysmal rebleeding after   0.3%
   lumbar drain is _____%.

46. **Complete the following:**   G7 p.1044:75mm
a. Hydrocephalus is more frequently   posterior fossa
   associated with aneurysms in what
   location?
b. Frequency of hydrocephalus in SAH is   15 to 20%
   _____%.
c. What aneurysm has a low incidence of   middle cerebral artery
   hydrocephalus?   aneurysms
d. Treat with _____,   ventriculostomy
e. which will be helpful in _____% of   80%
   patients.
f. Keep ICP in the range of _____.   15 to 25 mm Hg
g.
   i. Is rupture of aneurysm more likely in   probably
      patients with ventriculostomy?
   ii. If so probably because of an increase   transmural
      in _____ pressure

■ Vasospasm

47. **Vasospasm. List the components of**   G7 p. 1045:50mm
the "Triple H" therapy.
a. hypert_____   hypertension
b. hyperv_____   hypervolemia
c. hemo_____   hemodilution

48. Complete the following about vasospasm: G7 p.1045:95mm

a. also known as _____   delayed ischemic neurologic deficit (DIND)

b. True or False. Higher incidence occurs in:
   i. ACA aneurysm   true
   ii. MCA aneurysm   false

49. Complete the following: G7 p.1046:25mm

a. The incidence of radiographic cerebral vasospasm is _____%.   30 to 70%

b. The incidence of symptomatic cerebral vasospasm is _____%   20 to 30%

c. as measured on the _____ day   seventh

d. Produces infarction in _____%   7%

e. Produces mortality in _____%   7%

f. Onset never before day _____   3

g. Resolved by day _____   12

h. Radiographically resolves over _____ weeks.   3

50. Complete the following: G7 p.1046:80mm

a. Spasmogenic region on ACA and MCA is the _____.   proximal 9 cm

b. True or False. There is more vasospasm with
   i.   cigarette smoking   true
   ii. lower Hunt and Hess grade   false
   iii. amount of bleed on CT   true
   iv. advancing age of patient   true

51. Complete the following about vasospasm: G7 p.1046:147mm

a. True or False. Angiography has been shown to exacerbate cerebral vasospasm.   true

b. Describe the Fisher grading system.
   i.   grade 1   no blood
   ii. grade 2   slight—less than 1 mm
   iii. grade 3   localized clot—more than 1 mm
   iv. grade 4   intracerebral or intraventricular clot

c. Clinical vasospasm is essentially limited to Fisher grade _____.   3 G7 p.1046:155mm

52. What chemical has been identified as a critical mediator and cause of vasospasm?   endothelin 1 (ET 1) G7 p.1047:90mm

30

53. **What transcranial Doppler (TCD) values are consistent with vasospasm?**   G7 p.1048:20mm
   a. Velocity at MCA of more than _____.   120 cc/s
   b. Ratio of more than _____ between   3
   c. the _____ and the _____ indicates vasospasm.   MCA and the ICA mean MCA velocity MCA:ICA ratio (Lindegaard ratio)
   d. Velocity < than _____ and ratio <_____ is normal.   120 and ratio 3
   e. Velocity between _____ and _____ is mild.   120 and 200 cm/s
   f. Velocity above _____ is severe.   200 cm/s
   g. Ratio between _____ is mild vasospasm.   3 to 6
   h. Ratio above _____ is severe vasospasm.   6

54. **Complete the following:**   G7 p.1048:135mm
   a. Describe the treatment for vasospasm
      i. avoid h_____, a_____, and h_____   hypovolemia, anemia, and hypotension
      ii. surgery   do early
      iii. remove c_____   clots
      iv. drug   calcium channel blocker nimodipine
      v. catheter   dilatation
      vi. drain   bloody CSF
      vii. obtain Hct of _____%   30 to 35%
   b. Angioplasty produces clinical improvement of _____%.   60 to 80%   G7 p.1049:55mm
   c. Intra-arterial drugs   G7 p.1050:55mm
      i. P_____ is not effective   Papaverine
      ii. V_____–watch for hypotension   Verapamil
      iii. N_____ restores vessel diameter to at least _____%; _____% patients had no stroke   Nicardipine; 60%; 70%

55. **Complete the following regarding papaverine:**   G7 p.1050:36mm
   a. What does it do?   relaxes smooth muscle
   b. How does it work?   as a calcium channel blocker
   c. It is used to _____.   reverse mechanical vasospasm
   d. What is the amount to be used?   30 mg in 9 cc normal saline

56. **Complete the following:**   G7 p.1052:15mm
   a. What is "triple H" therapy?
      i. h_____v_____   hypervolemia
      ii. h_____t_____   hypertension
      iii. h_____d_____   hemodilution
   b. The fluid to use is _____.   normal saline, a crystalloid
   c. Maximum blood pressure (BP) for a(n)   G7 p.1052:90mm
      i. clipped aneurysm is _____   240 mm Hg
      ii. unclipped aneurysm is _____   160 mm Hg
   d. What do you do if triple H does not work?   endovascular techniques

30

e. Goals for hypervolemia
    i. clipped aneurysm: CVP _____   CVP 8 to 12 cm H_2O
    ii. unclipped aneurysm: CVP _____   CVP 6 to 10 cm H_2O
f. Hemodilution to _____Hct   30 to 35   G7 p.1051:170mm

57. Complete the following: G7 p.1053:50mm
a. complications of hyperdynamic therapy
    i. pulmonary edema _____%   17%
    ii. dilutional hyponatremia _____%   3%
b. benefits
    i. improved permanently _____%   81%
    ii. improved temporarily _____%   7%
    iii. no benefit _____%   16%
    iv. worse _____%   10%

58. Complete the following about dose for calcium channel blocker: G7 p.1053:150mm
a. name of antivasospasm medication/drug _____   nimodipine

b. dose _____ mg every _____ hours   60 mg every 4
c. route _____   by mouth or nasogastric tube
d. duration _____   21 days
e. unless _____   patient going home intact—if so may stop the calcium channel blocker

■ Neurogenic Stunned Myocardium

59. EKG changes that can occur after SAH are   G7 p.1054:120mm
a. T wakes may be i_____   inverted
b. QT may be p_____   prolonged
c.
    i. ST segments may be e_____   elevated
    ii. or d_____   depressed
d. Premature atrial or ventricular c_____   contraction
e. f_____   fib
f. b_____   bradycardia

60. The mechanism for the EKG changes are thought to be due to   G7 p.1054:135mm
a. h_____ i_____,   hypothalamic ischemic
b. which causes increased _____ tone,   sympathetic
c. which releases a surge of c_____,   catecholamines
d. which produces s_____ ischemia,   subendocardial
e. or c_____ a_____ vasospasm.   coronary artery

30

61. **Complete the following about cardiac problems and SAH:**   G7 p.1054:120mm
    a. Electrocardiographic (ECG) changes occur in _____%.   50%
    b. The mechanism is (Hint: hics)   G7 p.1054:135mm
        i.   h_____ i_____   hypothalamic ischemia
        ii. i_____ s_____ t_____   increased sympathetic tone
        iii. c_____ s_____   catecholamine surge
        iv. s_____ i_____   subendocardial ischemia

■ Cerebral Aneurysms

62. **Matching. What are ideas regarding the etiology of aneurysms? Match the lettered term with the numbered description.**   G7 p.1055:55mm
    Description:
    ① less elastica; ② less muscle; ③ more prominent; ④ less supportive connective tissue
    Term:
    a. tunica media   ②
    b. adventitia   ①
    c. internal elastic lamina   ③
    d. location—occur   ④

63. **Give the% incidence of cerebral aneurysm for each of the following:**   G7 p.130:130mm
    a. A-comm   30%
    b. P-comm   25%
    c. MCA   20%
    d. posterior circulation   15%
    e. basilar   10%
    f. multiple   20 to 30%

64. **Complete the following about intraventricular hemorrhage:**   G7 p.1056:25mm
    a. General
        i. True or False. It does not affect morbidity-mortality.   false
        ii. It has a mortality of _____%.   64%
    b. A-comm aneurysms rupture into the ventricle through the _____   lamina terminalis
        _____.
    c. Distal basilar artery aneurysms rupture through the _____ of the _____   floor of the third ventricle
        _____.
    d. PICA aneurysm may rupture through the
        i. _____ of _____   foramen of Luschka
        ii. and into the _____ _____.   fourth ventricle

30

65. **Third nerve palsy can occur with**   G7 p.1056:95mm

a. _____ or   aneurysm

b. _____.   diabetes

c. One can differentiate by examining the   pupils

_____.

  i. Pupil dilated in _____.   aneurysm

  ii. Pupil not dilated in _____.   diabetic

d. The mnemonic is _____ from the   "diabetes deletes the pupil"

third nerve palsy syndrome.

e. Aneurysms _____ the pupil.   include

f. NPSTN means _____ palsy.   non-pupil-sparing third nerve

66. **True or False. All of the following**   G7 p.1057:30mm

conditions may be associated with

SAH:

a. hypertension   true

b. Osler-Weber-Rendu syndrome   true

c. diabetes mellitus   false (Diabetes insipidus can

be associated.)

d. renal fibromuscular dysplasia   true

e. Ehlers-Danlos type IV   true

67. **The following conditions are**   G7 p.1057:31mm

associated with an increased incidence

of aneurysm:

a. a_____ d_____ p_____   autosomal dominant

k_____ d_____   polycystic kidney disease—

15%

b. a_____ m_____   arteriorvenous malformation

c. a _____   atherosclerosis

d. b_____ e_____   bacterial endocarditis

e. c_____ of the a_____   coarctation of the aorta

f. c_____ t_____ d_____   connective tissue disorders

g. Eh_____-Da_____   Ehlers-Danlos type IV

h. fib_____ d_____ r_____   fibromuscular dysplasia renal

d_____   disease—7%

i. f_____ o_____   familial occurrences   G7 p.1057:59mm

j. M_____ s_____   Marfan syndrome

k. m_____ d_____   moyamoya disease

l. O_____-W_____-R_____   Osler-Weber-Rendu syndrome

s_____

m. p_____ e_____   pseudoxanthoma elasticum

68. **Complete the following about**   G7 p.1057:87mm

aneurysms and polycystic kidney:

a. ADPKD stands for _____ _____   adult polycystic kidney

_____ _____.   disease

b. Incidence is 1 in _____ autopsies. 500

c. Prevalence of aneurysms in patients with 10 to 30% —15% a reasonable

ADPKD is _____%.   estimate

d. Risk of SAH in a person with ADPKD is   10 to 20 times

_____ the general population.

e. Screening protocol in a patient with   MRA every 2 to 3

ADPKD with a prior aneurysm or a

kindred with aneurysm is to perform

_____ every _____ years.

30

■ Treatment Options for Aneurysms

69. Complete the following: G7 p.1058:100mm

a. In trapping an aneurysm is it better to tie   common carotid occlusion is
   off the common carotid artery or the   better
   internal carotid artery?

b. It reduces the incidence of _____   thromboembolic
   _____.   phenomenon

70. True or False. Regarding treatment   G7 p.1058:115mm
options for aneurysms:

a. The following procedure(s) offers
   protection if the aneurysm can't be
   clipped or coiled:
   i.   wrapping with muscle   false
   ii.   wrapping with cotton   false
   iii. wrapping with muslin   false
   iv.   coating with plastic resin   false
   v.   coating with polymer   false
   vi.   coating with Teflon   false
   vii. coating with fibrin glue   false

b. In such cases you could consider   true
   trapping or bypass or carotid ligation.

71. True or False. Coils are not ideal for   G7 p.158:173mm

a. very small aneurysms   true
b. very large aneurysms   true
c. aneurysms with wide necks   true
d. If after coiling residual filling is noted you   false (Proceed with surgery.)
   should "recoil."

72. Data for Guglielmi detachable coils   G7 p.1059:125mm
indicate

a. morbidity _____%   4%
b. mortality _____%   1%
c. complete obliteration of aneurysm   40%
   _____%
d. subsequently required open surgical   20%
   repair _____%

■ Timing of Aneurysm Surgery

73. Complete the following about timing   G7 p.1060:105mm
for aneurysm surgery:

a. The definition of early surgery is less than   48 to 96 hours
   _____ to _____ hours.

b. Late surgery is after _____.   10 to 14 days
c. Timing of basilar artery aneurysm is   more likely to delay surgery
   _____.

d. Avoid doing surgery between days   4 and 10; vasospastic interval
   _____ and _____ because that is
   considered a _____ _____.

74. **Complete the following regarding vasospasm treatment:**

G7 p.1061:85mm

a. It peaks in incidence between days _____ and _____.

6 and 8

b. It never occurs before day _____.

3

c. Vasospastic interval during which surgery should be avoided is days _____ to _____.

4 to 10

■ General Technical Considerations of Aneurysm Surgery

75. **Complete the following:**

G7 p.1061:160mm

a. What is an aneurysmal rest?

residual unclipped part of aneurysm

b. Why are they dangerous?

they may bleed

c. What is the incidence of rebleeding?

3.7%

d. There is a risk per year of _____%.

0.4 to 0.8%

e. How should they be handled?

serial angiography

f. If they increase in size treat with _____ or _____ _____.

surgery or endovascular coiling

76. **Answer the following about CSF drainage during craniotomy:**

G7 p.1062:90mm

a. True or False. CSF should be drained before opening the dura.

false (This is associated with an increased incidence of rebleeding.)

b. True or False. CSF should be drained after opening the dura.

true

c. What is the rate of rebleeding with CSF drainage?

0.3%

77. **Complete the following:**

G7 p.1062:135mm

a. O_2 consumption by the neuron is for two functions:
   i. to maintain _____ _____

cell integrity

   ii. for conduction of _____ _____

electrical impulse

b. If there is occlusion of a vessel it produces _____

ischemia

c. due to _____ _____.

oxygen deficiency

d. This precludes
   i. a_____ g_____ and

aerobic glycolysis

   ii. o_____ p_____

oxidative phosphorylation

e. What happens to adenosine triphosphate (ATP) production?

it declines

f. What happens to the cell?

cell death occurs

30

78. **What can be done to protect against ischemia?**   G7 p.1062:165mm
   a. Tactics to reduce injury by ischemia include
      i. n_____   nimodipine—calcium channel blockers
      ii. b_____   barbiturates—free radical scavengers
      iii. m_____   mannitol
   b. Tactics to reduce the cerebral metabolic rate of oxygen consumption ($CMRO_2$) required include
      i. reducing electrical activity of the neuron with _____   barbiturates-etomidate
      ii. reducing maintenance energy of the neuron with _____   hypothermia

79. **Answer the following about temporary clipping during aneurysm surgery:**   G7 p.1064:23mm
   a. True or False. Under 5 minutes occlusion is well tolerated.   true
   b. If occluded 10 to 15 minutes must add _____.   5 mg/kg thiopental loading dose and drip titrated to burst suppression
   c. If occluded more than 20 minutes _____.   not tolerated

80. **Answer the following about postop angiography after aneurysm or AVM surgery:**   G7 p.1064:65mm
   a. True or False. It is not needed.   false
   b. Because _____% showed unexpected findings.   19%
   c. True or False. It is the standard of care.   false
   d. True or False. It is recommended.   true

81. **Complete the following:**   G7 p.1064:90mm
   a. What special medications should be used during temporary clipping of an aneurysm?   etomidate or propofol
   b. What do they do?   suppress neuronal activity by reducing neuronal metabolism
   c. By how much?   50%
   d. What is the side effect of etomidate?   lowers seizure threshold
   e. Guard against this side effect by _____.   using preoperative antiepileptic drugs

82. **Complete the following about intraoperative aneurysm rupture (IAR):**   G7 p.1064:138mm
   a. True or False. Intraoperative aneurysm rupture increases the morbidity and mortality of surgery threefold.   true

30

b. True or False. Techniques to decrease the probability of intraoperative rupture include

    i.   preventing hypertension   true

    ii.   minimizing brain retraction   true

    iii.   sharp vs blunt dissection   true

    iv.   radical removal of sphenoid wing   true

c. List the three general stages of aneurysm surgery during which intraoperative rupture is most likely to occur.   stage 1 = initial exposure, stage 2 = dissection of the aneurysm, and stage 3 = clip application

d. Of these, during which stage is intraoperative rupture most likely to occur?   dissection of aneurysm (stage 2)

83. True or False. During intraoperative rupture by clip application bleeding reduces as clip blades approximate.   false   G7 p.1065:130mm

■ Aneurysm Recurrence after Treatment

84. Complete the following about aneurysm recurrence after treatment: G7 p.1065:177mm

a. Can an incompletely clipped aneurysm bleed?   yes—0.4 to 0.8% per year

b. Can an incompletely coiled aneurysm bleed?   yes—0.16% per year

c. Can an aneurysm that has been completely obliterated recur and bleed?   yes—0.37% per year

■ Aneurysm Type by Location

85. Complete the following: G7 p.1066:90mm

a. The most common site of ruptured aneurysms is _____.   A-commA

b. Diabetes insipidus and/or hypothalamic dysfunction can be the presenting symptoms of an aneurysm of the _____.   A-commA

86. Complete the following about aneurysm type by location: G7 p.1066:105mm

a. The single most common site for an aneurysm is _____.   A-commA

b. Subarachnoid hemorrhage from an A-comm aneurysm rupture is associated with an intracerebral hematoma in what percentage of cases?   63%

c. The most common site for subarachnoid blood on a CT associated with A-comm aneurysm rupture is_____.   anterior interhemispheric fissure

d. In what percent of cases?   virtually 100%

30

87. Complete the following: G7 p.1066:120mm
a. Vasospasm from A-comm aneurysm   apathy and abulia
   rupture can cause bilateral ACA infarcts
   in the frontal lobes and result in the
   symptoms of _____ and _____.
b. Frontal lobe infarcts occur in _____%   20%
   of cases of A-comm aneurysm.
c. This results in a virtual _____   prefrontal
   lobotomy.

88. True or False. Regarding A-comm   G7 p.1066:175mm
aneurysms:
a. It is unnecessary to assess the side from   false
   which an A-comm aneurysm fills by
   angiography because all A-comm
   aneurysms should be approached from
   the right side.
b. Surgical approaches to an A-comm
   aneurysm include
   i.   pterional approach   true
   ii. anterior interhemispheric approach   true
   iii. transcallosal approach   true
   iv. subfrontal approach   true
c. The two most common sites for distal
   ACA aneurysms are
   i.   terminal pericallosal artery   false
   ii. terminal callosomarginal artery   false
   iii. frontopolar artery origin   true
   iv. bifurcation of pericallosal and   true
        callosomarginal arteries above the
        splenium of the corpus callosum

89. There are three indications for left   G7 p.1067:35mm
pterional craniotomy for A-commA
aneurysm.
a. pointing to _____   the right
b. feeder from _____   the left
c. multiple _____   additional left-sided
                           aneurysm(s)

90. Pericallosal aneurysms are   genu   G7 p.1068:30mm
anatomically close to which part of
the corpus callosum?

91. **True or False. Regarding ACA and A-commA aneurysms and approaches:**

G7 p.168:32mm

a.

i. The more distally located ACA aneurysms are generally due to posttraumatic, infectious, or embolic etiologies.

true

ii. Aneurysms up to 1 cm from the A-commA may be approached through a standard pterional craniotomy.

true

iii. Aneurysms > 1 cm distal to the A-commA may also be easily approached through a pterional craniotomy with partial gyrus rectus resection.

false (Aneurysms > 1 cm distal to the A-comm up to the genu of the corpus callosum may be approached frontally via a basal frontal interhemispheric route. A right-sided craniotomy is generally preferred unless the dome is buried in the right cerebral hemisphere.)

iv. ACA aneurysms distal to the genu of the corpus callosum may be approached via an interhemispheric route.

true

b. Prolonged retraction of the cingulate gyrus during an interhemispheric approach may result in a foot drop that is usually temporary.

false (may result in temporary akinetic mutism)

92. **Which approach should be used for aneurysms > 1 cm distal to A-comm?**

basal frontal interhemispheric approach, right side preferred

G7 p.1068:76mm

93. **Complete the following:**

G7 p.1068:160mm

a. Which aneurysm presents with a third nerve palsy?

posterior communicating artery

b. What is the status of the pupil?

dilated

c. There is another aneurysm that presents with a third nerve palsy; what is it?

carotid cavernous sinus aneurysm

d. What is the status of the pupil?

not dilated

e. This can be confused with what medical condition?

diabetes

f. What is the posterior fossa aneurysm that on occasion presents with a third nerve palsy?

basilar tip

g. What is the status of the pupil?

dilated

94. **Complete the following about third nerve palsy:**

G7 p.1068:160mm

a. What position does the eye have at rest?

"down and out"

b. If due to P-comm the pupil is _____

not spared—it is dilated in 99% of cases

c. because pupillary fibers run on the _____ of the third nerve.

surface—and can be compressed there

30

d. If due to diabetes the pupil is _____   spared—not dilated from the syndrome—diabetes deletes the pupil

e. because motor fibers run in the _____ part of the third nerve and are affected by pathology of the _____.   deeper; vasa nervorum

f. If due to cavernous carotid artery aneurysm pupil will be _____   spared—not dilated

g. because there is also paralysis of the _____, which _____ the pupil.   sympathetics; dilate

95. **True or False. Regarding P-comm aneurysms:**   G7 p.1068:161mm

a. Third nerve palsies associated with P-comm aneurysms are not pupil sparing in 99% of cases.   true

b. P-comm aneurysms most commonly occur at the junction of the P-comm with the PCA.   false (They arise at the junction of the P-comm with the ICA.)

c. Before clipping a P-comm aneurysm, the origin of the anterior choroidal artery must be identified and excluded from the clip.   true

d. Most P-comm aneurysms project laterally, inferiorly, and posteriorly.   true

96. **What congenital anomaly must be discovered on angiogram prior to surgery for P-comm aneurysm?**   whether there is fetal origin of the PCA, i.e., the posterior circulation is fed only though the P-comm   G7 p.1068:160mm

97. **What is the name of the dural constriction around the carotid artery**   G7 p.1070:90mm

a. as it exits the cavernous sinus?   proximal carotid ring

b. as it enters the subarachnoid space?   distal carotid ring or clinoidal ring

98. **Complete the following:**   G7 p.1070:95mm

a. List the supraclinoid branches of the ICA. Hint: ospa
   i. o_____   ophthalmic
   ii. s_____ h_____   superior hypophyseal
   iii. p_____ c_____   posterior communicating
   iv. a_____ c_____   anterior choroidal

b. What is the classification of supraclinoid aneurysms according to Rhoton and Day?
   i. _____ between _____ and _____   ophthalmic O and P between takeoff of ophthalmic and P-comm includes superior hypophyseal

   ii. _____ between _____ and _____   communicating segment P and A between takeoff of P-comm and anterior choroidal

   iii. _____ between _____ and _____   choroidal segment A and I between takeoff of anterior choroidal and ICA bifurcation

30

99. **Which segment is the largest in the supraclinoid ICA?**

ophthalmic segment

G7 p.1070:96mm

100. **Superior hypophyseal artery supplies**
  a. d_____ of c_____ s_____ and
  b. a_____ p_____ g_____ and
     s_____

dura of cavernous sinus
anterior pituitary gland and
stalk

G7 p.1070:115mm

101. **Ophthalmic artery aneurysms**
  a. arise just distal to the origin of the
     _____ and
  b. project _____.

ophthalmic artery

dorsomedially

G7 p.1070:165mm

102. **Name two major presentations of ophthalmic artery aneurysms.**
  a. S_____
  b. v_____ _____ _____

SAH (45%)
visual field defect (45%)

G7 p.1070:177mm

103. **Answer the following about ophthalmic artery aneurysms:**
  a. True or False. 45% present as SAH.
  b. True or False. 45% present as visual field defect.
  c. True or False. A superior nasal homonymous quadrantanopsia usually means impingement on the lateral portion of the optic nerve.

  d. True or False. An ipsilateral monocular inferior nasal field cut may result from compression of the optic nerve against the falciform ligament.
  e. List the two variants of superior hypophyseal artery aneurysms.
     i. p_____

     ii. s_____

true
true

false (An ipsilateral
monocular superior nasal
quadrantanopsia and not a
homonymous defect would
occur.)
true

paraclinoid—usually does not
produce visual symptoms
suprasellar—may compress
the stalk causing pituitary
dysfunction and the chiasm
causing a bitemporal
hemianopsia

G7 p.1070:180mm

104. **Complete the following:**
  a. What is the most common visual field defect with an ophthalmic artery aneurysm?
  b. What field defect occurs if the optic nerve is compressed by the falciform ligament?
  c. With optic nerve compression near the chiasm?

  d. Also known as j_____ s_____
  e. due to compression of the a_____
     k_____ of W_____.

ipsilateral monocular superior
nasal quadrantanopsia
(IMSNQ)
ipsilateral monocular inferior
nasal field cut (IMIN FC)

contralateral monocular
superior temporal quadrant
(CMSTQ) defect
junctional scotoma (i.e., pie
in the sky)
anterior knee of Willebrand

G7 p.1070:182mm

30

105.   **An ophthalmic artery aneurysm can cause a contralateral monocular superior temporal quadrant defect (CMSTQ), also called a junctional scotoma, by compression of the optic nerve n_____ the c_____.**

near the chiasm (Compression of the optic nerve near the chiasm can impinge on fibers that course anteriorly in the contralateral optic nerve after decussation and before entering the contralateral optic nerve. [anterior knee of Willebrand])

G7 p. X1071:28mm

106.   **Complete the following:**
   a.   Which variant of superior hypophyseal artery aneurysm can mimic pituitary tumor clinically and on CT?

suprasellar variant

   b.   Under what circumstances?

when it is a giant aneurysm

   c.   It may present clinically with _____

hypopituitarism

   d.   and visual symptoms of _____ _____.

bitemporal hemianopsia

G7 p.1071:58mm

107.   **Complete the following:**
   a.   On angiogram, a notch in a giant ophthalmic artery aneurysm is due to the _____ _____.

optic nerve

   b.   The notch if present is located in the _____-_____-_____ aspect.

anterior-superior-medial

G7 p.1071:75mm

108.   **Complete the following:**
   a.   What happens if you occlude the ophthalmic artery?

It is tolerated without loss of vision in most patients.

   b.   Ophthalmic artery aneurysms arise on what aspect of the internal carotid artery?

superomedial (dorsomedial)

   c.   And point _____

superiorly (toward the optic nerve)

   d.   True or False. A contralateral ophthalmic aneurysm is rare.

false (They are common.)

   e.   If present can both be clipped at the same surgery?

yes

G7 p.1071:105mm

109.   **Answer the following:**
   a.   Can you sacrifice a superior hypophyseal artery?

yes, the pituitary receives bilateral blood supply

   b.   Can you clip a contralateral superior hypophyseal aneurysm?

no, not technically feasible

G7 p.1071:140mm

110.   **Matching. Match the frequency of posterior circulation aneurysms compared with anterior circulation aneurysms to the lettered conditions.**
   ① same frequency; ② posterior is more frequent
   a.   clinical syndrome of SAH   ①
   b.   respiratory arrest   ②
   c.   neurogenic pulmonary edema   ②
   d.   midbrain syndrome from vasospasm ②
   e.   hydrocephalus   ②

G7 p.1071:174mm

30

111. Complete the following: G7 p.1072:25mm

a. True or False. 20% of patients with a   true
posterior fossa SAH will require
permanent ventricular shunting.

b. Regarding vertebral artery aneurysms:

   i. The preoperative angiogram should   contralateral vertebral artery
assess the patency of the _____
in the event that trapping is
necessary.

   ii. The Allcock test involves vertebral   carotid compression
angiography with _____
_____ to assess the patency of
the circle of Willis.

   iii. Vertebral artery (VA) aneurysms   VA with the posterior inferior
most commonly occur at the   cerebellar artery (PICA)
junction of the _____ with the

     _____.

   iv. True or False. Nontraumatic VA   false
aneurysms are more common than
dissecting, traumatic VA aneurysms.

112. Complete the following: G7 p.1072:55mm

a. What vessel is injected when performing   vertebral artery
the Allcock test?

b. What is compressed?   carotid arteries

c. What is being tested? Tolerance of   vertebral artery occlusion
_____ _____ _____

d. By assessing the patency of the   circle of Willis
_____ _____ _____

113. Complete the following regarding   G7 p.1072:80mm
PICA:

a. They represent _____% of cerebral   3%
aneurysms.

b. The most common site is at _____   VA-PICA
junction.

c. Aneurysms far more distal on PICA tend   fragile; promptly
to be _____ and therefore should be
treated _____.

114. PICA aneurysms most commonly occur   G7 p.1072:87mm
at the

a. superior angle between the v_____   vertebral artery
a_____ and the

b. P_____.   PICA

c. They lie in the anterolateral portion of   medullary cistern
the _____ _____

d. anterior to the _____ _____   first dentate ligament
_____.

e. PICA aneurysms distal to the VA-PICA   fragile
junction are different in that they are

   _____.

f. Blood from rupture is predominantly in   fourth ventricle
the _____ _____.

30

■ Basilar Bifurcation Aneurysms

115. **Complete the following:**   G7 p.1074:45mm

a. The most common site for a posterior   basilar tip (5% of all
    circulation aneurysm is the _____   intracranial aneurysms)
    _____.

b. True or False. Regarding basilar tip
    aneurysms:
    i.   Surgical treatment is associated with   true
         a 5% overall mortality rate.
    ii. Surgical approaches include   false (Surgical approaches
         pterional and supracerebellar   include pterional
         infratentorial routes.   subtemporal.)
    iii. Because of the technical difficulties   true
         associated with clipping basilar
         aneurysms many still recommend
         waiting up to 1 week prior to
         surgery.
    iv. The morbidity rate of 12% is mostly   true
         due to perforating vessel injury.

116. **On angiography the following**   G7 p.1074:90mm
characteristics should be noted about
basilar artery aneurysms:

a. points direction of the d_____,   dome, usually superiorly
    u_____ s_____
b.
    i.   P-comm _____   flow
    ii. may need _____ _____   Allcock test
c.
    i.   position of _____   bifurcation
    ii. in relation to _____   dorsum sella
    iii. if high use _____ _____   pterional transsylvian
         _____   approach
    iv. if low use _____ _____   subtemporal approach
d. Fill in the blanks after the letters.
    Hint: pPp
    i.   p_____   points
    ii. P-c_____   P-comm
    iii. p_____   position

117. **Matching. Match the numbered**   G7 p.1075:45mm
approaches to the conditions for the
basilar artery aneurysm surgical
approach.
Approach:
① subtemporal approach; ② pterional
approach
Conditions:
a. bifurcation is high   ②
b. aneurysm projects   ①
    posteriorly/posteriorly inferiorly
c. low bifurcation   ①
d. concomitant anterior circulation   ②
    aneurysms

30

e. for better visualization of P1 and   ②
    thalamoperforating vessels
f. for less temporal lobe retraction   ②
g. for shorter distance (by 1 cm)   ①
h. produces a risk to third nerve (mild and   ②
    temporary)

118. What are the approaches to basilar tip   G7 p. 1075:46mm
aneurysms?
a. Drake's approach is _____.   subtemporal
b. Yasargil's approach is _____.   pterional

119. What is the risk of oculomotor palsy   G7 p.1075:52mm
by the pterional approach?   30%

120. Complete the following about basilar   G7 p.1076:110mm
artery aneurysms:
a. Mortality is _____%.   5%
b. Morbidity is _____%.   12%

■ Unruptured Aneurysms

121. What is the incidence of incidental   5 to 10%   G7 p.1077:135mm
aneurysms in the population?

122. Complete the following about   G7 p.1078:57mm
unruptured aneurysms:
a. What is the annual risk of rupture for an   0.05%
    asymptomatic aneurysm < 10 mm?
b. What is the annual risk of rupture for an   1%
    asymptomatic aneurysm > 10 mm?
c. The surgical morbidity and mortality   2% mortality (2.6),
    rates for clipping an unruptured   6% morbidity
    aneurysm are MC _____% mortality
    and _____% morbidity.

123. How is surgical morbidity on cerebral   G7 p.1078:95mm
aneurysms related to aneurysm size,
patient age, and location of
aneurysm?
a. size
    i.   under 5 mm _____%   2.3%
    ii.   6 to 15 mm _____%   6.8%
    iii. 16 to 25 mm _____%   14%
b. age
    i.   under 45 years _____%   6.5%
    ii.   between 45 and 64 years   14%
          _____%
    iii. over 64 years _____%   32%
c. location
    i.   P-comm _____%   4.8%
    ii.   MCA _____%   8.1%
    iii. ophthalmic _____%   11.8%
    iv.   A-comm _____%   15.5%
    v.   carotid bifurcation _____%   16.8%

30

124. **For incidental aneurysms, recommending surgery is appropriate if the patient's life expectancy is at least _____ years.**   12   G7 p.1048:145mm

125. **Complete the following about a carotid cavernous sinus aneurysm (CCSA):**   G7 p.1079:150mm
   a. The segment most frequently involved is the h_____ s_____.   horizontal segment
   b. It usually presents with   G7 p.1079:170mm
       i.   c_____ c_____ f_____   carotid cavernous fistula (i.e., bruit, proptosis, and chemosis)
       ii. a_____ in h_____   ache in head
       iii. V t_____ n_____ p_____   V trigeminal neuralgia pain
       iv. e_____   emboli
       v.   r_____ and e_____   rupture and epistaxis via sphenoid sinus
       vi. m_____ b_____   monocular blindness
       vii. o_____   ophthalmoplegia
       viii. u_____ p_____   undilated pupil with a third nerve palsy (like diabetes)   G7 p.1079:175mm
       ix. s_____ h_____   subarachnoid hemorrhage (may occur with giant aneurysm)
       x.   Pupil is not dilated in CCSA because the _____ are also paralyzed.   sympathetics   G7 p.1079:182mm

126. **What are the indications for treatment of a cavernous carotid aneurysm (unruptured)?**   G7 p.1080:50mm
      Hint: gees
   a. g_____   giant aneurysm (esp. if straddling clinoidal ring)
   b. e_____   enlarging on serial images before carotid endarterectomy (controversial)
   c. e_____   symptomatic (pain, headache, visual)
   d. s_____

■ Multiple Aneurysms

127. **What% of SAH patients have multiple aneurysms?**   15 to 33.5%   G7 p.1080:120mm

128. **True or False.**   G7 p.1080:120mm
   a. Multiple aneurysms occur in 15 to 33% of cases of SAH.   true

30

b. When SAH is associated with multiple aneurysms, clues as to which aneurysm bled include
   i. epicenter of SAH relative to aneurysms   true
   ii. vasospasm distribution relative to aneurysms   true
   iii. irregularities in the shape of the aneurysm   true
   iv. largest aneurysm   true

129. When a patient presents with SAH and is found to have multiple aneurysms, which clues point to which aneurysm has bled?
Hint: evil

   a. e_____   epicenter of blood on CT/MRI
   b. v_____   vasospasm on angiogram
   c. i_____   irregularities in shape (Murphy's tit)
   d. l_____   largest aneurysm

G7 p.1080:133mm

■ Familial Aneurysms

130. Complete the following about familial aneurysms:

G7 p.181:20mm

   a. Should first-degree relatives undergo screening for cerebral aneurysms if a first-degree relative has a known aneurysm?   yes (MRI/MRA then angiography to confirm any suspected lesions. MRA has 16% false-positive rate.)

   b. What% of aneurysms are familial?   2%

   c. Most common relative to also have an aneurysm is a _____.   sibling

   d. Most common location if aneurysm is found in a relative is at the _____.   same or mirror location

   e. There is a lower incidence in familial aneurysm of _____ aneurysm.   A-comm

131. Complete the following:

G7 p.181:27mm

   a. What is the criterion for the familial aneurysm syndrome?   two or more relatives, third degree or closer, who harbor radiographically proven aneurysms

   b. True or False. Familial aneurysms tend to bleed at a smaller size and older age.   false (smaller size and younger age)

   c. True or False. First-degree relatives of patients found to have a familial aneurysm should not undergo any screening because the likelihood of harboring an aneurysm is no greater than in the general population.   false (MRI/MRA is recommended as a screening tool in first-degree relatives.)

G7 p.181:65mm

132. Magnetic resonance angiography (MRA) for aneurysms has a false-positive rate of _____%.   16%

G7 p.181:66mm

30

■ Traumatic Aneurysms

133. **Complete the following:**   G7 p.1081:90mm

a. Traumatic aneurysms represent _____% of aneurysms.   1%

b. They are not really aneurysms but are _____.   pseudoaneurysms

c. True or False. Traumatic aneurysms usually occur as a result of penetrating as opposed to closed head injuries.   false (Closed head injury is more common.)

d. True or False. They often occur where an artery abuts a dural edge or along the skull base associated with fractures.   true

e. True or False. They rarely rupture.   false (Traumatic aneurysms have a high rate of rupture.)

134. **What are the mechanisms of injury for traumatic aneurysm?**   G7 p.1081:100mm

a. p_____ _____   penetrating trauma: gunshot wound (GSW) > sharp object

b. c_____ _____ _____   closed head injury (more common)

   i. f_____   falcine edge peripheral vessel (distal ACA)

   ii. f_____   fractured skull distal cortical vessel

   iii. s_____ b_____   skull base: ICA (petrous, cavernous, supraclinoid)

c. i_____   iatrogenic: surgery (transsphenoidal, endovascular)

135. **Complete the following:**   G7 p.1082:20mm

a. Should traumatic aneurysms undergo surgical treatment?   yes (Direct treatment is recommended of traumatic aneurysms.)

b. If so, why?   They have high rate of rupture.

■ Mycotic Aneurysms

136. **Complete the following about mycotic aneurysms:**   G7 p.1082:45mm

a. True or False. The most common etiology for infections in aneurysms is a fungal infection; thus the term *mycotic*.   false

b. The most common etiology for mycotic aneurysm is _____ _____.   *Streptococcus viridans*— bacterial

c. The next most common is _____ _____.   *Staphylococcus aureus*

d. They are often associated with

   i. _____ _____ abuse.   IV drug

   ii. systemic _____ _____.   bacterial endocarditis

30

e. The most common location is the   distal MCA
    _____ _____.

f. Treat with
    i.   _____   antibiotics
    ii. and consider _____.   clipping

137. **Complete the following:**   G7 p.1082:67mm

a. What% of aneurysms are considered   4%
    mycotic?

b. What% of patients with subacute   3 to 15%
    bacterial endocarditis develop mycotic
    aneurysms?

c. They occur where?   usually distal MCA (75 to
                                            80%)

d. What percent of mycotic aneurysms are   20%
    multiple?

e. Workup should include
    i.   b_____ c_____   blood cultures
    ii. l_____ p_____   lumbar puncture
    iii. e_____   echocardiogram

■ Giant Aneurysms

138. **True or False. Complete the following**   G7 p.1082:175mm
     regarding giant aneurysms:

a. A giant aneurysm is defined as an   false (A giant
    aneurysm greater than 1.5 cm in   aneurysm => 2.5 cm = 1 inch
    diameter.   in diameter.)

b. Most giant aneurysms present as SAH.   false (35% present with
                                            hemorrhage. Most come to
                                            attention due to mass effect.)

c. They are more common in women.   true (A 3:1 female:male
                                            ratio.)

139. **Complete the following regarding**   G7 p.1083:70mm
     giant aneurysm treatment options:

a. c_____   clip
b. b_____ and c_____   bypass and clip
c. t_____   trap
d. h_____ l_____   hunterian ligation
e. w_____   wrap

■ SAH of Unknown Etiology

140. **Complete the following regarding**   G7 p.1083:105mm
     angiogram-negative SAH:

a. It occurs in _____%.   10%
b. It could be due to _____   inadequate
    angiography.
c. To be adequate angiography must show   PICA vessels
    both _____ _____.
d. What% of aneurysms occur at this site? 1 to 2%

30

e. To be adequate angiography must show cross-fill through the _____ _____ _____.

anterior communicating artery

f. Angiography should be repeated unless the blood is located in the _____ _____.

perimesencephalic cistern

g. This is also known as _____ _____ _____.

pretruncal nonaneurysmal SAH

141. **Complete the following regarding considerations for repeat angiography:**

G7 p.1084:50mm

a. Identification of an aneurysm not seen on the original study is _____%.

2 to 10% or 2 to 24%

b. The recommended time to repeat the angiogram series is _____ days.

10 to 14

c.
    i. There is no need to repeat if blood is restricted to the _____ _____.

perimesencephalic cistern

    ii. It is also known as PNSAH, which stands for _____.

pretruncal nonaneurysmal SAH

d. Name was changed because blood
    i. is actually in front of the _____ _____

G7 p.1084:50mm

brain stem

    ii. aka the _____ _____.

truancies cerebri

    iii. It is centered at the _____

pons

    iv. and not in the p_____ c_____.

perimesencephalic cistern

e.
    i. Rebleeding _____ _____ _____

does not occur

    ii. Aneurysm _____.

is not found on repeat angiogram

    iii. Bleeding is likely due to a _____ of a _____ _____.

rupture of a small vein

G7 p.1085:50mm

◼ Nonaneurysmal SAH

142. **Complete the following about nonaneurysmal SAH:**

G7 p.1085:100mm

a. The perimesencephalic cistern has the following segments:
    Hint: Iraq Icaq
    i. i_____

interpeduncular

    ii. c_____

crural

    iii. a_____

ambient

    iv. q_____

quadrigeminal

b.

i. A new name for perimesencephalic nonaneurysmal SAH is _____ _____ _____.

pretruncal nonaneurysmal SAH

ii. A new name is warranted because that is where the blood _____ _____ _____.

truly is located

143. Complete the following:

G7 p.1085:135mm

a. Subarachnoid blood in what cistern casts doubt on a diagnosis of nonaneurysmal SAH?

chiasmatic cistern

b. What is the anatomic basis for this doubt?

Liliequist membrane should form an effective barrier for blood not under high pressure

c. True or False. Repeat angiography is required.

false

d. Risk of permanent injury from angiogram is _____ to _____%.

0.2 to 05

G7 p.1086:40mm

◼ Pregnancy and Intracranial Hemorrhage

144. True or False. Intracranial hemorrhage of pregnancy is more commonly caused by

G7 p.1086:140mm

a. AVM

false (23% AVMs)

b. aneurysms

true (77% aneurysms)

145. True or False. The following is a correct recommendation for pregnant patients with SAH:

G7 p.1086:180mm

a. Do not perform CT or angiogram.

false (They are okay if the fetus is shielded.)

b. Mannitol, Nipride, and nimodipine can be used as usual.

false (They are not to be used during pregnancy.)

c. Delay surgery until pregnancy has come to term.

false (Clipping is recommended in the pregnant patient.)

d. Deliver by C-section.

false (There is no different fetal or maternal outcome by C-section vs vaginal delivery.)

e. MRI is safe in pregnancy.

true

f. Gadolinium is safe in pregnancy.

not yet studied

g. Angiographic contrast is safe.

true

h. Treatment recommendation is surgical clipping.

true

30

31

Vascular Malformations

■ Arteriovenous Malformations

1. True or False. Which of the following statements accurately describes an arteriovenous (AV) fistula?

G7 p.1098:70mm

a. They are low flow, high pressure lesions with a low incidence of hemorrhage.   false

b. They are high flow, high pressure lesions with a high incidence of hemorrhage.   false

c. They are high flow, high pressure lesions with a low incidence of hemorrhage.   true (Think: counterintuitive: low bleeding rates even though they are high flow and high pressure lesions.)

d. They are low flow, low pressure lesions with a high incidence of hemorrhage.   false

2. Complete the following about vascular malformations:

G7 p.1098:75mm

a. True or False? A vein of Galen aneurysm is actually:
   i. an arteriovenous malformation (AVM)   false
   ii. a cavernous malformation   false
   iii. an AV fistula   true
   iv. a venous malformation   false
b. Name the other AV fistulas:
   i. d_____ _____   dural AVM
   ii. c_____ c_____ f_____   carotid cavernous fistula

3. True or False. Regarding arteriovenous malformations:

G7 p.1098:100mm

a. AVMs are characterized by dilated arteries and veins with dysplastic vessels, no capillary bed, and no intervening neural parenchyma.   true

b. In adulthood, AVMs are medium to high pressure and high flow.   true

31

c. AVMs usually present with seizures, less often with hemorrhage.

false (They usually present with hemorrhage and less often with seizures.)

d. These are congenital lesions with a lifelong risk of bleeding of ~2 to 4% per year.

true

4. True or False. The average age of patients diagnosed with AVMs is
a. 11 years — false
b. 21 years — false
c. 33 years — true
d. 45 years — false

G7 p.199:18mm

5. True or False. AVMs can
a. cause bleeding — true
b. cause seizures — true
c. steal blood from surrounding parenchyma — true
d. cause heart failure — true
e. cause headache — true

G7 p.1099:35mm

6. Complete the following about AVMs:
a. What is the peak age for hemorrhage? — 15 to 20 years
b. What is the mortality for each bleed? — 10%
c. What is the morbidity for each bleed? — 30 to 50%
d. What is the average risk of rebleeding per year? — 4% (2 to 4%)
e. What is the risk of mortality per year? — 1%
f. What is the combined mortality and morbidity per year? — 2.7%

G7 p.1099:85mm

7. True or False. Regarding AVMs:
a. Small AVMs tend to present more often as hemorrhages than do large ones. — true (Hint: The little ones bleed more.)
b. Small AVMs are less lethal than large ones. — false

G7 p.1099:140mm

G7 p.1099:160mm

8. True or False. As with aneurysms there is an increased rate of rebleeding with AVMs that have ruptured.

false (Although some say rebleeding rate increases to 6% for every year after bleed, most agree the rates stay the same at 4%/yr.)

G7 p.1100:88mm

9. True or False. Regarding AVM bleeding rates:
a. Studies suggest a higher risk of bleeding depending on whether the initial presentation was hemorrhage (3.7%/yr) vs seizure (1 to 2%/yr). — true
b. The hemorrhage risk may be higher in pediatric or with posterior-fossa AVMs. — true

G7 p.1100:117mm

31

c. The younger the patient at diagnosis, the higher the risk of developing convulsions. — true

d. The accepted risk of major bleeding is 6% per year. — false (The accepted risk of major bleeding is 4% per year. A study of 166 symptomatic AVMs with long average follow-up found the risk of major bleeding was constant at 4% per year.)

10. **What is the risk of bleeding (at least once) from an AVM during the lifetime of a 35-year-old healthy male, assuming a 3% annual bleeding risk?** — 73% — G7 p.1100:90mm

11. **Complete the following about AVMs:** — G7 p.1100:165mm
    a. True or False. 11% of patients with AVM have aneurysms. — false (7% of patients with AVMs have aneurysms.)
    b. Aneurysms associated with AVMs usually arise from a _____ artery. — feeding (75%)
    c. If it is not clear which bled, the AVM or the aneurysm, it is usually the _____. — aneurysm
    d. Do aneurysms regress after AVM removal? — yes (66%)

12. **Matching. Match the pathology and the numbered magnetic resonance imaging (MRI) criterion.** — G7 p.1101:70mm
    ① tumor; ② AVM
    a. flow void on T1-weighted imaging (T1WI) or T2-weighted imaging (T2WI) — ②
    b. feeding arteries — ②
    c. edema — ①
    d. draining veins — ②
    e. complete ring of low density surrounding the lesion — ②

13. **Which magnetic resonance (MR) sequence best shows hemosiderin?** — gradient echo — G7 p.1101:95mm

14. **Complete the following about AVMs:** — G7 p.1101:105mm
    a. Presence of edema can help differentiate AVM from _____. — tumor (Edema is more likely in tumors.)
    b. True or False. A hemosiderin ring may suggest an AVM rather than a neoplasm. — true (The AVM may have bled in the past, whereas hemosiderin ring in tumors is rare.)

15. **True or False. Criteria for the Spetzler-Martin grading of AVMs include the following:** — G7 p.1101:100mm
    Hint: SED size eloquence drainage
    a. presence of associated aneurysm — false
    b. size — true
    c. pattern of venous drainage — true
    d. eloquence of adjacent brain — true

31

16. Complete the following about AVMs: G7 p.1101:161mm

a. True or False. The Spetzler-Martin grade of a 4 cm AVM that drains into the vein of Galen and is located in the visual cortex is

    i. grade 1 — false

    ii. grade 2 — false

    iii. grade 3 — false

    iv. grade 4 — true (size 4 cm = 2, eloquence = 1 drainage, deep = 1)

    v. grade 5 — true

b. and has a morbidity rate of _____% — 27%

    i. of which _____% is minor — 20%

    ii. and _____% is major — 7%

17. Complete the following about AVMs: G7 p.1101:102mm

a. Using the Spetzler-Martin AVM grading system, what grade is an AVM located in the visual cortex of a 38-year-old man that has a nidus measuring 2.5 cm in diameter and shows on angiogram high flow and drainage into a cortical vein? — size: < 3.0 cm size 1 point, eloquent brain 1 point, superficial venous drainage – 0 points = 2 points = grade 2

b. We expect a minor deficit of _____% — 5%

c. and a major deficit of _____%. — 0%

18. Complete the following about AVMs: G7 p.1101:103mm

a. True or False. An AVM that lies over the left motor cortex, is 5.9 cm, and drains superficially is a Spetzler-Martin grade:

    i. 6 — false

    ii. 3 — true (size: 3 to 6 cm 2 points, for eloquent area 1 point, for superficial drainage 0 points; 3 = 3 points)

    iii. 4 — false

    iv. 1 — false

b. and has a morbidity of _____% — 16%

    i. minor being _____% — 12%

    ii. major being _____% — 4%

19. True or False. Regarding AVMs: G7 p.1102:54mm

a. Conventional radiation is effective in less than 20% of cases. — true

b. Stereotactic radiosurgery eliminates the risk of bleeding almost immediately. — false (Stereotactic radiosurgery takes 1 to 3 years to work, during which the patient is still at risk of bleeding from the AVM.)

c. Surgery eliminates the risk of bleeding almost immediately. — true

d. Stereotactic radiosurgery should be considered for small AVMs in eloquent cortex. — true

31

20. **Complete the following about**   G7 p.1102:110mm
    embolization of AVM:
    a. Does not permanently _____ AVMs   obliterate
    b. Does _____ surgery   facilitate
    c. Induces acute _____ changes   hemodynamic
    d. May require _____ procedures   multiple
    e. Embolization prior to stereotactic
        i.   Radiosurgery _____ obliteration   reduces
             rate
        ii. From _____ to _____%   70 to 47%

21. **True or False. Endovascular**   G7 p.1102:155mm
    embolization is usually adequate by
    itself to treat
    a. conventional AVMs   false (Embolization alone is
                                                   inadequate to treat AVMs.)
    b. direct fistulas   true (It is usually adequate to
                                                   primarily treat direct fistulas
                                                   without the use of other
                                                   methods such as surgery and
                                                   stereotactic radiosurgery.)

22. **What can be predicted about the 2-**   G7 p.1103:110mm
    year result from the 6-month
    angiographic assessment after
    embolization?
    a. If no residual is seen, it will _____.   also not be seen at 2 years
    b. If residual is seen, it will _____.   not progress to obliteration;
                                                     that is, the AVM will not
                                                     progress on its own to
                                                     obliteration in 2 years

23. **What pretreatment can be used to**   propranolol 20 mg four times   G7 p.1103:125mm
    reduce the incidence of perfusion   a day for 3 days
    pressure breakthrough?

24. **True or False. Propranolol used for**   true   G7 p.1103:125mm
    3 days prior to AVM resection can
    minimize the incidence of postop
    normal perfusion pressure
    breakthrough.

■ Venous Angiomas

25. **True or False. Regarding venous**   G7 p.1104:133mm
    angiomas:
    a. They are usually demonstrable on   true
        angiography as a starburst pattern.
    b. Typically seizures are rare.   true

c.	Typically hemorrhage is rare.	true	
d.	Surgery is usually indicated to prevent bleeding.	false (Surgery is *not* indicated to prevent bleeding. Surgery is very rarely indicated. Surgery may be considered for documented bleeding or for intractable seizures definitely attributed to the lesion.)	
26.	True or False. Neural parenchyma is not found between the vessels of a venous angioma.	false	G7 p.1104:130mm
27.	True or False. Venous angiomas require prompt surgical attention.	false (Venous angiomas require no treatment.)	G7 p.1104:130mm
28.	True or False. Venous angiomas are low flow, low pressure lesions.	true	G7 p.1104:130mm

---

■ Angiographically Occult Vascular Malformations (AOVMs)

29.	True or False. The incidence of angiographically occult vascular malformations (AOVMs) among all cerebrovascular malformations is		G7 p.1105:120mm
a.	2%	false	
b.	5%	false	
c.	10%	true	
d.	4%	false	
30.	True or False. Angiographically occult vascular malformations most often present with hemorrhage.	false (seizures or headache)	G7 p.1105:130mm
31.	True or False. The following cerebrovascular malformations are the most common angiographically occult vascular malformations:		G7 p. 1105:170mm
a.	venous angioma	false	
b.	capillary telangiectasia	false	
c.	cavernous angioma	false	
d.	arteriovenous malformation	true (Arteriovenous malformation is the most common angiographically occult vascular malformations [AOVM]. AVM 44 to 60%; cavernous angioma 19 to 31%; venous angioma 9 to 10%; telangiectasias 4 to 12%; mixed or unclassified 11%.)	

31

32. **True or False. The following vascular malformations contain intervening brain tissue:** G7 p.1105:170mm

   a.   AVM   false
   b.   venous angioma   true
   c.   cavernous angioma   false
   d.   capillary telangiectasia   true

33. **True or False. Each of the following syndromes is associated with capillary telangiectasias except:** G7 p.1106:30mm

   a.   Sturge-Weber   true
   b.   Osler-Weber-Rendu   true
   c.   Louis-Barr   true
   d.   Myburn-Mason   true
   e.   Waardenburg   false

■ Cavernous Malformations

34. **True or False. The following is true regarding cavernous malformation:** G7 p.1106:140mm

   a.   They most often present with seizures.   true
   b.   They are angiographically occult.   true
   c.   They occur more commonly in the brain stem vs supratentorially.   false
   d.   They can occur sporadically or in a hereditary form.   true

35. **True or False. The following are characteristics of cavernous malformations (CMs):** G7 p.1106:140mm

   a.   high flow malformation   false
   b.   no intervening brain parenchyma   true
   c.   usually not demonstrable on angiogram   true
   d.   no large draining veins or arteries   true

36. **True or False. The percentage of central nervous system (CNS) vascular malformations that cavernous malformations represent is** G7 p. 1107:45mm

   a.   2%   false
   b.   20%   false
   c.   10%   true (10%, quoted prevalence is 5 to 13% of all CNS vascular malformations)
   d.   1%   false

37. Complete the following regarding cavernous malformations (CMs):   G7 p.1107:65mm

a. There are _____ genetic subtypes of CM.   three

b. They may present with   G7 p.1107:95mm
   i.   s_____ in 60%   seizures
   ii. p_____ n_____ deficit in 50%   progressive neurological
   iii. h_____ in 20%   hemorrhage
   iv. i_____ finding in 50%   incidental

c. Risk of significant bleeding is   G7 p.1107:106mm
   i.   _____ to _____% per year.   2 to 3%
   ii. True or False. It is higher in females.   true
   iii. Risk in females is _____%.   4.2%
   iv. Risk in males is _____%.   0.9%
   v.   True or False. Risk is increased by
        prior bleed   controversial
        pregnancy   false
        parturition   false

38. Complete the following regarding cavernous malformations: G7 p.1107:160mm

a. The risk of bleeding is _____.   low (and only rarely significant)

b. The best test is _____ _____.   T2WI MRI
c. Radiologic appearance is _____.   pathognomonic
d. New onset seizures
   i.   may be an indication for _____ _____   surgical resection
   ii. because removal before _____ may reduce future seizures.   kindling

e. Stereotactic radiosurgery
   i.   may have a limited place in cavernous malformation treatment (True or False.)   true (but very limited)
   ii. except in r_____ h_____.   recurrent hemorrhage

39. True or False. Venous angiomas may be seen adjacent to   G7 p.1107:168mm

a. solitary cavernous malformations   true
b. multiple cavernous malformations   false

■ Dural AVM

40. True or False. The most common location of dural AVM is   G7 p.1109:132mm

a. superior sagittal sinus   false
b. tentorial   false
c. transverse sinus   true
d. torcula   false

31

41. **True or False. Dural AVMs are most commonly found in**
G7 p.1109:158mm

  a. men > 40 years of age   false
  b. men < 40 years of age   false
  c. women > 40 years of age   true
  d. women < 40 years of age   false

42. **Complete the following about dural AVMs:**
G7 p.1109:170mm

  a. True or False. Etiology is thought to be related to
   i.   trauma   false
   ii. congenital cause   false
   iii. thrombosis and revascularization true
   iv. chronic infection   true
  b. True or False. The sinus that is most commonly occluded is
   i.   superior sagittal   false
   ii. straight   false
   iii. transverse   false
   iv. sigmoid   true
   v.   confluens   false
  c. Which artery is the dominant feeder in most cases?   occipital
G7 p.1109:180mm

43. **True or False. Each of the following is a common presenting sign or symptom of dural AV fistula (AVF), also known as dural AV malformation:**
G7 p.1110:15mm

  a. hydrocephalus   false
  b. bruit   true
  c. headache   true
  d. tinnitus   true
  e. visual impairment   true
  f. papilledema   true
  g. blindness   true

■ Vein of Galen Malformation

44. **True or False. Vein of Galen malformations cause symptoms by**
G7 p.1112:85mm

  a. causing obstructive hydrocephalus   true
  b. hemorrhage   false
  c. congestive heart failure   true
  d. seizures   false

45. **Complete the following regarding vein of Galen malformations:**
G7 p.1112:125mm

  a. If untreated mortality is _____%.   60 to 100%
  b. Hydrocephalus usually presents at age _____ _____.   1 year
G7 p.1112:147mm

31

■ Carotid-Cavernous Fistula

46. **Describe Barrow-Spector classification of spontaneous carotid-cavernous fistulas.**

G7 p.1113:55mm

a. type 1 _____   traumatic

b. type 2 _____   spontaneous (Type A = direct high flow shunt between cavernous ICA and cavernous sinus, frequently due to ruptured aneurysm. B = dural shunts between meningeal branches of ICA and cavernous sinus. C = dural shunts between meningeal branches of ECA and cavernous sinus [CS]. D = dural shunts between meningeal branches of ICA and ECA and cavernous sinus.)

i. type 2A _____ flow between _____ and _____   high flow between ICA aneurysms and CS

ii. type 2B _____ flow between_____ and _____   low flow between meningeal branches of ICA and CS

iii. type 2C _____ flow between _____ and _____   low flow between meningeal branches of ECA and CS

iv. type 2D _____ flow between _____ and _____ and _____   low flow between meningeal branches of ICA and ECA and CS

47. **True or False. The following is an example of a low-flow carotid-cavernous fistula:**

G7 p.1113:56mm

a. internal carotid artery (ICA) → cavernous sinus type 2A   false (Direct ICA-cavernous fistulas occur from aneurysmal rupture and are high flow fistulas.)

b. ICA meningeal branch → cavernous sinus type 2B   true (Connections between meningeal branches of either ICA or ECA and cavernous sinus are low flow fistulas.)

c. external carotid artery (ECA) meningeal branch → cavernous sinus type 2C   true (Connections between meningeal branches of either ICA or ECA and cavernous sinus are low flow fistulas.)

48. **Complete the following about carotid-cavernous fistulas (CCFs):**

G7 p. 1113:60mm

a. What is the frequency in the head trauma patient?   0.2%

b. True or False. Low flow CCFs may thrombose spontaneously.   true (in ~50% of patients)

c. What pain-relieving procedure may produce a CCF as a complication?   percutaneous trigeminal procedures

31

49. True or False. The percentage of patients with craniocerebral trauma that develop carotid-cavernous fistulas is:

G7 p. 1113:60mm

a. 0.02%   false
b. 0.2%   true
c. 2%   false

50. True or False. According to Barrow-Spector, a carotid-cavernous fistula that is a low flow shunt between meningeal branches of the external carotid artery and the cavernous sinus is a type

G7 p.1113:82mm

a. 2A   false
b. 2C   true
c. 2B   false
d. 2D   false

51. True or False. The following is the most important factor in treating a carotid-cavernous fistula:

G7 p.1114:15mm

a. progressive diplopia   false
b. progressive exophthalmos   false
c. worsening headaches   false
d. progressive visual loss   true (Progressive visual loss is G7 p.1114:33mm overwhelmingly the most important factor influencing the decision to treat a carotid-cavernous fistula. Diplopia can be ameliorated with frosted glasses, whereas vision loss cannot be ameliorated.)

52. True or False. Regarding carotid-cavernous fistula:

G7 p.1114:22mm

a. Surgery is the treatment of choice for carotid-cavernous fistulas.   false (Endovascular embolization is the treatment of choice.)

b. Low flow CCFs thrombose spontaneously
    i.   80% of the time   false
    ii.   50% of the time   true
    iii. 20% of the time   false
    iv.   They don't thrombose spontaneously.   false

31

32

Intracerebral Hemorrhage

■ Intracerebral Hemorrhage in Adults

1. **Intracerebral hemorrhage (ICH) accounts for _____ to _____% of strokes.**

   15 to 30%

   G7 p.1118:73mm

2. **Complete the following regarding incidence of intracerebral hemorrhage in adults:**

   G7 p.1118:130mm

   a. In 100,000 people incidence is _____ to _____ cases per year.

   12 to 15

   b. Relative to subarachnoid hemorrhage (SAH) it is _____ times as frequent.

   2

   c. More cases occur in which sex?

   males

3. **True or False. The following are risk factors for ICH:**

   G7 p.1118:140mm

   a. age — true
   b. gender — true (M > F)
   c. race — true (black > white)
   d. recent ETOH — true
   e. chronic ETOH — true
   f. cigarettes — false

4. **True or False. The following increases the incidence of cerebral hemorrhage:**

   G7 p.1118:141mm

   a. alcohol, amyloid angiopathy, age — true
   b. birefringence — true
   c. Charcot-Bouchard aneurysms — true
   d. carotid disease — true
   e. central nervous system (CNS) infection — true
   f. cerebrovascular accident (CVA) previously — true
   g. street drugs — true
   h. male gender — true
   i. liver disease — true
   j. race — true
   k. smoking — false

5. **For hypertensive hemorrhage sites of predilection are**
G7 p.1119:40mm
a. s_____; _____%
striate body (basal ganglia); 50% (putamen, lenticular nucleus, internal capsule, globus pallidus)

b. t_____; _____%
thalamus; 15%

c. p_____; _____%
pons; 10%

d. c_____; _____%
cerebellum; 10%

e. c_____ w_____ m_____; _____%
cerebral white matter; 10%

f. b_____ s_____; _____%
brain stem; 5%

6. **Complete the following regarding intracerebral hemorrhage in adults:**
G7 p.1119:41mm
a. The number one location for deep ICH is _____
putamen

b. from rupture of _____ _____.
lenticulostriate arteries

7. **Complete the following regarding intracerebral hemorrhage in adults:**
G7 p.1119:78mm
a. Incidence of lobar hemorrhages is _____ to _____%.
10 to 30%

b. Is lobar or deep more fatal?
deep

c. Which is more related to alcohol?
lobar

8. **Complete the following regarding lobar hemorrhage:**
G7 p.1119:80mm
a. Incidence per 100,000 is _____ to _____.
2 to 10 (10 to 30% of the 15 to 30% of hemorrhagic CVAs)

b. Compared with deep hemorrhages, lobar hemorrhages have a _____ prognosis.
better

c. Hemorrhagic transformation may occur in
i. _____% of CVAs
43%

ii. in time from _____ to _____.
1 day to 1 month

9. **List the causes of lobar hemorrhage.**
Hint: teach it
G7 p.1119:95mm
a. t_____
tumor

b. e_____
extension of deep ICH

c. a_____
amyloid angiopathy

d. c_____
cerebrovascular malformation or aneurysm

e. h_____
hemorrhagic conversion of ischemic stroke

f. i_____
idiopathic

g. t_____
trauma

10. **Hemorrhagic transformation of an ischemic infarct**
G7 p.1120:69mm
a. is estimated to occur in _____%
43%

b. within the first _____
month

c. and may occur within _____ hours.
24

32

11. **True or False. The incidence of symptomatic ICH within 36 hours of tissue plasminogen activator (t-PA) treatment for acute ischemic CVA is approximately**

a. < 1%

false

b. 6%

true (The incidence is 6.4% versus 0.6% for placebo.)

c. 15%

false

d. 30%

false

12. **What types of infection predispose to cerebral hemorrhage?**

a. f_____

fungal

b. g_____

granulomas

c. h_____ s_____

herpes simplex

13. **True or False. Cocaine/amphetamine can cause**

a. ischemic CVA

true

b. ICH

true

14. **Complete the following regarding intracerebral hemorrhage in adults:**

a. Hypertension is a risk factor for hemorrhage in which locations?

   i. p_____

pontine ICH

   ii. c_____

cerebellar ICH

   iii. b_____ g_____ h_____

basal ganglia hemorrhages (65%)

b. Not a risk factor for _____%

35% of basal ganglia hemorrhages

15. **Complete the following regarding intracerebral hemorrhage in adults:**

a. Lobar hemorrhages are associated with _____ _____

amyloid angiopathy

   i. also known as _____ _____

congophilic angiopathy

   ii. deposit of _____ _____

beta amyloid

   iii. appears on polarized light as _____

birefringent—apple green color

b. Responsible for _____% of cases of ICH

10%

c. Any genetic factors?

yes

d. If so, what?

Apoli protein E e4 allele

e. How does this affect patients clinically?

those with APOE have hemorrhage 5 years earlier

16. **True or False. Cerebral amyloid angiopathy is associated with systemic amyloidosis.**

false (It does not require systemic amyloidosis.)

17. **Recurrent lobar hemorrhages should suggest a diagnosis of c_____ a_____ a_____.**

cerebral amyloid angiopathy

32

18. **Malignant tumors associated with ICH include**   G7 p.1123:60mm
    a. primary (name two)
       i. g_____ m_____   glioblastoma multiforme
       ii. l_____   lymphoma
    b. metastatic (name four)
       i. l_____   lung (Only approximately 9% hemorrhage but is so much more common than the others that it is seen the most.)
       ii. ch_____   choriocarcinoma (approximately 60% bleed)
       iii. m_____   melanoma (approximately 40% bleed)
       iv. r_____   renal cell carcinoma

19. **Complete the following regarding anticoagulation preceding ICH:**   G7 p.1123:125mm
    a. Incidence of bleeding complications in patients on anticoagulation is _____% per year.   10%
    b. Incidence of ICH is _____.   0.3 to 1.8% per year; 3 to 18/1000
    c. Mortality in the ICH group is _____.   65%; 2 to 12/1000 die each year

20. **True or False. Transient ischemic attack (TIA)–like symptoms precede lobar ICH in patients with amyloid angiopathy ~50% of the time.**   true (But these have Jacksonian-March-style numbness, weakness, or tingling.)   G7 p.1124:15mm

21. **What is the most common site for intracerebral hemorrhage?**   putamen   G7 p.1124:45mm

22. **Complete the following regarding ICH with thalamic hemorrhage:**   G7 p.1124:60mm
    a. Clinically usually found to have _____ loss.   hemisensory loss (contralaterally)
    b. Any motor function loss?   yes (hemiparesis if internal capsule compressed)
    c. Any eye signs such as anisocoria or miosis?   yes (with upper brain stem extension)
    d. Beyond what size has high mortality?   3.3 cm in diameter (i.e., 18 cc)   G7 p.1124:78mm

23. **True or False. Cerebellar hematomas**   G7 p.1124:106mm
    a. produce hemiparesis before coma   false
    b. produce coma before hemiparesis   true (because of compression of the brain stem)
    c. do not produce coma or hemiparesis   false

24. **Answer the following about rebleeding after intracerebral hematoma:** G7 p.1124:160mm

a. True or False. It occurs more frequently in basal ganglia hemorrhages than lobar. true

b. True or False. It occurs most frequently on the second day. false (most commonly within the first hour)

c. True or False. Incidence increases with time. false (decreases with time)

d. True or False. It is more common with small hemorrhages. false (more common with large hemorrhages)

e. True or False. It is more likely if there is a coagulopathy. true

f. Early rebleeding can occur in _____%. 33 to 38% (in 1 to 3 hours)

g. Late rebleeding can occur in _____%. 1.8 to 5.3%

25. **The component that is released by clot and presumed to be the most likely cause of surrounding delayed edema and deterioration is _____.** thrombin G7 p.1125:45mm

26. **What is the formula for volume of a hematoma?** G7 p.1125:105mm

a. sphere V = _____

b. ellipse V = _____

c. modified V = _____

$V = \pi D3 \div 6$ for a sphere
$V = \pi (h \times w \times d) \div 6$ for ellipse
$V = h \times w \times d \div 2$ modified

27. **What equation can be used to estimate the volume of an ICH?** $(A \times B \times C) \div 2$ modified ellipsoid volume where A, B, and C are the diameters of the clot in each of the three dimensions G7 p.1125:106mm

28. **Complete the following regarding intracerebral hemorrhage in adults:** G7 p.1125:113mm

a. An average size of a clot decreases at the rate of _____ mm/day. 0.75

b. The density decreases by _____ Hounsfield units (HU) per day. 2

c. There is _____ change for the first little

d. _____ weeks. 2

29. **List the sequence of hemoglobin evolution after intracerebral hemorrhage.** G7 p.1125:125mm

Hint: On days my mom's home

a. o_____ 0 to 1 day oxyhemoglobin

b. d_____ 1 to 3 deoxyhemoglobin

c. m_____ 3 to 7 methemoglobin

d. m_____ 7 to 14 methemoglobin

e. h_____ 14-plus hemosiderin

32

30. Give the ICH scores for the following:

G7 p.1126:35mm

a. Glasgow coma scale (GCS)
   i.   finding 3 to 4 points _____   2
   ii. finding 5 to 12 points _____   1
   iii. finding 13 to 15 points _____   0
b. location
   i.   finding infratentorial points   1
        _____
   ii. finding supratentorial points   0
        _____
c. age
   i.   finding > 80 years points _____   1
   ii. finding < 80 years points _____   0
d. volume
   i.   finding > 30 cc points _____   1
   ii. finding < 30 cc points _____   0
e. intraventricular
   i.   finding yes points _____   1
   ii. finding no points _____   0

31. ICH score vs mortality

G7 p.1126:35mm

a. points 0 mortality in 30 days _____ rounded out _____   points 0, mortality in 30 days 0%, rounded out 0
b. points 1 mortality in 30 days _____ rounded out _____   points 1, mortality in 30 days 13%, rounded out 10
c. points 2 mortality in 30 days _____ rounded out _____   points 2, mortality in 30 days 26%, rounded out 30
d. points 3 mortality in 30 days _____ rounded out _____   points 3, mortality in 30 days 72%, rounded out 70
e. points 4 mortality in 30 days _____ rounded out _____   points 4, mortality in 30 days 97%, rounded out 90
f. points 5 mortality in 30 days _____ rounded out _____   points 5, mortality in 30 days 100%, rounded out 100
g. points 6 mortality in 30 days _____ rounded out _____   points 6, mortality in 30 days rounded out 100

32. Complete the following about management of ICH:

G7 p.1126:118mm

a. Blood pressure (BP) permissible to reduce mean arterial pressure (MAP) by _____%.   20%
b. Target level BP is _____ and diastolic _____.   140 and diastolic; 90

33. Matching. Match the percent yield for finding AVM or aneurysm on angiogram in the following patients:

G7 p.1127:88mm

   ① 0%; ② 10%; ③ 65%
a. patient > 45 years old + hypertension (HTN) lobar ICH   ②
b. patient > 45 years old + HTN thalamic putamen ICH cerebellar/pons   ①
c. patient with intraventricular hemorrhage (IVH) without parenchymal hemorrhage   ③

34. **When is it appropriate to restart anticoagulation after cerebral hemorrhage?**

G7 p.1128:45mm

a. If there is a strong indication restart in _____ days.

5

b. If Coumadin is stopped for 10 days the chance of stroke within 30 days in a patient with
   i.   prosthetic heart value is _____%
   ii. atrial fibrillation is _____%
   iii. cardioembolic stroke is _____%

2.5%
2.6%
4.8%

c. The basic recommendation is to stay off blood thinners for _____.

2 weeks

d. If the patient needs dialysis, use h_____-f_____ d_____.

heparin-free dialysis

35. **True or False. The volume of hematoma on which it is usually most appropriate to operate is**

G7 p.1129:125mm

a. < 10 cc

false (< 10 cc too small; no major mass effect)

b. 10 to 30 cc

true

c. > 30 cc

false (usually a poor outcome)

d. > 85 cc

false (no survivors)

36. **True or False. Surgical treatment for cerebellar ICH is recommended for**

G7 p.1130:35mm

a. GCS 14, hematoma 3 cm diameter

false (may treat conservatively 14 cc)

b. GCS 13, hematoma 4 cm diameter

true (Surgical treatment is recommended for GCS ≤ 13 or hematoma ≥ 4 cm diameter = 32 cc.)

c. GCS 3

false (not in the face of complete neurologic destruction where the outcome will be poor [i.e., flaccid, no brain stem reflex])

d. hematoma plus hydrocephalus

true

37. **With cerebral hemorrhage, the possible mortality in 30 days for the following conditions is**

G7 p.1131:44mm

a. SAH _____%
b. ICH-basal ganglia thalamus _____%
c. ICH-lobar _____%

46%
44%
11%

32

■ ICH in Young People

38. **Name the top five causes of nontraumatic ICH in patients 15 to 45 years old (other than "undetermined," which is ~ 1/4).**
     Hint: AHadt

     G7 p.1131:70mm

     a. A_____   AVM (~30%)
     b. H_____   HTN (~15%)
     c. a_____   aneurysm (~10%)
     d. d_____   drugs (~7%)
     e. t_____   tumor (~4%)

■ Intracerebral Hemorrhage in the Newborn

39. **Synonyms are**

     G7 p.1131:143mm

     a. SEH _____   subependymal hemorrhage
     b. GMH _____   germinal matrix hemorrhage
     c. IVH _____   intraventricular hemorrhage

40. **True or False. The germinal matrix normally involutes around**

     G7 p.1131:170mm

     a. 26 to 28 weeks gestation   false
     b. 28 to 30 weeks gestation   false
     c. 30 to 32 weeks gestation   false
     d. 32 to 36 weeks gestation   true

41. **Complete the following about intracerebral hemorrhage in the newborn:**

     G7 p.1131:180mm

     a. True or False. Extremely early (< 28 weeks gestation) germinal matrix hemorrhage is most likely to occur at the
         i.   head of caudate   false
         ii. body of caudate   true (Most hemorrhages, however, occur at the head of the caudate at a later age of gestation.)

         iii. tail of caudate   false
         iv. choroid plexus   false
     b. Sequence the preceding responses according to the following ages:
         i.   Premature under 28 weeks gestation bleed in _____   body of caudate
         ii. Infants 32 to 34 weeks gestation bleed in _____   head of caudate
         iii. Mature infants bleed from the _____   choroid plexus

32

G7 p.1132:70mm

42. **True or False. The following is most important for risk of developing a germinal matrix hemorrhage:**
    a. ↑ CO_2
    b. ↑ cerebral blood flow (CBF)
    c. ↑ temperature
    d. ↑ cerebral perfusion pressure (CPP)

true
true
false
true (The most common denominators for all risk factors for germinal matrix hemorrhage are increased cerebral blood flow and increased cerebral perfusion pressure. Specific risk factors include asphyxia, hypervolemia, seizures, pneumothorax, cyanotic heart disease, extracorporeal membrane oxygenation [ECMO] ventilation, and maternal cocaine abuse.)

G7 p.1132:85mm

43. **List the risk factors for germinal matrix (subependymal) hemorrhage.**
    Hint: vespacc
    a. v_____
    b. e_____

    c. s_____
    d. p_____
    e. a_____
    f. c_____
    g. c_____

volume expansion
extracorporeal membrane oxygenation (ECMO)
seizures
pneumothorax
asphyxia
cyanotic heart disease
cocaine abuse (maternal)

G7 p.1133:150mm

44. **Complete the following regarding intracerebral hemorrhage in the newborn:**
    a. What% of babies with germinal matrix hemorrhage (GMH) will develop hydrocephalus?
    b. Grading system of _____
    c. List the criteria for the four grades.
       i. grade I

       ii. grade II

       iii. grade III

       iv. grade IV

20 to 50%

Papile

subependymal hemorrhage (SE)
intraventricular hemorrhage without ventricular enlargement (IVH without VE)
IVH + ventricular enlargement (IVH with VE)
IVH + parenchymal hemorrhage (IVH with PH)

32

d. Hydrocephalus occurs in _____ to _____%.

20 to 50%

G7 p.1134:70mm

e. Hydrocephalus usually occurs _____ to _____ weeks after the subependymal hemorrhage (SEH).

1 to 3

G7 p.1134:82mm

45. True or False. A germinal matrix hemorrhage that extends into the ventricle but does not cause ventricular dilation is the following grade, according to the Papile grading system:

G7 p.1133:150mm

a. grade I

false

b. grade II

true

c. grade III

false

d. grade IV

false

46. Complete the following regarding intracerebral hemorrhage in the newborn:

G7 p.1136:163mm

a. CSF protein above _____ mg/cc will prevent spontaneous reabsorption.

100

b. Additional concerns regarding high protein include

i. m_____ by the p_____

malabsorption by the peritoneum

ii. i_____

ileus

iii. o_____ of s_____ t_____

occulsion of shunt tubing

47. Indications for converting an Ommaya to a VP shunt are

G7 p.1137:35mm

a. CSF protein below _____

100 mg/cc

b. Weight of the child is at least _____

2500 g

48. Give the germinal matrix hemorrhages outcome.

G7 p.1137:70mm

a. mortality _____%

5 to 65%

b. hydrocephalus _____%

15 to 100%

c. IQ _____

75% (normal)

d. ambulatory _____%

100% (all survivors ambulatory)

33

Occlusive Cerebrovascular Disease

■ Vaso-occlusive Disease

1. **True or False. A transient ischemic attack (TIA) is a focal neurological deficit lasting 24 hours but not more than 48 hours.**

   false (A TIA, by definition, lasts ≤ 24 hours.)

   G6 p.869:50mm

2. **Complete the following about transient ischemic attack (TIA):**

   G7 p.1010:55mm

   a. TIA is usually _____.

   short

   b. Most last only _____ _____.

   10 minutes

   c. 70% last only _____ _____.

   10 minutes

   d. 90% last less than _____ _____.

   4 hours

   e. If a deficit lasts more than 60 minutes, only _____% resolve in 24 hours.

   14%

3. **Complete the following about RIND:**

   G6 p.869:60mm

   a. RIND stands for r_____ i_____ n_____ d_____.

   reversible ischemic neurologic deficit

   b.
   i. It is defined as a n_____ d_____

   neurologic deficit

   ii. that lasts > _____ hours but less than _____ _____.

   24 hours; 1 week

   iii. Frequency of occurrence is _____%.

   2.5%

4. **With atherosclerotic cerebrovascular disease (CVA), atherosclerotic plaques**

   G7 p1144 :70mm

   a. begin to form as early as age _____

   20

   b. begin on the back wall of the _____ _____ _____

   common carotid artery

   c. risk of CVA correlates with

   i. s_____

   stenosis

   ii. u_____

   ulcerations

   iii. h_____

   hypercoagulable

   iv. v_____

   viscosity

5. **True or False. Patients with a depressed level of consciousness or an acute fixed deficit should undergo emergency carotid endarterectomy.**

   false (These are two contraindications to emergency CEA.)

   G6 p.880:20mm

33

■ Atherosclerotic Cerebrovascular Disease

6. Carotid artery lesions   G7 p.1144:95mm
a. are considered symptomatic if
　　i.   there is _____ or _____   one or more
　　　　ischemic episodes
　　ii. in the _____ of the vessel.   distribution
b. True or False. They are considered
　　asymptomatic if the patient only has
　　i.   visual complaints   true
　　ii. dizziness   true
　　iii. syncope   true

7. In a patient with carotid plaque   G7 p.1144:95mm
categorize the following:
a. blurred vision   asymptomatic
b. aphasia for less than 24 hours   symptomatic
c. weakness of arm for 10 min   symptomatic
d. dizziness   asymptomatic

8. True or False. The stroke rate in a   G7 p.1144:108mm
patient with asymptomatic carotid
bruit is approximately
a. 0%   false
b. 2%   true
c. 8%   false
d. 22%   false

9. True or False. The central retinal artery G7 p.1144:126mm
is often insufficient in cerebrovascular
disease. This artery is a branch of the
following:
a. posterior cerebral artery   false
b. orbital artery   false
c. ophthalmic artery   true
d. M2   false
e. anterior communicating artery   false

10. Retinal insufficiency can manifest by   G7 p.1144:126mm
a. temporary loss of vision, aka _____   amaurosis fugax
　　_____
b. True or False. Such loss of vision is
　　i.   bilateral   false
　　ii. contralateral   false
　　iii. ipsilateral   true
　　iv. homonymous   false

c. There are four types.

    i. Type I is called "black curtain" due to _____.   emboli   G7 p.1144:136mm

    ii. Type III is called "gray vision" due to _____.   hypoperfusion

    iii. Type III is associated with migraines and the cause is _____.   vasospastic

    iv. Type IV is associated with anti cardio lipin antibodies, and the cause is _____.   miscellaneous

    v. Blindness may be _____.   permanent

11. What are Hollenhorst plaques?   cholesterol crystal emboli seen on funduscopic examination in patients with carotid artery disease   G7 p.1145:178mm

12. Complete the following about the classification of carotid ulcerations: G7 p.1145:18mm

a. Type A is s_____ s_____ s_____.   small smooth shallow

b. Type B is l_____ d_____.   large deep

c. Type C is c_____ c_____.   complex cavitated

d. Annual stroke rate for type A is _____%.   0.5%

e. Annual stroke rate for type B is _____%.   0.4 to 4.5%

f. Annual stroke rate for type C is _____%.   5 to 7%

13. What is the gold standard for evaluation of carotid artery disease?   angiography   G7 p.1145:63mm

14. In the arteriosclerotic patient what is the risk that angiography will cause a cerebrovascular accident (CVA)?   Less than 1% risk of CVA   G7 p.1145:71mm

15. Complete the following about Nascet study: G7 p.1145:90mm

a. Nascet stands for _____.   North American Symptomatic Carotid Endarterectomy Trial

b. It measures degree of c_____ s_____.   carotid stenosis

c. Formula is _____ =% stenosis $\left(x = \dfrac{N}{D}\right) \times 100$ =% stenosis

d. where N is measured at maximal _____   narrowing

e.

    i. where D is measured _____   distal

    ii. to the _____ _____   carotid bulb

    iii. where the walls become _____   parallel

f. Surgery is not indicated for less than _____%.   40%

33

16. **Complete the following about duplex Doppler ultrasound limitations:**   G7 p.1145:165mm
    a. It can't scan above the angle of the _____.   mandible
    b. It performs poorly with the _____ _____.   string sign
    c. Depth of penetration is greater with _____ _____.   lower frequencies
    d. Signal definition is better with _____ _____.   higher frequencies

17. **True or False. Ultrasound of the carotid artery is excellent for evaluating patients with "the string sign."**   false (Ultrasound is very poor for evaluation of such low flow states.)   G7 p.1145:168mm

18. **The use of magnetic resonance angiography**   G7 p.1145:180mm
    a. may demonstrate a flow _____   gap
    b. which obviates the need for _____.   angiography
    c. It may _____ the degree of carotid stenosis.   underestimate

19. **True or False. The following irreversibly inhibits cyclooxygenase:**   G7 p.1146:166mm
    a. ticlodipine   false
    b. aspirin   true (Aspirin irreversibly inhibits cyclooxygenase preventing synthesis of vascular prostacyclin and platelet thromboxane A2. Platelets cannot resynthesize cyclooxygenase, whereas the vascular tissues do so rapidly.)
    c. clopidogrel   false
    d. prednisone   false

20. **Aspirin**   G7 p.1147:16mm
    a. The optimal dose for cerebrovascular ischemia is _____.   debated
    b.
       i. Risk of stroke after TIA can be reduced by _____ to _____%   25 to 30%
       ii. by the use of _____ mg PO per day.   325
    c. True or False. More mg of ASA is better after TIA.   false
    d. Daily doses of 81 or 325 mgm were _____ than higher doses.   better
    e. CVA, MI and death were reduced to _____% from _____%.   6.2 from 8.2

21. **Complete the following about Plavix:**   G7 p.1147:55mm
    a. Has a lower incidence of _____   neutropenia
    b. Needs to be taken _____ per day   once
    c. Requires _____ days off the drug to reverse   5

22. **Complete the following about asymptomatic carotid artery stenosis:**

G7 p.1147:120mm

a. stroke rate of _____% per year

2%

b. percent that are not disabling is _____%

50%

c. Carotid endarterectomy may be beneficial for stenosis of more than _____%.

60%

23. **True or False. The annual stroke rate for patients with symptomatic carotid stenosis is**

G7 p.1148:95mm

a. 30%

false

b. 5%

false

c. 1 to 3.4%

true

d. 1%

false

24. **True or False. The Asymptomatic Carotid Atherosclerosis Study (ACAS) found that surgery is moderately beneficial for asymptomatic carotid stenosis ≥ 60%.**

true

G7 p.1149:20mm

■ Carotid Endarterectomy

25. **True or False. The North American Symptomatic Carotid Endarterectomy Trial (NASCET) found that in patients with a recent TIA and ipsilateral stenosis > 70%, carotid endarterectomy (CEA) reduced the risk of CVA by**

G7 p.1150:85mm

a. 17%

true (at 18 months follow-up)

b. 80%

false

c. 60%

false

d. It did not reduce the risk.

false

26. **The general trend in carotid endarterectomy surgery is to wait only _____ days after CVA to perform an endarterectomy.**

7

G7 p.1151:26mm

27. **True or False. Aspirin and dipyridamole have been shown unequivocally to reduce the rate of restenosis after CEA.**

false (The use of these medications has not been shown to reduce the rate of restenosis after CEA.)

G7 p.1152:145mm

28. **Complete the following about postop check after carotid endarterectomy:**

G7 p.1152:165mm

a. Pronator drift to rule out _____ _____

new hemiparesis

b. Dysphasia to rule out _____ _____ _____

dominant hemisphere CVA

c. Pupil size to rule out _____ _____

Horner syndrome

   d. STA pulsations to rule out _____   external carotid occlusion
       _____ _____

   e. Tongue deviation to identify _____   XII nerve injury
       _____ _____

   f.
       i.   Hoarseness consider _____   laryngeal edema
            _____

       ii. Or _____ _____ nerve injury   recurrent laryngeal
   g. Tracheal deviation to identify postop   hematoma
       _____

29. **List postop complications of carotid**   G7 p.1153:35mm
    endarterectomy.
    Hint: c-h$_4$arm$_2$s$_2$

    a. c_____   cranial nerve injury
    b. h_____   headache
    c. h_____   hoarseness
    d. h_____   hyperperfusion
    e. h_____   hypertension
    f. a_____   arteriotomy disruption
    g. r_____   restenosis
    h. m_____   morbidity
    i. m_____   mortality
    j. s_____   seizures
    k. s_____   stroke

30. **Complete the following about carotid**   G7 p.1153:40mm
    endarterectomy:
    a. Morbidity: absolute upper limit is   3%
        _____%.
    b. Mortality in hospital is _____%.   1%

31. **Complete the following about**   G7 p.1153:41mm
    arteriotomy disruption:
    a. Most immediate danger is _____   asphyxiation
    b. Symptoms and signs
        i.   Swelling of _____   neck
        ii.   Swallowing _____   difficulty
        iii. Deviation of _____   trachea
        iv.   Air _____   hunger
        v.   Late _____ _____   false aneurysm

32. **Complete the following about stroke:**   G7 p.1153:83mm
    a. Infarction incidence: _____%   5%
    b. Hemorrhagic incidence: _____%   0.6%

33. **What is the most common cause of**   G7 p.1153:102mm
    a. minor post-CEA CVA?   emboli
    b. major post-CEA CVA?   postoperative ICA occlusion

34. **Risk of stroke is related to**   G7 p.1153:107mm
    a. t_____   technique
    b. h_____ state   hypercoaguable
    c. h_____ reaction   heparin
    d. Endarterectomy site is t_____   thrombogenic

33

35. **Complete the following about seizures:**   G7 p.1153:139mm
   a. Most occur postop day _____ to _____   5 to 13
   b. Usually _____   focal
   c. Incidence _____%   1%

36. **Complete the following about restenosis after CEA surgery:**   G7 p.1153:150mm
   a. within 2 years is usually due to _____   fibrous hyperplasia
   b. after 2 years is usually due to _____   atherosclerosis

37. **Complete the following about late restenosis:**   G7 p.1153:152mm
   a. It occurs within the first year in _____%.   25%
   b. If it occurs within 2 years, it is due to f_____ h_____.   fibrous hyperplasia
   c. If it occurs after 2 years, it is due to a _____.   atherosclerosis

38. **Complete the following about cerebral hyperperfusion syndrome:**   G7 p.1153:158mm
   a. Due to return of blood to area of lost _____   autoregulation
   b. Usually from chronic cerebral _____   ischemia
   c. Secondary to high-grade _____   stenosis
   d. May result in _____ _____   intracerebral hemorrhage

39. **True or false. Hoarseness is most likely caused by**   G7 p.1153:175mm
   a. superior laryngeal nerve injury   false
   b. laryngeal edema   true
   c. recurrent laryngeal nerve injury   false

40. **Complete the following about hypoglossal nerve injury:**   G7 p.1154:16mm
   a. Incidence is _____%.   1%
   b. Tongue deviates _____ _____ _____ of the injury.   toward the side
   c. Unilateral injury causes problem with
      i. sp_____   speaking
      ii. sw_____   swallowing
      iii. c_____   chewing
   d. Bilateral injury can cause a_____ o_____.   airway obstruction
   e. It may last as long as _____ months.   4 months
   f. Palsy is a contraindication to doing endarterectomy.   contralaterally

41. Complete the following about endarterectomy and vocal cord paralysis:

G7 p.1154:30mm

   a. Incidence is _____%.
       1%

   b. Which side would be affected?
       ipsilateral

   c. Due to injury to
     i. v_____ nerve
       vagus
     ii. r_____ l_____ nerve
       recurrent laryngeal

42. Damage to which nerve could cause postoperative lip asymmetry following CEA? (i.e., not due to stroke)
   marginal mandibular branch of facial nerve MMB-VII (usually a retraction injury with the nerve being retracted against the mandible)

G7 p.1154:37mm

43. Complete the following about hypertension:

G7 p.1154:42mm

   a. May develop _____ to _____ days after CEA
       5 to 7
   b. Due to loss of the carotid s_____ b_____ reflex
       sinus baroreceptor

44. True or False. Immediately following CEA (i.e., in the post-anesthesia care unit), a patient who developed neurologic deficit in the distribution of the endarterectomized carotid should undergo immediate computed tomography/magnetic resonance imaging (CT/MRI) or angiogram.
   false (The patient should be emergently reexplored. There is no deficit if flow is reestablished in 45 minutes.)

G7 p.1154:40mm

45. True or False. When performing CEA, the order of removing clamps after completion of endarterectomy is

G7 p.1154:80mm

   a. internal, common, external carotid
       false
   b. internal, external, common carotid
       false
   c. external, common, internal carotid
       true (This ensures that any embolic material will be flushed to the external carotid circulation.)
   d. The order of removal does not matter.
       false

46. True or False. When performing reexploration of a CEA occlude in the following order:

G7 p.1154:84mm

   a. Internal, common, external
       false
   b. Internal, external, common
       false
   c. External, common, internal
       false
   d. Common, external, internal
       true

47. Complete the following about arteriotomy disruption:

G7 p.1154:125mm

   a. If you notice difficulty breathing _____ _____
       open wound

33

  b. then i_____.

  c. This may be difficult if the _____ is deviated.

intubate
trachea

48. **True or False. A patient with disruption of arteriotomy closure following carotid surgery should never be intubated.**

false (Intubation is a high priority.)

G7 p.1154:137mm

49. **Complete the following about anesthesia and monitoring:**

  a. Hemodynamic intolerance to clamping occurs in _____%.

  b. If identified, place a vascular _____.

  c. Which is safer: local or general anesthesia?

  d. Add thiopental to general anesthesia until EEG burst suppression lasts for _____ to _____ seconds.

G7 p.1154:165mm

1 to 4%

shunt

no difference

15 to 30

50. **True or False. A shunt is commonly used in carotid surgery when the stump pressure is less than**

  a. 100 mm Hg

  b. 25 mm Hg

  c. 1 mm Hg

  d. Never use a shunt

G7 p.1155:48mm

false
true
false
false

51. **Surgical results correlate best with _____ neurologic status.**

presenting

G7 p.1157:75mm

52. **Totally occluded carotid and patient presents with mild neurologic deficit.**

  a. Assume _____ occlusion

  b. Have stroke rate of _____ to _____% per year

G7 p.1157:165mm

chronic

3 to 5%

53. **Complete the following about acute carotid occlusion:**

  a. Some neurologic deficit in _____ to _____%

  b. Mortality: _____ to _____%

  c. Good recovery in _____ to _____%

G7 p.1157:165mm

40 to 70%

15 to 55%

2 to 12%

54. **Six of the symptoms of vertebrobasilar insufficiency (VBI) begin with the letter "d." They are**

  a. dr_____ _____

  b. di_____

  c. dy_____

  d. de_____ _____ _____

  e. diz_____

  f. de_____ b_____

G7 p.1158:110mm

drop attack
diplopia
dysarthria
defect in vision
dizziness
deficit bilaterally (motor and/or sensory)

33

55. Answer the following about vertebrobasilar insufficiency (VBI):   G7 p.1158:125mm

a. Clinical diagnosis of VBI requires how many of those criteria?   2 or more

b. Which symptom suggests:
  i. Ischemia to the brain?   diplopia near ocular nuclear
  ii. Ischemia to lower brain stem?   dysarthria
  iii. Ischemia to occipital cortex?   homonymous hemianopsia

56. Complete the following about vision symptoms: G7 p.1158:140mm

a.
  i. Carotid artery vision symptoms are _____   unilateral
  ii. For example, a_____ f_____   amaurosis fugax
b.
  i. Vertebral artery symptoms are _____   bilateral
  ii. For example, h_____ h_____   homonymous hemianopsia

57. If a patient has transient episodes of vertigo you may suspect _____.   VBI   G7 p.1158:146mm

58. The most common cause of VBI   G7 p.1158:185mm

a. is s_____ s_____   subclavian steal
b.
  i. which is r_____ f_____ in the VA   reversed flow
  ii. due to p_____ s_____   proximal stenosis
  iii. of the s_____ a_____.   subclavian artery

59. The mainstay treatment of VBI is a_____.   anticoagulation   G7 p.1159:70mm

60. Complete the following regarding bow hunter's stroke: G7 p.1159:105mm

a. Bow hunter's stroke is caused by occlusion of the _____ _____   vertebral artery

b. resulting from _____ _____.   head rotation

c. Can this occur from forceful treatment by a chiropractor?   yes

d. The vessel occluded is _____ to the direction of head rotation.   contralateral

e. It is more likely in patients with incompetent _____ _____ arteries.   posterior communicating

f. An appropriate test for this condition is _____ _____ _____.   dynamic cerebral angiography (DCA)

g. If condition is proved treatment of choice is _____ _____ _____.   decompression of VA at C1-2

h. If still symptomatic treatment is _____ _____.   C1-2 fusion

■ Cerebral Arterial Dissections

61. True or False. The following are features of cerebral arterial dissections:

a. Hemorrhage into medial layer — true

b. Presentation includes pain, subarachnoid hemorrhage (SAH), TIA, and Horner syndrome. — true

c. Extracranial dissection is treated surgically. — false

d. Intracranial dissections with SAH are treated surgically. — false

G7 p.1160:125mm

62. True or False. Regarding arterial dissection:

a. Hemorrhage can occur outside the vascular lumen due to transintimal extravasation of hematoma. — true

b. The hematoma may dissect the internal elastic membrane from the intima. — true

c. Subintimal dissection is more common with extracranial lesions. — false (Subintimal dissection is more common with intracranial dissection—sub*inti*mal = *intr*acranial.)

d. Dissection of the internal elastic membrane results in luminal narrowing. — true

G7 p.1161:22mm

63. Matching. Match the dissection with its location.
① media; ② subintima; ③ between media and adventitia

a. intracranial dissection — ②

b. extracranial dissection — ①, ③

G7 p.1161:38mm

64. Matching. Rank the following dissection sites in order of frequency of occurrence and give their approximate percentages:
① first; ② second; ③ third

a. ACA/PCA/PICA _____% — ③ 10%

b. basilar/ICA/MCA _____% — ② 30%

c. vertebral _____% — ① 60%

G7 p.1161:103mm

65. True or False. Headache usually precedes neurologic deficits by less than 1 hour. — false (Headache usually precedes deficits by days to weeks.)

G7 p.1162:22mm

66. **True or False. The most reliable finding on radiographic examination of suspected arterial dissections is**   G7 p.1162:90mm
  a. direct visualization on CT   false
  b. crescent sign on T2-weighted (T2W) axial imaging   false
  c. string sign on angiography   false
  d. double lumen sign on angiography   true (Double lumen sign on angiography is considered pathognomonic.)

67. **True or False. In cerebral arterial dissection the angiographic configuration is expected**   G7 p.1162:105mm
  a. to remain stable   false
  b. to resolve or worsen   true
  c. to often change   true

68. **Mortality in cerebral arterial dissections is higher in**   G7 p.1162:150mm
  a. _____ lesions   carotid
  b. carotid _____%   49%
  c. vertebrobasilar artery (VBA) _____%   22%
  d. subarachnoid hemorrhage _____%   24
  e. non-SAH patients _____%   29

69. **Complete the following regarding carotid dissection:**   G7 p.1163:15mm
  a. True or False. The most frequent presenting symptom of spontaneous ICA dissection is
      i.   neck pain   false (Pain is 9% more common in VBA.)
      ii. neck swelling   false (swelling 2%)
      iii. headache   true (headache 59%)
      iv. oculosympathetic palsy (partial Horner syndrome)   false (30%)

70. **Complete the following about vertebral artery dissection:**   G7 p.1163:85mm
  a. Categories:
      i.   s_____   spontaneous
      ii. a_____   aneurysmal
      iii. t_____   traumatic
  b. True or False. Frequency:
      i.   Carotid dissections are more common.   true
      ii. Vertebral dissections are more common.   false

71. **Complete the following regarding cerebral arterial dissections:**   G6 p.885:150mm

a. True or False. Posttraumatic ICA dissection injury mechanisms include
   i. chiropractic manipulation — true
   ii. attempted strangulation — true
   iii. postangiography — true
   iv. hyperextension of neck with ICA stretch — true (compress ⇒ stretch ⇒ dissection risk poke ⇒ tweak ⇒)

b. After trauma symptoms manifest within _____ hours _____%. — 24 hours; 75%   G6 p.885:180mm

c. The most frequent presenting symptom of posttraumatic ICA dissection is _____ _____. — ischemic symptoms

d. Which is more common: traumatic or spontaneous ICA dissection? — traumatic

72. **True or False. Persistent embolic complications of ICA dissection are indications for the following interventions:**   G6 p.886:50mm

a. interposition venous grafting — true

b. EC/IC bypass with maintenance of ICA luminal integrity — false (Extracranial/intracranial [EC/IC] bypass is okay, but once you bypass the clot, close the ICA off to reduce further embolic risk.)

c. carotid ligation alone — true

d. heparin-warfarin-based anticoagulation with close angiographic observation — true

73. **Complete the following about traumatic dissections:**   G7 p.1163:97mm

a. Occur where VA crosses _____ _____ — bony prominences

b. Typically the _____ - _____ junction — C1-2

c. Can result from
   i. Manipulation of _____ — neck
   ii. Automobile a_____ — accidents
   iii. C_____ treatment — chiropractic
   iv. Sudden head _____ — turning
   v. Blow to _____ of _____ — back of neck

d. Can produce massive _____ hematomas — neck   G7 p.1164:15mm

e.
   i. Angiography demonstrates lesion posterior to the _____ — atlas
   ii. Which is the distal extracranial _____ _____ — third segment

f. The first and third portions of the VA are _____. — movable

g. The second and fourth portions are immobilized by _____. — bone

33

h. Most commonly angiography
    i. demonstrates _____ _____   irregular stenosis
    ii. of the horizontal loops as they pass   C1
        _____.

74. **Complete the following about**   G7 p.1163:112mm
    spontaneous dissection:
    a. Tends to be _____   intracranial
    b. Occur on the _____VA   dominant

    c. Associated with
        i.   f_____ d_____   fibromuscular dysplasia
        ii. m_____   migraine
        iii. o_____ c_____   oral contraceptives
    d. More common in _____ _____   young adults
    e. Have other sites of dissection _____% 36%
    f. Have bilateral VA dissection _____% 21%

75. **True or False. Dissecting aneurysms of**   G7 p.1163:125mm
    the vertebrobasilar arteries commonly
    present as
    a. saccular aneurysms   false
    b. fusifom aneurysms   true
    c. subarachnoid hemorrhage   true
    d. are ameniable to clipping   may be
    e. altered consciousness   true

76. **Although most spontaneous vertebral** occipital pain   G7 p.1163:155mm
    artery dissections are intracranial,
    those that are extracranial present
    with _____ _____.

77. **True or False. Dissecting aneurysms of**   G7 p.1163:175mm
    the vertebrobasilar arteries commonly
    present as
    a. saccular aneurysms   false
    b. fusiform dilatation   true
    c. subarachnoid hemorrhage   true

78. **Matching. Match the treatment with**   G7 p. 1164:70mm
    the condition.
    Treatment:
    ① medical-anticoagulation; ② surgical
    Condition:
    a. subarachnoid hemorrhage   ②
    b. intradural dissection   ②
    c. extradural dissections that progress   ②
        clinically or angiographically despite
        anticoagulation
    d. non-hemorrhagic small infarction   ①   G6 p. 886:116mm

■ Cerebrovascular Venous Thrombosis

79. **True or False. The following are conditions associated with dural sinus thrombosis formation:**   G7 p.1166:80mm

a. oral contraceptives — true
b. ulcerative colitis — true
c. dehydration — true
d. peripheral vascular disease — false
e. infection — true
f. hypercoagulable state — true
g. pregnancy — true
h. trauma — true

80. **Hypercoagulable state includes (Hint: a^2p^4rs):**   G7 p.1166:135mm

a. a_____ III deficiency — antithrombin
b. a_____ antibodies — antiphospholipid
c. p_____ C deficiency — protein
d. p_____ S deficiency — protein
e. p_____ _____ hemoglobinuria — paroxysmal nocturnal
f. p_____ deficiency — plasminogen
g. r_____ to activated protein C — resistance
h. s_____ lupus erythematosis — systemic

81. **Complete the following about cerebrovascular venous thrombosis:**   G7 p.1167:15mm

a. Incidence is 1 in _____ births. — 10,000
b. Period of highest risk of cerebrovascular venous thrombosis during the puerperium is within the first _____ _____ after delivery. — 2 weeks

82. **True or False. Dural sinus thrombosis occurs more often in the superior sagittal sinus and the**   G7 p.1167:40mm

a. right transverse sinus — false
b. left transverse sinus — true
c. straight sinus — false
d. inferior sagittal sinus — false

83. **Incidence of dural sinus thrombosis (DST)**   G7 p.1164:47mm

a. in the superior sagittal sinus is _____% — 70%
b. in the left transverse sinus is _____% — 70%
c. in multiple sinuses is _____% — 71%

84. **Complete the following about clinical symptoms from superior sagittal sinus thrombosis (SSS):**   G7 p.1167:125mm

a. No symptoms _____ _____ — anterior third
b. Spastically, increased muscle tone _____ _____ — middle third
c. Cortical blindness or edema, or death _____ _____ — posterior third

33

85. **What are the clinical symptoms of thrombosis of SSS?**   G7 p.1167:126mm
   a. Anterior third: may produce _____   no symptoms
      _____
   b. Middle third: may produce _____   spasticity
   c. Thrombosis of posterior third: may   blindness, edema, death
      produce _____, _____, _____

86. **Thrombosis of the jugular bulb may produce the following syndrome:**   G7 p.1167:152mm
   a. symptoms (Hint: bash)
      i.   b_____   breathlessness
      ii. a_____   aphonia
      iii. s_____   swallowing difficulties
      iv. h_____   hoarseness
   b. named _____ _____   Vernet syndrome   also see
                                                       G6 p.86:140mm
   c. nerves involved are _____ _____   9, 10, 11
      _____
   d. due to compression of the pars   nervosa
      _____

87. **The best way to diagnose thrombosis of a venous sinus is by**   G7 p.1167:175mm
   a. M_____ or   MRI
   b. a_____.   angiography

88. **With dural sinus thrombosis and plain CT scan, suspect the diagnosis of DST.**   G7 p.1168:20mm
   a. May be _____ in 20%   normal
   b. Intraparenchymal f_____   flame; 20%
      hemorrhage _____%
   c. Small v_____ in _____%   ventricles; 50%
   d. White matter e_____   edema
   e. Above changes occurring b_____   bilaterally

89. **Thrombosis of the superior sagittal sinus**   G7 p.1168:44mm
   a. may produce a configuration on CT scan   delta sign
      called a _____ _____,
   b. which represents _____ _____ in   clotted blood in the sinus
      the _____
   c. or on a CT with contrast it may produce   empty delta sign
      an _____ _____ _____.

90. Complete the following about delta sign types: G7 p1168 :46mm

33

a. Delta sign—a triangular-shaped configuration—is seen on
   i.   CT _____ contrast   without
   ii.   Represents _____ _____   clotted blood
   iii. _____ the sinus   within

b. Pseudo delta sign is
   i.   CT _____ contrast   without
   ii.   Represents _____ around SSS   SAH

c. Empty delta sign is seen in
   i.   CT _____ contrast   with
   ii.   Represents enhancement of _____   dura

   iii. More so than the intra sinus _____   clot

91. True or False. The following are benefits of assessing thrombosis of the superior sagittal sinus with MRI: G7 p.1168:95mm

a. preferred diagnostic procedure   true
b. can demonstrate vascular changes   true
c. can demonstrate parenchymal changes   true
d. can identify congenital absence of sinus   true
e. shows cerebral edema   true
f. can estimate age of thrombosis   true
g. more advantageous than angiography   true

92. Complete the following regarding cerebrovascular venous thrombosis: G7 p.1169:65mm

a. True or False. Heparin is the treatment of true
   choice for dural venous sinus thrombosis
   with associated intracranial hemorrhage.

b. Must not treat
   i.   with _____   steroids
   ii.   because they reduce _____ and fibrinolysis; thrombosis
       thereby increase _____

c. Should also correct
   i.   _____ _____   underlying abnormality (i.e., use antibiotics)
   ii.   and control _____   hypertension

d. continue anticoagulation for _____ 3 to 6   G7 p.1169:175mm
   to _____ months

93. What is the prognosis of superior sagittal sinus (SSS) thrombosis? G7 p.1170:65mm

a. Mortality is _____%.   5 to 70% (approximately 30%)

b. Poor prognostic indicators are
   i.   e _____ of a_____   extremes of age (infancy or old age)

   ii.   c_____   coma
   iii. n_____ d_____   neurological deterioration (rapid)

c. Treatment for visual loss from   optic nerve sheath   G7 p.1169:170mm
   papilledema is o_____ n_____ fenestration
   s_____ f_____.

33 ■ Moyamoya Disease

94. Complete the following regarding moyamoya disease: G7 p.1170:125mm

a. *Moyamoya* means p_____ o_____ s_____. puff of smoke

b. Skull base arteries are _____ narrowed

c. due to a thickened _____. intima

d. _____ deposits occur Lipid

e. without evidence of _____. inflammation

f. The other vascular abnormality that occurs is _____, which aneurysms (intracranial) G7 p.1171:65mm

g. may be due to a _____ defect in the wall. congenital

h. Aneurysms occur in unusual sites.
   i. Cerebral arteries at their _____ periphery
   ii. Posterior/anterior _____ choroidal
   iii. Recurrent artery of _____ Heubner
   iv. Frequency of VB aneurysms is _____% 62%

i. The country with highest incidence is _____. Japan

j. If untreated the prognosis of major deficit or death in 2 years is _____%. 73%

k. Treated prognosis is good in _____%. 58%

95. Presentation in G7 p.1171:150mm

a. children is by _____ attacks ischemic

b. adults is by _____ hemorrhage

c. Diagnose with
   i. a_____ angiography
   ii. M_____ MRA

d. The best medical treatment is _____. none known to be beneficial

e. Surgical treatments all involve _____. revascularization G7 p.1173:100mm

f. The surgical procedure of choice is _____ _____ _____. superficial temporal artery–middle cerebral artery (STA-MCA) bypass

96. What is the treatment for moyamoya disease? G7 p.1173:120mm

a. EMS = _____ encephalomyosynangiosis

b. EDAS = _____ encephaloduroarterio-synangiosis

c. OPT = _____ omental pedicle transplantation

34

Outcome Assessment

■ **Outcome Assessment**

1. **Matching. Match the following outcome scores with the condition they are designed to assess.**
   Outcome scores:
   ① Karnofsky; ② Rancho Los Amigos; ③ Glasgow Outcome; ④ Modified Rankin; ⑤ Barthel; ⑥ Functional Independence Measure
   Condition:
   a. cerebrovascular   ④, ⑤
   b. spinal cord   ⑥
   c. cancer   ①
   d. head injury   ②, ③

   G7 p.1182:45mm

2. **True or False. A higher number indicates better function.**
   a. Karnofsky scale   true
   b. Rancho Los Amigos scale   true
   c. Glasgow Outcome scale   true
   d. Modified Rankin scale   false
   e. Barthel scale   true
   f. Functional Independence Measure   true

   G7 p.1182:60mm

3. **True or False. On the Karnofsky scale, which score represents the transition from being able to engage in normal activity to only caring for self?**
   a. 80%   false
   b. 85%   false
   c. 75%   false
   d. 70%   true (There are no 75 or 85 scores. 70 cares for self, unable to carry on normal activity or work; 50 requires considerable care; and 40 is disabled.)

   G7 p.1182:75mm

35

Differential Diagnosis (DDx) by Location

■ Differential Diagnosis (DDx) by Signs and Symptoms

1. True or False. The following are potential causes of myelopathy: G7 p.1186:15mm
a. stenosis, cervical, or thoracic   true
b. anemia, chronic   true
c. Cushing disease   true
d. Lyme disease   true
e. acquired immunodeficiency syndrome (AIDS)   true

2. How does anemia produce myelopathy?   G7 p.1186:15mm
a. chronic: e_____ h_____, b_____ m_____ h_____, and c_____ c_____   extramedullary hematopoiesis, bone marrow hypertrophy, and cord compression
b. pernicious: s_____ c_____ d_____   subacute combined degeneration

3. How does Cushing disease produce myelopathy?   G7 p.1186:55mm
a. e_____ l_____   epidural lipomatosis

4. True or False. The following are neoplastic masses causing myelopathy, in order of most common to least common: G7 p.1186:95mm
a. extradural, intradural extramedullary, intramedullary   true (It follows anatomically outside to inside, most to least common.)
b. intradural extramedullary, extradural, intramedullary   false
c. intramedullary, extradural, intradural extramedullary   false
d. extradural, intramedullary, intradural extramedullary   false

5. What is the frequency of spinal cord tumors?   G7 p.1186:96mm and G7 p.728:60mm
a. Extradural: _____%   55%
b. Intradural extramedullary: _____%   40%
c. Intradural intramedullary: _____%   5%

6. **Complete the following regarding spinal cord infarction:**   G7 p.1186:166mm

a. The most common artery involved is _____ _____ _____.   anterior spinal artery

b. The most common level of involvement is _____.   T4

c. Why?   watershed area
d. It spares _____ _____   posterior columns
e. caused by _____ and   hypotension
f. due to
  i.   ath_____   atherosclerosis
  ii. emb_____   embolization
  iii. cla_____ a_____   clamping aorta
  iv. aor_____ d_____   aortic dissection
  v.   s_____ p_____ in the presence of s_____ s_____.   sitting position in the presence of spinal stenosis   G7 p.1186:166mm

7. **Necrotizing myelopathy associated with spontaneous thrombosis of a spinal cord arteriovenous malformation (AVM) presenting as spastic → flaccid paraplegia with ascending sensory level is called _____.**   Foix-Alajouanine   G7 p.1187:50mm

8. **True or False. Regarding acute (idiopathic) transverse myelitis:**   G7 p.1187:85mm

a. Clinical onset is indistinguishable from acute spinal cord compression.   true

b. Normal imaging is expected, including CT, myelogram and MRI.   true

c. Cerebrospinal fluid (CSF) analysis shows pleocytosis and hyperproteinemia.   true

d. The thoracic region is the most common level.   true

e. The most common onset is 20 to 40 years of age.   false (Most common onset is first 2 decades of life, other answers define the disease.)

f. Usually results in a diagnosis of multiple sclerosis   false (MS is diagnosed in only 7%.)   G7 p.1187:100mm

9. **Abdominal cutaneous reflexes are almost always absent in _____ _____.**   multiple sclerosis   G7 p.1187:110mm

10. **True or False. Regarding Devic syndrome:**   G7 p.1187:113mm and G7 p.728:60mm

a. It is characterized by acute bilateral retinitis and transverse myelitis.   false (acute bilateral optic neuritis, not retinitis, and myelopathy)

b. The transverse myelitis can be a cause of complete block on myelography.   true

c. It is more common in Asia than in the United States.   true

d. It is a variant of multiple sclerosis (MS).   true

11. **What is another name for Devic syndrome?** neuromyelitis optica G7 p.1187:114mm

12. **True or False. The following are part of the correct mechanism responsible for pernicious anemia:** G7 p.1187:148mm

a. malabsorption of B_{12} in the proximal ileum false (malabsorption of B_{12} in distal ileum)

b. lack of secretion of intrinsic factor by pancreas false (lack of secretion by gastric parietal cells)

c. dysfunction of gastric parietal cells true (malabsorption of B_{12} in the distal ileum due to lack of secretion of intrinsic factor, a small polypeptide, by gastric parietal cells)

d. downregulation of cyclic adenosine monophosphate (cAMP)—mediated transport of B_{12} false

13. **Matching. Match the disease with the important feature.** G7 p.1187:162mm
and
G7 p.1188:120mm
and
G7 p.1188:150mm

G7 p.1187:162mm

Disease:
① pernicious anemia; ② Guillain-Barré; ③ ALS
Important feature:

a. Ascending weakness ②
b. Atrophic weakness of hands ③
c. Symmetrical paresthesias ①
d. Posterior column involvement ①
e. Normal sensation ②
f. Dementia ①
g. Areflexia ②
h. Serum B_{12} levels ①
i. Fasciculations ③
j. Shilling test ①
k. Preserved sphincter control ③
l. Treat with B_{12} ①
m. Proprioception difficulty ①

14. **How might AIDS produce myelopathy?** vacuolization of spinal cord G7 p.1188:78mm

15. Complete the following about sciatica: G7 p.1188:183mm

a. The sciatic nerve contains roots from _____ to _____.   L4 to S3

b.

   i. The nerve passes out of the _____   pelvis

   ii. through the g_____ s_____ f_____.   greater sciatic foramen

c.

   i. In the lower third of the thigh it divides into the t_____   tibial

   ii. and the c_____ _____ nerves.   common peroneal

16. Complete the following about herpes zoster: G7 p.1189:87mm

a. Rarely it might mimic _____.   radiculopathy

b. Lumbosacral dermatomas are involved in _____ to _____%.   10 to 15%

c. Significantly, pain is independent of _____.   position

d. Typical herpetic skin lesions follow pain in _____ to _____ days.   3 to 8

e. True or False. Motor weakness can occur.   true

f. True or False. Urinary retention can occur.   true

g. If so, it is due to _____ paralysis.   detrusor

h.

   i. If motor symptoms occur _____% have good recovery   55%

   ii. and _____% have fair to good recovery.   30%

17. Complete the following regarding differential diagnosis by signs and symptoms: G7 p.1189:170mm

a. Pain produced in the sciatic distribution with weakness of external rotation and abduction of the hip is called _____.   piriformis syndrome due to sciatic nerve entrapment by piriformis muscle. (Symptoms are exacerbated by Freiberg test [forced internal rotation of hip with thigh extension]).

b. The Friedberg test consists of forced _____ _____ of _____   internal rotation of hip

c. and thigh _____.   extension

d. Significance of the Frieberg test is that it _____ the symptoms of the   exacerbates

e. p_____ s_____.   piriformis syndrome

35

18. Complete the following about extraspinal tumors causing sciatica: G7 p.1190:60mm

a. Pain is almost always
  i.   i_____   insidious
  ii.   p_____   progressive
  iii. c_____   constant
  iv.   not affected by _____   position
  v.   worse at _____ in 80% and   night
  vi.   not benefited by _____ therapy   conservative

b. Diagnosis is best made by
  i.   h_____   history
  ii.   r_____   radiographs
  iii. of the entire p_____   pelvis
  iv.   and p_____ f_____   proximal femur

19. Femoral neuropathy is often mistakenly identified as a radiculopathy at what level?   L4   G7 p.1190:120mm

20. Answer the following about femoral neuropathy: G7 p.1190:125mm

a. Femoral neuropathy may be mistaken for radiculopathy at what level?   L4

b. That mistake can occur because both share weakness of the _____ muscle.   quadriceps

c. That mistake should be avoided because sensory distribution is different.
  i.   Femoral nerve serves the _____ _____.   anterior thigh
  ii.   L4 serves the knee to the _____ _____ and   medial malleolus
  iii. spares the _____ _____ motor weakness is different.   anterior thigh
  iv.   Femoral nerve has weak _____.   iliopsoas
  v.   Femoral nerve has strong _____.   thigh adductors
  vi.   L4 has strong _____.   iliopsoas
  vii. L4 has weak _____ _____.   thigh adductors

21. Peroneal nerve palsy may be mistaken for radiculopathy at what level?   L5   G7 p.1190:133mm

22. Complete the following regarding differential diagnosis by signs and symptoms: G7 p.1191:32mm

a. Congenital degeneration of anterior horn cells leading to weakness, areflexia, tongue fasciculations, with normal sensation is W_____-H_____ d_____   Werdnig-Hoffmann disease

b. also known as s_____ m_____ a_____   spinal muscular atrophy

c. also known as f_____ i_____ s_____   floppy infant syndrome

23. **The most common etiology for pure motor hemiplegia without sensory loss is**
    a. l_____ i_____ of the
    b. c_____ i_____ c_____.

    lacunar infarct
    contralateral internal capsule

G7 p.1192:50mm

24. **Can hypoglycemia be associated with hemiparesis?**

    yes, treat with glucose— hemiparesis may clear

G7 p.1192:68mm

25. **Complete the following about back pain:**
    a. Will patients with abdominal or vascular etiology of back pain keep still, or writhe in pain?
       i. example: a_____ a_____ a_____
    b. Pain at bed rest. Think: _____ _____
    c. Relieved by aspirin. Think: _____
    d. Back pain on percussion. Think: _____

    writhe in pain

    abdominal aortic aneurysm

    spine tumor

    osteoid osteoma
    infection

G7 p.1192:120mm

26. **Complete the following regarding differential diagnosis by signs and symptoms:**
    a. Nocturnal back pain relieved by aspirin is suggestive of _____ _____.
    b. Morning back stiffness, hip pain, hip swelling, failure to get relief at rest, and improvement with exercise is suggestive of _____ or _____ _____.

    osteoid osteoma (or benign osteoblastoma)
    sacroiliitis or early ankylosing spondylitis

G7 p.1192:145mm

27. **Complete the following regarding cauda equina. Cauda equina syndrome has the following criteria:**
    a. p_____ a_____
    b. u_____ i_____
    c. p_____ w_____

    perineal anesthesia
    urinary incontinence
    progressive weakness

G7 p.1193:62mm

28. **Complete the following regarding annular tears:**
    a. assymptomatic in 50- to 60-year-old patients in _____%
    b. assymptomatic in 60- to 70-year-old patients in _____%

    40%

    75%

G7 p.1193:103mm

29. **Complete the following regarding Schmorl nodes:**
    a. defined as d_____ h_____
    b. through the c_____ e_____ p_____
    c. into the v_____ b_____
    d. seen in _____% of asymptomatic patients

    disc herniation
    cartilaginous end plate

    vertebral body
    19%

G7 p.1193:179mm

35

30. Complete the following about chronic low back pain: G7 p. 1194:19mm

a. Symptoms persist after 3 months in _____%.   5%

b. Structural diagnosis is possible in only _____% of these.   50%

c. Erosive changes adjacent to sacroiliac (SI) joint and positive test for human leukocyte antigen-B27 (HLA-B27) suggest the diagnosis of a_____ s_____.   ankylosing spondylitis   G7 p. 1194:40mm

d. In foot drop of unknown etiology, which muscle strength tests help differentiate peroneal nerve palsy from L4/L5 radiculopathy?   G7 p. 1194:85mm

i. p_____ t_____ (f_____ i_____)   posterior tibialis (foot inversion)

ii. g_____ m_____ (i_____ r_____ f_____ h_____)   gluteus medius (internal rotation flexed hip)(Both are spared in a peroneal nerve palsy, and both are involved with radiculopathy.)

e. Which division of the sciatic nerve is more sensitive to injury, the peroneal or the tibial division?   peroneal division is more sensitive to injury   G7 p. 1195:16mm

31. For a patient with foot drop, lesion could be at   G7 p.1195:26mm

a. main trunk of _____ _____   sciatic nerve

b. p_____ d_____   peroneal division

c. L_____ or L_____ radiculopathy   L4 or L5

d. c_____ p_____ nerve   common peroneal

e. s_____ p_____ nerve   superficial peroneal

f. d_____ p_____ nerve   deep peroneal

32. Study Chart. Examine the following functions tests and the muscles for a patient with foot drop: G7 p.1195:27mm

a. Adduct thigh   Adductors L2-3

b. Extend knee   Quadriceps L2-3-4

c. Internally rotate thigh   Gluteus medius L4-5 S1

d. Dig heel into bed   Gluteus maximus L5 S1-2

e. Flex knee with thigh flexed   Biceps femoris L5 S1-2

f. Foot planter flexion   Gastrocnemius

g. Invert plantar flexed foot   Tibialis posterior L4-5

h. Evert foot   Peroneus longus and brevis L5 S1

33. Adduct thigh.   G7 p.1195:35mm

a. Utilizes _____ muscles   adductor

b. Nerve: _____   obturator

c. Roots: _____   L2, 3

d. If weak means lesion includes more than the _____ _____   sciatic roots

34. **Extend knee.**   G7 p.1195:35mm
   a. Utilizes _____ muscles   quadriceps
   b. Nerve: _____   femoral
   c. Root:_____   L2, 3, 4
   d. If weak means lesion includes more than   sciatic roots
      _____ _____

35. **Internally rotate thigh.**   G7 p.1195:62mm
   a. Utilizes _____ _____ muscles   gluteus maximus
   b. Nerve: _____   superior gluteal
   c. Root: _____   L4, 5, S1
   d. If weak means lesion is very _____   proximal

36. **Dig heel into bed.**   G7 p.1195:62mm
   a. Utilizes _____ _____ muscles   gluteus maximus
   b. Nerve: _____   inferior gluteal
   c. Roots: _____ _____ and   L5-S1, 2
      _____
   d. If weak the injury is very _____   proximal

37. **Flex knee with thigh flexed.**   G7 p.1195:76mm
   a. Utilizes _____ _____ muscles   lateral hamstrings
   b. Nerve: _____   sciatic
   c. Roots: _____ _____ and   L5, S1, 2
      _____
   d. If weak there is injury to the _____   sciatic nerve
      _____

38. **Foot plantar flexion.**   G7 p.1195:76mm
   a. Utilizes _____ _____ muscles   gastrocnemius
   b. Nerve: _____   sciatic
   c. Roots: _____   L5
   d. If weak there is injury to the _____   sciatic nerve
      _____

39. **Invert plantar flexed foot.**   G7 p.1195:92mm
   a. Utilizes _____ _____ muscles   posterior tibial
   b. Nerve: _____   tibial
   c. Roots: _____ and _____   L4, 5
   d. If weak there is injury to the _____   tibial nerve
      _____
   e. If strong but there is foot drop, it means   common peroneal
      that there is injury distal to the take-off
      of the _____ _____

40. **Evert the foot.**   G7 p.1195:92mm
   a. Utilizes _____ _____ muscles   peroneus longus and brevis
   b. Nerve: _____   superficial peroneal
   c. Roots: _____ and _____   L5, S1
   d. Preservation of these with foot drop   deep peroneal
      means lesion is in the _____
      _____ nerve

35

41. **What are ways to differentiate foot drop from injury to the**   G7 p.1195:162mm
a. deep peroneal nerve?
  i. motor weakness manifests by _____ _____   foot drop (weak foot extension)
  ii. muscle that is weak is the _____ _____   anterior tibial (dorsiflexion)
  iii. sensory loss _____ _____   web space
b. common peroneal nerve?
  i. deficit is a _____ _____   foot drop
  ii. muscles involved are a_____ t_____ and p_____ l_____ and b_____   anterior tibial and peroneus longus and brevis
  iii. weakness of _____ and _____ _____   eversion and foot drop
  iv. sensory loss of _____ _____ and _____   lateral leg and foot

42. **List the ways to differentiate.**   G7 p.1195:182mm
a. plexus lesions on electromyography (EMG) _____ _____   paraspinals normal
b. root lesion on EMG _____ _____   paraspinals abnormal
c. superficial peroneal nerve
  i. motor weakness of _____   eversion
  ii. muscles that are weak are the _____ _____ and _____   peroneus longus and brevis
  iii. Any foot drop?   no
  iv. sensory loss at the _____ _____ and _____   lateral leg and foot

43. **Complete the following regarding differential diagnosis by signs and symptoms:**   G7 p.1196:29mm
a. Painless foot drop is likely due to _____ _____.   peroneal palsy
b. Painful foot drop is likely due to _____.   radiculopathy
c. Painless foot drop with no sensory loss could be due to _____ _____.   parasagittal lesion
d. If so how might the reflexes be?   hyperactive
e. This is called the _____ _____.   spastic foot drop

44. **A central nervous system (CNS) cause of foot drop is**   G7 p.1196:60mm
a. the result of a _____ lesion   parasagittal
b. and may produce a _____ reflex   Babinski
c. or a hyperactive _____ reflex.   Achilles (= spastic foot drop)

45. **Complete the following regarding symptoms in the hands:**   G7 p.1196:155mm
   a. Central cord syndrome shows more involvement in _____ than _____.   UE; LE
   b. Syringomyelia has b_____ d_____ in the hands.   burning dysesthesias

46. **Complete the following regarding lesion location and findings in "cruciate paralysis":**   G7 p.1196:180mm
   a. Physical exam shows _____ _____ _____   atrophy of hands
   b. due to pressure on the _____ _____   pyramidal decussations
   c. at the level of the _____ _____.   foramen magnum

47. **Complete the following about radiculopathy, upper extremity:**   G7 p.1197:120mm
   a. The "empty can" test suggests s_____ p_____.   shoulder pathology
   b. Interscapular pain suggests c_____ r_____.   cervical radiculopathy   G7 p.1197:135mm

48. **Myocardial infarction (MI) may present with symptoms similar to a radiculopathy at what level?**   left C6   G7 p.1197:142mm

49. **Matching. Match the symptom with the position of the disc most likely to produce it.**   G7 p.1198:23mm
   Disc:
   ① central cervical disc; ② lateral cervical disc
   Symptom:
   a. pain   ② lateral
   b. myelopathy   ① central
   c. bilateral symptoms   ① central
   d. upper extremity symptoms   ② lateral
   e. lower extremity symptoms   ① central
   f. numb clumsy hands   ① central

50. **Electric shock-like sensation radiating up or down the spine, usually with flexion and attributed to dysfunction of posterior columns is called the _____ _____.**   Lhermitte sign   G7 p.1198:170mm

35

51. **True or False. Lhermitte's sign can be seen in**   G7 p.1198:180mm
Hint: mc$_5$rs
a. multiple sclerosis   true
b. cervical spondylosis   true
c. cervical disc   true
d. cervical cord tumor   true
e. Chiari I   true
f. central cord syndrome   true
g. radiation myelopathy   true
h. subacute combined degeneration   true

52. **Complete the following regarding one or more episodes of brief loss of consciousness (LOC):**   G7 p.1199:70mm
a. referred to as s_____   syncope
b. prevalence is _____   ≈ 50% (higher in elderly)
c. presumed etiology is _____   vasovagal

53. **What are the causes of syncope?**   G7 p.1199:112mm
a. Disorder of AV node conduction is called   Stokes-Adams
_____ _____

b. Tight short collar, shaving, passing out is   carotid sinus syncope
called _____ _____ _____
c. Fainting aka _____ syncope   neurocardiogenic
d.
  i.   Micturition, cough called _____   triggered syncope
  _____
  ii. Usually associated with elevation of   intra-thoracic
  _____-_____ pressure
e. Orthostatic hypotension defined as a   25
drop in BP of _____mm Hg on
standing
f. Unknown etiology occurs in _____%   40%

54. **Complete the following about transient neurological deficit (TIA):**   G7 p.1200:175mm
a. By definition it lasts less than _____   24
hours
b. but usually subsides within _____   20 minutes
_____.
c. They are _____.   temporary
d. They are a result of _____.   ischemia

55. **Complete the following regarding the etiology of diplopia secondary to VI nerve palsy:**   G7 p.1201:85mm
a. i_____ _____ _____   ↑ ICP (pseudotumor cerebri)
b. s_____ _____   sphenoid sinusitis
c. t_____   tumor/mass etc.

56. **Complete the following regarding transient ischemic attacks (TIAs):**

G7 p.1200:175mm

a. By definition TIAs last less than _____.   24 hours

b. Most resolve within _____.   20 minutes

c. Migraine paresis differs from TIA in that it _____ over several minutes.   progresses (marches)

d. TIA-like symptoms from cerebral amyloid angiopathy (CAA) require avoidance of _____ or _____ drugs   antiplatelet or anticoagulation

G7 p.1201:29mm

e. because the CAA patient is more prone to _____.   hemorrhage

57. **Complete the following about anosmia:**

G7 p.1202:80mm

a. Most common cause is s_____ r_____ infection.   severe respiratory

b.

   i. Second most common cause is _____ _____.   head injury

   ii. For severe such cases _____ to _____% occurence.   7 to 15%

58. **Complete the following about cranial neuropathies:**

G7 p.1202:52mm

a. Congenital facial diplegia is also known as _____ _____.   Möbius syndrome

b. It affects which half of the face more?   upper

c. True or False. It may also involve other cranial nerves. If so, which ones?   true CN VI, III, or XII

d. Lyme disease can cause _____.   unilateral or bilateral seventh nerve palsy

e. Affects which half of the face?   lower (as in Bell palsy)

f. True or False. It may also involve other cranial nerves.   false

59. **Complete the following about cavernous sinus syndrome:**

G7 p.1204:60mm

a. A cavernous sinus aneurysm can compress the third nerve and cause _____   diplopia

b. due to _____.   ophthalmoplegia

c. In this form of third nerve palsy the pupil will be _____ _____   not dilated

d. because the _____ that dilate the pupil   sympathetics

e. are _____ _____.   also paralyzed

60. **Complete the following about osteopetrosis:**

G7 p.1204:75mm

a. It is also known as _____ _____   marble bone

b. a _____ disorder   genetic

c. of defective _____ resorption of bone   osteoclastic

d. resulting in increased _____ bone density
_____.

e. The most common neurologic blindness
manifestation is _____.

f. Treatment consists of bilateral _____ optic nerve
_____ decompression.

61. Complete the following about G7 p1204 :178mm
monocular blindness:

a. Giant cell arthritis aka t_____ temporal arthritis
a_____

b. Usually due to ischemia of the
    i. o_____ n_____ or optic nerve
    ii. o_____ t_____ optic tract
    iii. less likely the c_____ r_____ central retinal
         artery

62. Complete the following about G7 p. 1205:73mm
exophthalmos:

a. aka p_____ proptosis

b. Following trauma, think: c_____ carotid cavernous
    c_____ fistula

c. Following frontal-orbital surgery, think: defect in orbital roof
    _____ in _____ _____

63. Complete the following about G7 p.1207:40mm
arachnoid cyst: Also see

a. aka _____ _____ leptomeningeal cyst G7 p. 222
b. Due to a d_____ of the _____ duplication; arachnoid
c. Reach maximum size in _____ 1 month
    _____

d. Need surgery in about _____% 30%

64. Complete the following regarding G7 p.1208:87mm
differential diagnosis by signs and
symptoms:

a. Hemifacial spasm may produce tinnitus stapedial muscle
    because of s_____ m_____
    spasms.

b. High cervical lesion may cause facial spinal trigeminal tract G7 p.1208:40mm
    sensory changes due to compression of
    the s_____ t_____ t_____

c. at cervical levels down to _____. C2-C4

d. Causes of mutism include injury to
    i.   f_____ l_____ frontal lobes
    ii. c_____ g_____ cingulate gyrus
    iii. c_____ c_____ t_____ corpus callosum plus
                                         thalamus
    iv. c_____ cerebellum

e. Swallowing difficulties can be caused by anterior longitudinal ligament G7 p.1209:53mm
    ossification of the _____ _____
    _____.

65. **Complete the following about CPA lesions:**
Hint: amem

G7 p.1210:133mm

a.
  i.   Acoustic neuroma more accurately known as v_____ s_____   vestibular schwannoma
  ii. Occurs in _____ to _____%   80 to 90%
b.   Meningioma occurs in _____ to _____%.   5 to 10%
c.   Epidermoid occurs in _____ to _____%.   5 to 7%
d.   Metastatic _____   rarely

66. **Matching. Match the characteristic with the condition.**
Condition:
① vestibular schwannoma;
② meningioma
Characteristic:

G7 p.1211:120mm

a.   Hearing loss occurs early in _____.   ①
b.   Facial weakness occurs early in_____.   ②
c.   Internal auditory canal (IAC) is enlarged in _____.   ①
d.   Calcification is seen in_____.   ②
e.   It represents 90% of cerebellopontine angle (CPA) tumors.   ①
f.   It represents 5 to 10% of CPA tumors.   ②

67. **Complete the following about posterior fossa tumor:**

G7 p.1209:134mm

a.   Most likely a solitary lesion in an adult is a _____.   metastasis
b.   Most likely primary tumor is the _____.   hemangioblastoma
c.   Radiologic characteristics include
  i.   v_____ n_____   vascular nodule
  ii. c_____   cyst
  iii. s_____ _____ on _____   serpentine vessels on surface
d.   The tumor that is common in young adults is p_____ a_____.   pilocytic astrocytoma

68. **Complete the following regarding differential diagnosis by location:**

G7 p.1210:60mm

a.   The modern name for medulloblastoma is _____ _____ _____.   primitive neuroectodermal tumor (PNET)
b.   It usually begins at the _____,   fastigium
c.   which is located at the _____.   roof of the fourth ventricle
d.   The consistency is _____.   solid

69. **For posterior fossa tumors in children, give types and percentage.**

G7 p.1210:87mm

a.   a_____ (p_____), _____%   astrocytoma (pilocytic), 27%
b.   b_____ _____ _____, _____%   brain stem glioma, 28%
c.   P_____ (i.e., m_____), _____%   PNET (i.e., medulloblastoma), 27%

35

70. Complete the following about atlantoaxial subluxation: G7 p.1230:144mm
a. Incompetence of the _____ ligament   transverse
b. Results in increased _____ _____ interval   atlantodental

71. Complete the following regarding differential diagnosis by location: G7 p.1231:23mm
a. Morquio syndrome is hypoplasia of the _____   dens
b. due to a m_____.   mucopolysaccharidosis
c. It may result in _____ subluxation.   atlantoaxial

72. Complete the following about multiple intracranial lesions on CT or MRI: G7 p.1212:103mm
a. Glioma—what % are multicentric? _____%   6%
b. Herpes simplex usually occurs in the _____ lobe.   temporal   G7 p.1213:117mm
c. MS lesions are p_____.   periventricular   G7 p.1213:25mm
d. Dural sinus thrombosis cause multiple _____ _____.   venous infarcts   G7 p.1213:721mm
e. Multiple hypertensive hemorrhages is likely _____ _____.   amyloid angiopathy   G7 p.1213:110mm

73. Name the ring-enhancing lesions on computed tomography and magnetic resonance imaging (CT/MRI).   G7 p.1214:100mm
Hint: haam
a. h_____   hematoma
b. a_____   astrocytoma
c. a_____   abscess
d. m_____   metastases

74. Complete the following about ring-enhancing lesions on CT/MRI: G7 p.1214:100mm
a. A continuous ring suggests r_____ h_____.   resolving hematoma
b. An interrupted ring suggests m_____.   malignancy

75. List the conditions that cross the corpus callosum.   G7 p.1215:70mm
Hint: ms-glld
a. m_____ s_____   multiple sclerosis
b. g_____   glioblastoma
c. l_____   lymphoma (primary CNS)
d. l_____   lipoma
e. d_____   diffuse axonal injury

76. **Complete the following regarding sellar and paraseller lesions:**   G7 p.1215:95mm
   a. Adults: most common is _____
   _____   pituitary adenoma
   b.
      i. Children: most common are c_____   craniopharyngioma
      ii. and g_____   germinoma

77. **Complete the following regarding sellar lesions:**   G7 p.1215:150mm
   a. Pituitary pseudotumor is due to _____,   hypothyroidism
   b. which causes chronic pituitary stimulation by _____-_____ _____.   thyrotropin-releasing hormone

78. **Germ cell tumors in the suprasellar area are**   G7 p.1215:150mm
   a. more common in_____.   women
   b. have a triad of
      i. d_____ _____   diabetes insipidus
      ii. v_____ _____ _____   visual field defects
      iii. p_____   panhypopituitarism

79. **Complete the following about juxtasellar masses:**   G7 p.1216:16mm
   a. Craniopharyngioma
      i. In this region account for _____% of tumors in adults   20%
      ii. and _____% in children   54%
   b. Meningioma. To differentiate from pituitary macroadenoma use gadolinium. Meningiomas have:
      i. b_____ h_____ e_____   bright homogeneous enhancement
      ii. Epicenter is _____   suprasellar
      iii. Tapered extension aka _____ _____   dural tail
      iv. Sella is usually _____ _____   not enlarged
      v. Rarely produce _____ disturbances   endocrine
      vi. Tend to _____ carotid artery   encase

80. **True or False. Regarding lymphocytic hypophysitis:**   G7 p.1212:15mm
   a. It is rare.   true
   b. It may cause hypopituitarism.   true
   c. Most cases occur in women.   true
   d. It tends to selectively affect a single hormone.   true
   e. It requires surgery.   false (self-limiting or Rx with steroids)
   f. It may produce diabetes insipidus (DI).   true

35

81. Complete the following about cavum septum pellucidum (CSP):
   a. It is present in all _____ _____.   premature babies
   b. Adults have them in _____%.   10%
   c. It is commonly seen in _____.   boxers

G7 p.1218:45mm

82. Complete the following about cavum vergae:
   a. posterior to _____   CSP
   b. often communicates with the _____   CSP

G7 p.1218:45mm

83. Complete the following about cavum velum interpositum:
   a. due to separation of the _____   crura
   b. of the _____   fornix
   c. with the _____ above and   thalami
   d. the _____ _____ below   third ventricle
   e. present under 1 year of age in _____%   60%
   f. present between 1 and 10 years old in _____%   30%

G7 p.1218:45mm

84. True or False. The most common benign primary intraorbital neoplasm is
   a. capillary hemangioma   false
   b. lymphangioma   false
   c. optic nerve sheath meningioma   false
   d. cavernous hemangioma   true
   e. optic glioma   false

G7 p.1218:128mm

85. Matching. Match characteristics of orbital lesions with pathology (may match with more than one).
Pathology:
① capillary hemangioma;
② lymphangioma; ③ lymphoma;
④ thyroid ophthalmoplegia
Characteristic:
   a. infantile proptosis   ①, ②
   b. regresses spontaneously   ①
   c. does not regress   ②
   d. painless proptosis   ③, ④
   e. bilateral (80% of the time)   ④

G7 p.1218:145mm

86. The most common primary ocular malignancy of childhood is _____.   melanoma

G7 p.1218:152mm

87. Complete the following about skull lesions:
   a. Multiplicity suggests _____.   malignancy, especially if six or more
   b. Expansion of diploë suggests _____.   a benign lesion
   c. Peripheral sclerosis suggests _____.   a benign lesion
   d. Full-thickness lesions suggest _____.   malignancy
   e. Sharply demarcated, punched-out defects suggest _____.   myeloma

G7 p.1220:27mm

35

88. **Complete the following about skull lesions:**
    a. Name the skull lesion that shows a
       i.   trabecular pattern
       ii. sunburst pattern
       iii. islands of bone pattern
       iv. site of tenderness to palpation
    b. Another name for Paget disease that is only osteolytic is _____ _____.
    c. Eosinophilic granuloma is the mildest form of _____ _____.

hemangioma
hemangioma
fibrous dysplasia
eosinophilic granuloma
osteoporosis circumscripta

histiocytosis X

G7 p.1220:80mm

G6 p.930:120mm

G7 p.1221:87mm

89. **Complete the following about skull lesions:**
    a. There is no _____ lesion
    b. that grows out of the _____.

intra-axial
skull

G7 p.1223:35mm

90. **Choroid plexus calcification has the following characteristics:**
    a. % calcified between age 40 and 50 is _____
    b. rare under age _____
    c. Under age 10 consider choroid plexus _____.
    d. If you see calcified choroid plexus in the temporal horn consider _____.

75%

3
papilloma

neurofibromatosis

G7 p.1224:45mm

91. **Complete the following about basal ganglia calcifications:**
    a. Are common in the _____
    b. May be due to _____
    c. Or long-term use of _____
    d. Or _____ disease
    e. Correlated with psychiatric diseases if > _____ cm

elderly
hyperparathyroidism
anticonvulsants
Fahr
0.5

G7 p.1224:55mm

92. **Complete the following about Fahr disease:**
    a. Cause is _____
    b. Course is _____
    c. What do we see in x-rays?
    d. Where?
       i.   b_____ g_____
       ii. s_____
       iii. d_____ n_____

idiopathic
progressive
intracranial calcifications

basal ganglia
sulci
dentate nuclei

G7 p.1224:75mm

35

93. What are the characteristics of intraventricular lesions? Which: G7 p.1224:150mm
a. is most common?   astrocytoma
b. is at foramen of Monro?   colloid cyst
c. has punctate calcification?   craniopharyngioma
d. fills the fourth ventricle?   medulloblastoma
e. is the most common fourth ventricle low epidermoid
density lesion?
f. has free-floating fat in ventricles?   dermoid
g. has fat and calcification?   teratoma
h. is at the septum pellucidum?   central neurocytoma

94. Intraventricular meningiomas are fed by the G7 p.1224:180mm
a. a_____ c_____ a_____   anterior choroidal artery
b. and less commonly by the
i.   m_____ p_____ c_____   medial posterior choroidal
a_____   artery
ii. l_____ p_____ c_____   lateral posterior choroidal
a_____   artery
c. and are thought to arise from the   arachnoidal cap cells
_____ _____ _____.

95. True or False. The following intraventricular lesion is least likely to be found in the frontal horn: G7 p.1225:130mm
a. astrocytoma   false
b. meningioma   false
c. dermoid   false
d. choroid plexus papilloma   true

96. Matching. Match most common tumor type with location. G7 p.1225:125mm
Location:
① frontal horn; ② body; ③ atrium;
④ third ventricle; ⑤ fourth ventricle
Tumor type:
a. Colloid cyst   ④
b. Medulloblastoma   ⑤
c. Meningioma   ③
d. Ependymoma   ②
e. Astrocytoma   ①
f. Choroid plexus papilloma   ②
g. Choroid plexus carcinoma   ③
h. Subependymoma _____ or _____   ① or ⑤
i. teratoma   ④

97. Complete the following about tumors within the lateral ventricles. In adults all enhance except G7 p.1226:65mm
a. c_____ and the   cysts
b. s_____.   subependymoma

98. **Periventricular enhancing mass lesions. First consideration should be _____.**

lymphoma

G7 p.1227:138mm

99. **With periventricular low density, consider:**
    a. t_____ edema
    b. m_____ s_____
    c. acute arteriosclerotic encephalopathy aka _____ _____
    d. leukoaraiosis
        i. representing _____ _____
        ii. or w_____ i_____

G7 p.1227:138mm

transependymal
multiple sclerosis
Binswanger disease

normal aging
watershed infarction

100. **Ependymal enhancement can be due to**
    a. v_____

    b. l_____
    c. m_____
    d. g_____

G7 p.1227:142mm

ventriculitis (pyogenic or viral)
lymphoma
metastasis
granuloma (TB)

101. **What does the pattern of enhancement suggest?**
    a. Thin linear suggests v_____.
    b. Nodular suggests l_____.

G7 p.1228:35mm

virus (CMV)
lymphoma

102. **Complete the following about intraventricular hemorrhage:**
    a. Extension from
        i. t_____ in hypertensive adult
        ii. p_____ in hypertensive adult
        iii. s_____ in premature newborn
    b. True or False. Occurs commonly with aneurysm of the
        i. MCA
        ii. A-comm
        iii. P-comm
        iv. distal basilar
        v. vein of Galen
        vi. carotid bifurcation
        vii. pericallosal
        viii. vertebral
        ix. PICA
        x. dissecting vertebral type

G7 p.1228:95mm

thalamus
putamen
subependyma

false
true
false
false
false
true
false
true
true
true

103. **The most common medial temporal lobe lesions are**
    a. h_____
    b. m_____ t_____ s_____
    c. g_____

G7 p.1128:145mm

hamartoma
mesial temporal sclerosis
glioma (low grade)

35

35

104. **True or False. Esthesioneuroblastoma most commonly presents with**   G7 p.1230:42mm
a. pain   false
b. nasal obstruction   false
c. epistaxis   true
d. tearing   false
e. proptosis   false

105. **To differentiate:**   G7 p.1230:80mm
① nasal encephalocele
② nasal glioma in the newborn
a. pulsatile   ①
b. swells with Valsalva   ①
c. hypertelorism   ①
d. attachment to CNS   ①

106. **Destructive spondylo-arthropathy is**   G7 p.1233:30mm
a. the name for bone changes seen in   chronic renal failure
    c_____ r_____ f_____.
b. It resembles i_____.   infection

107. **True or False. Destruction of the disc space is highly suggestive of**   G7 p.1233:70mm
a. tumor   false
b. infection   true
c. degenerative disease   false
d. metabolic disease   false

108. **Matching. Match the destructive lesion of the spine with its cause.**   G7 p.1233:71mm
Cause:
① infection; ② tumor; ③ Paget disease
Destructive lesion:
a. Destruction of disc space suggests_____.   ①
b. Disc space not destroyed suggests _____.   ②
c. Single-level involvement suggests _____.   ①
d. Multiple-level involvement suggests _____.   ②
e. Dense vertebra on x-ray suggests _____.   ③

109. **True or False. Pott disease is confined to the disc space.**   false (The disc may be relatively resistant to tuberculous involvement.)   G7 p.1233:88mm